CHILDHOOD CANCER AND NUCLEAR INSTALLATIONS

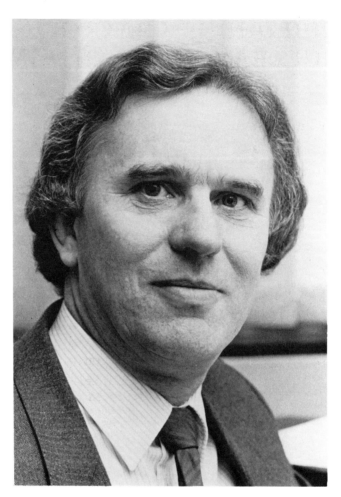

Martin John Gardner, PHD, FFOM, DIPMATHSTAT

CHILDHOOD CANCER AND NUCLEAR INSTALLATIONS

Papers, abstracts, letters, editorials, reports published since 1984
edited by

Valerie Beral and Eve Roman

Imperial Cancer Research Fund
Cancer Epidemiology Unit
Oxford University
and

Martin Bobrow

Paediatric Research Unit
Division of Medical and Molecular Genetics
United Medical and Dental Schools of Guy's and St Thomas's Hospitals
London

This book is dedicated to the late Martin J Gardner

Medical Research Council Environmental Epidemiology Unit
University of Southampton

Published by the BMJ Publishing Group
Tavistock Square, London WC1H 9JR

British Library Cataloguing in Publication Data
A catalogue record for this book is available from the British
Library

ISBN
0–7279–0815–4

Typeset, printed, and bound in Great Britain by
Latimer Trend & Company Ltd, Plymouth

Contents

List of contributors

Stoke Mandeville Hospital, Aylesbury, Buckinghamshire HP21 8AL
Anne Watson

Department of Haematology, Basingstoke District Hospital, Basingstoke
D Lynn Aston

Information and Statistics Division, Scottish Health Service, Common Services Agency, Edinburgh EH5 3SQ
Roger J Black
M A Heasman
David Adams Jones
I W Kemp
Stephen W Kendrick
Margaret Maxwell
Michael J Muirhead
Linda Sharp
James D Urquhart
Jan Warner

MRC Human Genetics Unit, Western General Hospital, Crewe Road, Edinburgh EH4 2XU
H John Evans

Radiation Oncology Research Group, Beatson Oncology Centre, Belvidere Hospital, Glasgow G31 4PG
A Barrett
R Mairs
T E Wheldon

West of Scotland Cancer Surveillance Unit, Greater Glasgow Health Board, Ruchill Hospital, Glasgow G20 9NB
C R Gillis
D J Hole

The Surgery, Kendal LA9 4BD
Jennifer Buckler

Department of Pathology, Lancaster Moor Hospital, Lancaster LA1 3JR
Jane M Edwards
J A Morris

Geography Department, Lancaster University, Lancaster LA1 4YW
R Butler
R Flowerdew
A C Gatrell

Leukaemia Research Fund Centre for Clinical Epidemiology, University of Leeds, Leeds LS2 9NG
R A Cartwright

Leukaemia Research Fund Centre, Institute of Cancer Research, Chester Beatty Laboratories, London SW3 6JB
Melvyn F Greaves

Department of Epidemiology and Population Sciences, London School of Hygiene and Tropical Medicine, London WC1E 7HT
Peter G Smith

Department of Paediatric Oncology, St Bartholomew's Hospital, London EC1A 7BE
O B Eden

Paediatric Research Unit, Division of Medical and Molecular Genetics, United Medical and Dental Schools of Guy's and St Thomas' Hospitals, London SE1 9RT
Martin Bobrow

Yorkshire Television Limited, London WC1
Michael Burke
James Cutler

Christie Hospital and Holt Radium Institute, Manchester
Michael Palmer

Children's Department, Royal Victoria Infirmary, Newcastle upon Tyne NE1 4LP
A W Craft

University Library, Newcastle upon Tyne NE2 4HQ
John Urquhart

xii

Cancer Research Campaign Epidemiology Unit, University of Oxford, Oxford OX2 6HE
A Balkwill
K Clarke
Leo J Kinlen
F O'Brien

Childhood Cancer Research Group, University of Oxford, Oxford OX2 6HJ
Kathryn J Bunch
G J Draper
C A Stiller
T J Vincent

Imperial Cancer Research Fund, Cancer Epidemiology Unit, University of Oxford, Oxford OX2 6HE
Krys Baker
Valerie Beral
Diana Bull
Paula Cook-Mozaffari
Sarah Darby
Gwyneth Davey
Sir Richard Doll
David Forman
C Hermon
Eve Roman
Irene Stratton

Department of Public Health and Primary Care, Oxford University
Lucy Carpenter

Department of Haematology, Royal Berkshire Hospital, Reading
Carol Barton
Sandra Buckle
Hilary Ryder

MRC Environmental Epidemiology Unit, University of Southampton, Southampton General Hospital, Southampton SO9 4XY
S Downes
Martin J Gardner
Andrew J Hall
Caroline A Powell
Michael P Snee
P D Winter

Division of Epidemiology, Institute of Cancer Research, Sutton, Surrey SM2 5NG
F Matthews

West Cumbria District Health Authority, West Cumberland Hospital, Whitehaven, Cumbria CA28 8JG
John D Terrell

Miscellaneous UK contributors

Derek Jakeman, *Weymouth, Dorset DT3 6NL*

Old Cottage, Wexham Street, Stoke Poges, Buckinghamshire SL3 6NB
Robin Russell Jones

R H Mole, *Oxford OX1 5DF*

Overseas contributors

Bureau of Radiation and Medical Devices, Department of National Health and Welfare, Ottawa, Ontario, Canada
J Patrick Ashmore

Division of Epidemiology and Statistics, Ontario Cancer Treatment and Research Foundation, Toronto, Ontario, Canada
E Aileen Clarke
Will D King
John R McLaughlin

Department of Health Care and Epidemiology, University of British Columbia, Vancouver, British Columbia, Canada
Terence W Anderson

Public Health Department, Regional Hospital of Metz, 57038 Metz, Cedex 1, France
J F Viel

Department of Biostatistics and Epidemiology, Institut National de la Santé et de la Recherche Medicale, and Institut Gustave Roussy, 94807 Villejuif Cedex, France
Catherine Hill
Agnes Laplanche
S T Richardson

Institut für Medizinische Statistik und Dokumentation, D-6500 Mainz, Germany
Gunter Haf
Peter Kaatsch
Birgit Keller
Jorg Michaelis

Biomedical Group, Bhabha Atomic Research Centre, Trombay, Bombay 400 085, India
N K Notani

Epidemiology and Health Services Evaluation Unit, Occupational Epidemiology Section, Faculty of Health Sciences, Ben Gurion University of the Negev, Beer Sheva, Israel
John R Goldsmith

Department of Radiation Biology, Faculty of Medicine, Osaka University, Nakanoshima, Kita-ku, Osaka 530, Japan
Iaisei Nomura

Department of Pathology, Academic Hospital, 3508 GA Utrecht, Netherlands
W DenOtter
J W Koten

Radiation Epidemiology Branch, Epidemiology and Biostatistics Program, National Cancer Institute, Bethesda, Maryland 20892, USA
John D Boice junior
Zdenek Hrubec
Seymour Jablon

Boston, USA
Seth Shulman

Department of Preventive Medicine, University of Southern California Medical School, Los Angeles, California 90033, USA
M C Pike

Massachusetts Cancer Registry, Massachusetts, USA
Richard W Clapp

Harvard University, Cambridge, Massachusetts, USA
C K Chan
Sidney Cobb

LIST OF CONTRIBUTORS

School of Public Health, Columbia University, New York, NY 10032, USA
Maureen C Hatch
Jeri W Nieves
Mervyn Suser
Sylvan Wallenstein

National Audubon Society, New York, NY, USA
Jan Beyea

State University of New York, Albany, New York, USA
Bailus Walker junior

Chronic Disease Epidemiology Section, Division of Public Health ED-13, Washington State Department of Social and Health Services, Olympia, Washington 98504, USA
Samuel Milham junior

Acknowledgements

We thank the following publishers for permission to reprint the papers listed: the **American Medical Association** for (ch 53) Jablon S, Hrubec Z, Boice JD junior. Cancer in populations living near nuclear facilities: a survey of mortality nationwide and incidence in two states. *JAMA* 1991;**265**:1403; the **American Public Health Association** for (ch 52) Hatch MC, Wallenstein S, Beyea J, Neives JW, Susser M. Cancer rates after the Three Mile Island nuclear accident and proximity of residence to the plant. *Am J Public Health* 1991;**81**:719; **Blackwell Scientific Publishers** for (ch 18) Gardner MJ. Review of reported increases of childhood cancer rates in the vicinity of nuclear installations in the United Kingdom. *Journal of the Royal Statistical Society [Series A]* 1989;**152**:307–25; the **Bureau of Hygiene and Tropical Diseases, CAB International**, for (ch 27) Smith PG. Comments on the case-control study of Gardner *et al* of leukaemia and lymphoma among young people in west Cumbria. *Abstracts on Hygiene and Communicable Disease* 1990;**65**:1–6; the Controller of **Her Majesty's Stationery Office** for (ch 41) Excerpts from: Black D for the Independent Advisory Group. *Investigation of the possible increased incidence of cancer in west Cumbria.* London: HMSO, 1984. (Black report), (ch 42) Excerpts from: Committee on Medical Aspects of Radiation in the Environment. *First report. The implications of the new data on the releases from Sellafield in the 1950s for the conclusions of the report on the investigation of the possible increased incidence of cancer in west Cumbria.* London: HMSO, 1986, (ch 43) Excerpts from: Committee on Medical Aspects of Radiation in the Environment. *Second report. Investigation of the possible increased incidence of childhood cancer in young persons near the Dounreay nuclear establishment, Caithness, Scotland.* London: HMSO, 1988; and (ch 44) Excerpts from: Committee on Medical Aspects of Radiation in the Environment. *Third report. Investigation of the possible increased incidence of childhood cancer in the west Berkshire and north Hampshire area, in which are situated the Atomic Weapons Research Establishment, Aldermaston, and the Royal Ordnance Factory, Burghfield.* London: HMSO, 1989 (all four Crown copyright), the **Johns Hopkins University School of Hygiene and Public Health** for (ch 47) Hatch MC, Beyea J, Nieves JW, Susser M. Cancer near the Three Mile Island nuclear plant: radiation emissions. *Am J Epidemiol* 1990;**132**:397, the **Lancet Ltd** for: (ch 1) Gardner MJ, Winter PD. Mortality in Cumberland during 1959–78 with reference to cancer in young people around Windscale. *Lancet* 1984;**i**: 216–7; (ch 2) Urquhart J, Palmer M, Cutler J. Cancer in Cumbria: the Windscale connection. *Lancet* 1984;**i**:217–8; (ch 4) Barton CJ, Roman E, Ryder H, Watson A. Childhood leukaemia in west Berkshire. *Lancet* 1985;**ii**:1248–9; (ch 5) Heasman MA, Kemp IW, Urquhart JD, Black R. Childhood leukaemia in northern Scotland. *Lancet* 1986;**i**:266 and 358 (correction to preceding paper); (ch 6) Urquhart J, Cutler J, Burke M. Leukaemia and lymphatic cancer in young people near nuclear installations. *Lancet* 1986;**i**:384; (ch 7) Hole DJ, Gillis CR. Childhood leukaemia in the west of Scotland. *Lancet* 1986;**ii**:524–5; (ch 13) Kinlen L. Evidence for an infective cause of childhood leukaemia: comparison of a Scottish new town with nuclear reprocessing sites in Britain. *Lancet* 1988;**ii**:1323–7; (ch 14) Jones RR. Infective cause of childhood leukaemia. *Lancet* 1989;**i**:94; (ch 15) Wheldon TE, Mairs R, Barrett A. Germ cell injury and childhood leukaemia clusters. *Lancet* 1989;**i**:792–3: (ch 17) Cook-Mozaffari P, Darby S, Doll R. Cancer near potential sites of nuclear installations. *Lancet* 1989;**ii**:1145–7; (ch 45) Clapp RW, Cobb S, Chan CK, Walker B junior. Leukaemia near Massachusetts nuclear power plant. *Lancet* 1987;**ii**:1324–5; and (ch 46) Goldsmith JR and Milham S junior. Childhood leukaemia mortality before 1970 among populations near two United States nuclear installations. *Lancet* 1989;**i**:793, 1443, and 1444, **Macmillan Magazines Limited** for: (ch 12) Forman D, Cook-Mozaffari P, Darby S, Davey G, Stratton I, Doll R, Pike M. Cancer near nuclear installations. *Nature* 1987;**329**:499–505; (ch 22) Evans HJ. Leukaemia and radiation. *Nature* 1990;**345**:16–7; (ch 25) Nomura I. Of mice and men? *Nature* 1990;**345**:671; (ch 50) Shulman S. Cancer around nuclear plant. *Nature* 1990;**347**:604–5; and (ch 51) Hill C, Laplanche A. Overall mortality and cancer mortality around French nuclear sites. *Nature* 1990;**347**:755–7. Reprinted by permission from *Nature* vol **329**, pp 499–505; vol **345**, pp 16–7; and vol **347**, pp 604–5 and 755–7. © 1987 and 1990 Macmillan Magazines Limited, **Macmillan Press Ltd** for (ch 16) Cook-Mozaffari PJ, Darby SC, Doll R, Forman D, Hermon C, Pike MC, Vincent T. Geographical variation in mortality from leukaemia and other cancers in England and Wales in relation to proximity to nuclear installations, 1969–78. *Br J Cancer* 1989;**59**:476–85; (ch 28) Gardner MJ. Childhood cancer and nuclear installations. *Public Health* 1991;**105**:277–85; and (ch 32) Kinlen LJ, Hudson CM, Stiller CA. Contacts between adults as evidence for an infective origin of childhood leukaemia: an explanation for the excess near nuclear establishments in west Berkshire? *Br J Cancer* 1991;**64**:549–54, the **National Cancer Institute,** USA, for (ch 33) Gardner MJ. Leukaemia in children and paternal radiation exposure at the Sellafield nuclear site. *J Natl Cancer Inst Monogr* 1992;**12**:133–5, **Oxford University Press** for (ch 48) Hatch M, Susser M. Background γ radiation and childhood cancers within 10 miles of a United States nuclear plant. *Int J Epidemiol*

1990;19:546, **Rapid Communications of Oxford Ltd** for (ch 54) Michaelis J, Keller B, Haaf G, Kaatsch P. Incidence of childhood malignancies in the vicinity of West German nuclear power plants. *Cancer Causes and Control* 1992;3:255, **US Department of Health and Human Services, National Institute of Environmental Health** for (ch 29) Gardner MJ. Father's occupational exposure to radiation and the raised level of childhood leukaemia near the Sellafield nuclear plant. *Environ Health Perspect* 1991;94:5–7, **Williams and Wilkins** for (ch 24) Greaves MF. The Sellafield childhood leukaemia cluster: are germ line mutations responsible? *Leukemia* 1990;4:391–6.

LIST OF ALL ORIGINAL PUBLICATIONS, BY CHAPTER NUMBER

1 Gardner MJ, Winter PD. Mortality in Cumberland during 1959–78 with reference to cancer in young people around Windscale. *Lancet* 1984;i:216–7.
2 Urquhart J, Palmer M, Cutler J. Cancer in Cumbria: the Windscale connection. *Lancet* 1984;i:217–8.
3 Jakeman D. New estimates of radioactive discharges from Sellafield. *BMJ* 1986;293:760.
4 Barton CJ, Roman E, Ryder H, Watson A. Childhood leukaemia in west Berskhire. *Lancet* 1985;ii:1248–9.
5 Heasman MA, Kemp IW, Urquhart JD, Black R. Childhood leukaemia in northern Scotland. *Lancet* 1986;i:266.
5a Heasman MA, Kemp IW, Urquhart JD, Black R. Childhood leukaemia in northern Scotland. *Lancet* 1986;1:385. (Correction to preceding paper.)
6 Urquhart J, Cutler J, Burke M. Leukaemia and lymphatic cancer in young people near nuclear installations. *Lancet* 1986;i:384.
7 Hole DJ, Gillis CR. Childhood leukaemia in the west of Scotland. *Lancet* 1986;ii:524–5.
8 Roman E, Beral V, Carpenter L, Watson A, Barton C, Ryder H, Aston DL. Childhood leukaemia in the West Berkshire and Basingstoke and North Hampshire District Health Authorities in relation to nuclear establishments in the vicinity. *BMJ* 1987;294:597–602.
9 Darby DC, Doll R. Fallout, radiation doses near Dounreay, and childhood leukaemia. *BMJ* 1987;294:603–7.
10 Gardner MJ, Hall AJ, Downes S, Terrell JD. Follow up study of children born elsewhere but attending schools in Seascale, west Cumbria (schools cohort). *BMJ* 1987;295:819–21.
11 Gardner MJ, Hall AJ, Downes S, Terrell JD. Follow up study of children born to mothers resident in Seascale, west Cumbria (birth cohort). *BMJ* 1987;295:822–7.
12 Forman D, Cook-Mozaffari P, Darby S, Davey G, Stratton I, Doll R, Pike M. Cancer near nuclear installations. *Nature* 1987;329:499–505.
13 Kinlen L. Evidence for an infective cause of childhood leukaemia: comparison of a Scottish new town with nuclear reprocessing sites in Britain. *Lancet* 1988;ii:1323–7.
14 Jones RR. Infective cause of childhood leukaemia. *Lancet* 1989;i:94.
15 Wheldon TE, Mairs R, Barrett A. Germ cell injury and childhood leukaemia clusters. *Lancet* 1989;i:792–3.
16 Cook-Mozaffari PJ, Darby SC, Doll R, Forman D, Hermon C, Pike MC, Vincent T. Geographical variation in mortality from leukaemia and other cancers in England and Wales in relation to proximity to nuclear installations, 1969–78. *Br J Cancer* 1989;59:476–85.
17 Cook-Mozaffari P, Darby S, Doll R. Cancer near potential sites of nuclear installations. *Lancet* 1989;ii:1145–7.
18 Gardner MJ. Review of reported increases of childhood cancer rates in the vicinity of nuclear installations in the United Kingdom. *Journal of the Royal Statistical Society [Series A]* 1989;152:307–25.

19 Gardner MJ, Snee MP, Hall AJ, Powell CA, Downes S, Terrell JD. Results of case-control study of leukaemia and lymphoma among young people near Sellafield nuclear plant in west Cumbria. *BMJ* 1990;**300**:423–9.

20 Gardner MJ, Hall AJ, Snee MP, Downes S, Powell CA, Terrell JD. Methods and basic data of case-control study of leukaemia and lymphoma among young people near Sellafield nuclear plant in west Cumbria. *BMJ* 1990;**300**:429–34.

21 Gardner MJ. Paternal occupations of children with leukaemia. *BMJ* 1992;**305**:715. (Correction to preceding chapter.)

22 Evans HJ. Leukaemia and radiation. *Nature* 1990;**345**:16–7.

23 Notani NK. Leukaemia and lymphoma among young people near Sellafield. *BMJ* 1990;**300**:877–8.

23a Koten JW, DenOtter W. Leukaemia and lymphoma among young people near Sellafield. *BMJ* 1990;**300**:878.

23b Mole RH. Leukaemia and lymphoma among young people near Sellafield. *BMJ* 1990;**300**:878.

23c Gardner MJ, Snee MP. Leukaemia and lymphoma among young people near Sellafield. *BMJ* 1990;**300**:878.

24 Greaves MF. The Sellafield childhood leukaemia cluster: are germ line mutations responsible? *Leukemia* 1990;**4**:391–6.

25 Nomura I. Of mice and men? *Nature* 1990;**345**:671.

26 Morris JA, Edwards JM, Buckler J. Retinoblastoma in grandchildren of workers at Sellafield nuclear plant. *BMJ* 1990;**301**:1257.

27 Smith PG. Comments on the case-control study of Gardner *et al* of leukaemia and lymphoma among young people in west Cumbria. *Abstracts on Hygiene and Communicable Disease* 1990;**65**:1–6.

28 Gardner MJ. Childhood cancer and nuclear installations. *Public Health* 1991;**105**:277–8.

29 Gardner MJ. Father's occupational exposure to radiation and the raised level of childhood leukaemia near the Sellafield nuclear plant. *Environ Health Perspect* 1991;**94**:5–7.

30 Urquhart JD, Black RJ, Muirhead MJ, Sharp L, Maxwell M, Eden OB, Jones DA. Case-control study of leukaemia and non-Hodgkin's lymphoma in children in Caithness near the Dounreay nuclear installation. *BMJ* 1991;**302**:687–92.

31 Smith PG. Case-control studies of leukaemia clusters: children of parents receiving higher doses of radiation than most nuclear workers should be studied now [Editorial]. *BMJ* 1991;**302**:672–3.

32 Kinlen LJ, Hudson CM, Stiller CA. Contacts between adults as evidence for an infective origin of childhood leukaemia: an explanation for the excess near nuclear establishments in west Berkshire? *Br J Cancer* 1991;**64**:549–54.

33 Gardner MJ. Leukaemia in children and paternal radiation exposure at the Sellafield nuclear site. *J Natl Cancer Inst Monogr* 1992;**12**:133–5.

34 Black RJ, Urquhart JD, Kendrick SW, Bunch KJ, Warner J, Jones DA. Incidence of leukaemia and other cancers in birth and schools cohorts in the Dounreay area. *BMJ* 1992;**304**:1401–5.

35 Draper GJ, Stiller CA, Cartwright RA, Craft AW, Vincent TJ. Cancer in Cumbria and in the vicinity of the Sellafield nuclear installation, 1963–90. *BMJ* 1993;**306**:89–94.

36 Roman E, Watson A, Beral V, Buckle S, Bull D, Baker K, Ryder H, Barton C. Case-control study of leukaemia and non-Hodgkin's lymphoma among children aged 0–4 years living in west Berkshire and north Hampshire health districts. *BMJ* 1993;**306**:615–21.

37 Morris JA, Butler R, Flowerdew R, Gatrell AC. Retinoblastoma in children of former residents of Seascale. *BMJ* 1993;**306**:650.

38 Kinlen LK, O'Brien F, Clarke K, Balkwill A, Matthews F. Rural population mixing and childhood leukaemia: effects of the North Sea oil industry in Scotland, including the area near Dounreay nuclear site. *BMJ* 1993;**306**:743–8.

39 Kinlen LJ, Clarke K, Balkwill A. Paternal preconceptual radiation exposure in the nuclear industry and leukaemia and non-Hodgkin's lymphoma in young people in Scotland. *BMJ* 1993;**306**:1153–8.

40 Kinlen LJ. Can paternal preconceptional radiation account for the increase of leukaemia and non-Hodgkin's lymphoma in Seascale? *BMJ* 1993;**306**:1718–21.

41 Excerpts from: Black D for the Independent Advisory Group. *Investigation of the possible increased incidence of cancer in west Cumbria.* London: HMSO, 1984. (Black report.)

42 Excerpts from: Committee on Medical Aspects of Radiation in the Environment. *The implications of the new data on the releases from Sellafield in the 1950s for the conclusions of the report on the investigation of the possible increased incidence of cancer in west Cumbria.* London: HMSO, 1986. (COMARE 1st report.)

43 Excerpts from: Committee on Medical Aspects of Radiation in the Environment. *Investigation of the possible increased incidence of childhood cancer in young persons near the Dounreay nuclear establishment, Caithness, Scotland.* London: HMSO, 1988. (COMARE 2nd report.)

44 Excerpts from: Committee on Medical Aspects of Radiation in the Environment. *Investigation of the possible increased incidence of childhood cancer in the west Berkshire and north Hampshire area, in which are situated the Atomic Weapons Research Establishment, Aldermaston, and the Royal Ordnance Factory, Burghfield.* London: HMSO 1989. (COMARE 3rd report.)

Abstracts and letters relating to non-United Kingdom cancer and nuclear sites

45 Clapp RW, Cobb S, Chan CK, Walker B junior. Leukaemia near Massachusetts nuclear power plant. *Lancet* 1987;ii:1324–5.

46 Goldsmith JR. Childhood leukaemia mortality before 1970 among populations near two United States nuclear installations. *Lancet* 1989;i:793.

46a Milham S junior. Childhood leukaemia mortality before 1970 among populations near two United States nuclear installations. *Lancet* 1989;i:1443.

46b Goldsmith JR. Childhood leukaemia mortality before 1970 among populations near two United States nuclear installations. *Lancet* 1989;i:1444.

47 Hatch MC, Beyea J, Nieves JW, Susser M. Cancer near the Three Mile Island nuclear plant: radiation emissions. *Am J Epidemiol* 1990;132:397.

48 Hatch M, Susser M. Background γ radiation and childhood cancers within 10 miles of a United States nuclear plant. *Int J Epidemiol* 1990;19:546.

49 Viel JF, Richardson ST. Childhood leukaemia round the La Hague nuclear waste reprocessing plant. *BMJ* 1990;300:580.

50 Shulman S. Cancer around nuclear plant. *Nature* 1990;347:604–5.

51 Hill C, Laplanche A. Overall mortality and cancer mortality around French nuclear sites. *Nature* 1990;347:755.

52 Hatch MC, Wallenstein S, Beyea J, Nieves JW, Susser M. Cancer rates after the Three Mile Island nuclear accident and proximity of residence to the plant. *Am J Public Health* 1991;81:719.

53 Jablon S, Hrubec Z, Boice JD junior. Cancer in populations living near nuclear facilities: a survey of mortality nationwide and incidence in two states. *JAMA* 1991;265:1403.

54 Michaelis J, Keller B, Haaf G, Kaatsch P. Incidence of childhood malignancies in the vicinity of West German nuclear power plants. *Cancer Causes and Control* 1992;3:255.

55 McLaughlin JR, King WD, Anderson TW, Clarke AE, Ashmore JP. Paternal radiation exposure and leukaemia in offspring: the Ontario case-control study. *BMJ* 1993;307: (16 October).

Introduction

VALERIE BERAL, EVE ROMAN, MARTIN BOBROW

Childhood leukaemia in the vicinity of nuclear establishments has been one of the most intensely discussed issues in British medical research in the past 10 years. The late Professor Martin Gardner, an eminent medical statistician, was a central figure in this debate. His publications on this topic, and a selection of those of others who have carried out research in this area, are collected together in this volume.

This book chronicles the events of the past 10 years, beginning in early 1983 when James Cutler, a producer with Yorkshire Television, went to west Cumbria to gather information for a programme on the health of employees at the British Nuclear Fuels reprocessing plant at Sellafield. His questioning led him to Seascale, a small village two miles from Sellafield, where he learnt that several local children had been diagnosed as having leukaemia. His research team ultimately discovered that seven children and young adults had had leukaemia diagnosed between 1956 and 1983, whereas fewer than one case of leukaemia would normally be expected among residents at those ages. These findings were presented in the Independent Television documentary *Windscale – the Nuclear Laundry* (Sellafield was previously called Windscale) on 1 November 1983, and further discussed in the correspondence columns of the Lancet in January the following year (chapters 1–2). Public interest was intense and it was widely believed that discharges from the Sellafield site had caused the cancers.

Sellafield and the "Black report"

Government response to the documentary was prompt. The minister of health asked Sir Douglas Black to head an independent inquiry. Extracts of what is commonly referred to as the "Black report" are reproduced in chapter 41. The committee concluded that the incidence of leukaemia in people under 25 years of age living in Seascale was indeed increased, and that the excess was neither explained by the unorthodox methods that the documentary team had used to identify cases nor by the age and time categories used. It also concluded that the amount of radiation in the environment and estimated doses of radiation received by the local population were, according to conventional knowledge, insufficient to account for the excess. Finally, it remained possible that the "cluster" had arisen by chance. The further research the committee recommended was the subject of many of the publications reprinted in this book.

On the recommendation of the Black Advisory Group the Committee on the Medical Aspects of Radiation in the Environment (COMARE) was established in 1985. Its first report dealt with new information about discharges from the Sellafield site, of which the Black Advisory Group had been unaware. Jakeman, who had worked as a physicist at Sellafield, drew attention to a number of substantial releases which occurred during the 1950s from the Sellafield nuclear reactor chimneys (chapter 3). COMARE concluded that there had indeed been substantial undisclosed releases during the 1950s, but that they were still insufficient to account for the extra cases of leukaemia found at Seascale (chapter 42).

Is there an excess of cancer near other nuclear establishments?

Detailed studies of the incidence of leukaemia in children and young adults have so far been reported only for certain selected nuclear sites in the United Kingdom—Sellafield, Dounreay, and Aldermaston and Burghfield. Although a report is expected soon, no comprehensive analysis of cancer incidence in the small areas in the immediate vicinity of each nuclear establishment in Britain has yet been published.

DOUNREAY

Dounreay is the only other reprocessing plant in the United Kingdom, and although the amount of radioactive material reprocessed is much smaller than at Sellafield, its mode of operations and the nature of its discharges are more similar to those at Sellafield than at other nuclear plants. Dounreay therefore offered an independent opportunity to investigate some of the questions which had been raised about the incidence of childhood cancer in the vicinity of Sellafield.

Heasman and colleagues (from the Information and Statistics Division of the Scottish Health Service Common Services Agency) found that six people aged under 25 who lived within 25 km of the Dounreay plant had had leukaemia diagnosed between 1968 and 1984, whereas between one and two cases would normally be expected. All six cases occurred after 1979, whereas fewer than one would be expected (chapter 5).

COMARE concluded that the evidence indicated a raised incidence of leukaemia in young people near Dounreay but, on the basis of existing radiobiological knowledge, the authorised radioactive discharges from the site could not account for the excess. The committee recommended that several alternative explanations should be considered, including other mechanisms by which the authorised discharges could be implicated, the possibility that parental occupational exposure could be relevant, and that other factors not related to radiation, such as chemicals or viruses, might be involved (chapter 43).

ALDERMASTON AND BURGHFIELD

The Atomic Weapons Establishments at Aldermaston and Burghfield in Berkshire differ in many ways from the reprocessing plants at Sellafield and Dounreay. The substances handled and the nature of the work performed is different, and the amount of radioactive material discharged into the environment is considerably smaller. Furthermore, the surrounding area is relatively densely populated and includes Reading and several other large towns and villages.

Concern about a possible excess of childhood leukaemia in the vicinity of the nuclear plants at Aldermaston and Burghfield was first expressed by Carol Barton, a consultant haematologist at the Royal Berkshire Hospital in Reading, and her colleagues. They thought they might be seeing more children with leukaemia than would normally be expected at their clinic, and asked epidemiologists at the London School of Hygiene and Tropical Medicine to investigate their suspicions. Their preliminary findings confirmed a small excess of childhood leukaemia in the area (chapter 4). A more detailed report showed that the excess was confined to children under 5 years of age who lived within 10 km of the nuclear establishments at Aldermaston and Burghfield (chapter 8).

The third COMARE report examined data on other childhood cancers, as well as leukaemia, in the vicinity of Aldermaston and Burghfield (chapter 44). The committee concluded that there was a small but significantly increased incidence of leukaemia and of other cancers in children aged under 5 living within 10 km of the nuclear establishments at Aldermaston and Burghfield. COMARE reiterated several recommendations made in earlier reports and further suggested that the health of children of workers in the nuclear industry should be investigated.

OTHER NUCLEAR ESTABLISHMENTS

United Kingdom—Several researchers have used routinely collected data to look at mortality from cancer in broad areas around nuclear establishments, and their findings have suggested that there may be any increase in childhood lymphoid leukaemia in the surrounding area (chapters 12, 16, 17).[12] The data analysed in these studies tended to be assembled for other purposes and usually covered comparatively large geographical areas, so that if there were an increase confined to people who lived very close to the plants this would be diluted by the rates for the substantial numbers who lived further away. Moreover, many researchers studied mortality statistics, which do not necessarily reflect cancer incidence, especially for childhood lymphoid leukaemia: in the early 1960s only 5% of children with lymphoid leukaemia survived for five years but by the mid-1980s the five year survival had increased to around 70%.[34]

Outside Britain—Prompted by the findings in Britain, researchers began to investigate the occurrence of cancer in the vicinity of nuclear establishments in other countries. Existing evidence does not suggest an increase in childhood leukaemia near certain installations in France (chapters 49, 51), Germany (chapter 54), or the United States (chapters 45, 46–8, 50, 52, 53). Most studies from outside Britain have relied on the collation of routinely collected mortality statistics over comparatively large areas, which, for the reasons described above, may mask any increase in risk for people who live close to the nuclear establishments.

Summary—Careful investigations have indicated that there are real increases in the incidence of childhood leukaemia around Sellafield, Dounreay, and Aldermaston and Burghfield. There are differences between these installations and between the details of the increases observed, and the reasons for the excesses remain unclear. Studies of cancer incidence near other nuclear establishments in Britain and elsewhere in the world have not been as detailed but suggest no major increase in risk.

Detailed studies of cancer in people living near nuclear installations

The geographical studies described so far compared number of cases of cancer and leukaemia in people living near the plants with the number that would have been expected had national or regional rates applied. The only information used for these studies was the age and sex of the individuals concerned. Subsequently epidemiological studies were set up which collected detailed information about the characteristics of these individuals. The results of these studies are discussed in this section.

SELLAFIELD

The Black Advisory Group recommended a series of studies on individuals who had lived near Sellafield, three of which were undertaken by Gardner (chapters 10, 11, 19, and 20). The first was to identify all people born in Seascale since 1950, to follow them even if they moved from Seascale, and find out how many had developed cancer. The second was to identify children who had gone to school in Seascale, but who had been born elsewhere and follow them in a similar way. The third (chapters 19 and 20) was to conduct a case-control study of leukaemia and non-

Hodgkin's lymphoma in west Cumbrian residents under 25 years of age to investigate whether there were any characteristics of the children with leukaemia or their parents which might explain the excess.

In their study of children born in Seascale, Gardner and his colleagues identified 1068 children born in the village between 1950 and 1983. They found that the children were 10 times more likely to develop leukaemia than the average, and three times more likely to develop other cancers (chapters 11, 28, 29, 33). There were six cases of leukaemia, compared with 0·6 expected in the children born in Seascale (observed to expected (O/E) ratio 10·0, 95% confidence interval (CI) 3·7 to 21·8). In addition, there were six other cancers (lymphosarcoma, retroperitoneal sarcoma, carcinoma of the tongue, melanoma, non-Hodgkin's lymphoma, and Wilms's tumour) compared with 2·2 expected (O/E 2·7, 1·0 to 5·0). By contrast, there was no increase in leukaemia or other cancers in the 1546 children who went to school in Seascale but were born elsewhere (chapters 10, 28, 29, 33).

In their case-control study Gardner and his colleagues set out to investigate whether the excess leukaemia and lymphoma diagnosed in children and young adults near the Sellafield plant was associated with established risk factors or with factors related to the plant. Information was gathered about each of the 107 people with a diagnosis of leukaemia or lymphoma before their 25th birthday during 1950–85, who were born in the west Cumbrian health district and were resident there when their cancer was diagnosed. For comparative purposes 1001 controls of the same age and sex as those with cancer, and who were born in the same area and resident there when their corresponding case was diagnosed, were also studied (chapters 19, 20, 21). This painstaking study, which is often called the "Gardner report," took six years to complete and is acknowledged to have been well planned, well executed, and well analysed (chapter 27). The main finding was that the risk of childhood leukaemia increased in relation to father's exposure to external sources of ionising radiation before his child was conceived. The authors reported an eightfold increase in risk (relative risk (RR) 8·38, 1·4 to 52·0), based on four fathers with a recorded cumulative dose of 100 mSv or more (the same four fathers had accumulated a dose of 10 mSv or more in the six months before conception). Three of the four fathers of children with the highest exposures to radiation lived in Seascale, and Gardner suggested that fathers' exposure to external sources of ionising radiation could, if correct, explain the excess leukaemia and non-Hodgkin's lymphoma in young people living in Seascale.

DOUNREAY

On the recommendation of COMARE Black and colleagues identified 4144 children born between 1969 and 1988 in the Dounreay area. Five cancers were diagnosed (O/E 0·9, 0·3 to 2·0), and all five cancers were leukaemia, (O/E 2·3, 0·7 to 5·4). Among the 1641 children who attended school in the area but were not born there, three cancers were diagnosed, (O/E 2·1, 0·4 to 6·2), and all were leukaemia, (O/E 6·7, 1·4 to 19·5). All eight children with leukaemia were resident in the area at the time their cancer was diagnosed (chapter 34).

A case-control study of leukaemia and non-Hodgkin's lymphoma in young people living in Caithness in the vicinity of the Dounreay nuclear reprocessing plant was carried out by Urquhart and his colleagues. Its aims were similar to those of Gardner's study. The number of individuals studied was much smaller. Fourteen children under 15 years diagnosed as having leukaemia or non-Hodgkin's lymphoma in Caithness between 1970 and 1986 were compared with 55 control children, matched for sex, date of birth, and area of residence within Caithness at the time of birth. No reason for the excess was found, and their results neither supported nor contradicted those of the Gardner report (chapter 30).

ALDERMASTON AND BURGHFIELD

The case-control study of children diagnosed as having leukaemia or non-Hodgkin's lymphoma before their fifth birthday in west Berkshire and north Hampshire (the age group in which the excess had been noted) was set up in 1987. The main aim was to investigate the role of parental employment in the nuclear industry. The characteristics of 54 children diagnosed as having leukaemia or non-Hodgkin's lymphoma during 1972–89 were compared with those of 324 control children of the same sex, date of birth, and area of residence within west Berkshire and north Hampshire health districts. The main positive finding, based on only three fathers of case children and two of control children, was a ninefold higher risk of leukaemia in children whose father had been monitored for exposure to ionising radiation at work before their child was conceived (RR 9·0, 1·0 to 107·8). Neither this observation, nor any other factor examined in the study, could account for the above average incidence of leukaemia in the area (chapter 36).

OTHER STUDIES

In response to the Gardner report new research was set up in the United Kingdom and abroad to link, on an individual basis, fathers' recorded exposure to ionising radiation at work with their children's health. The results of three such studies, all of which have found no associations, have recently been published (chapters 39, 40, 55) and another is in press.[5]

In Scotland Kinlen and colleagues searched nuclear industry databases with the aim of comparing employment characteristics of fathers of 1261 children diagnosed as having leukaemia or non-Hodgkin's lymphoma before the age of 25 during 1950–90 with three times as many controls. That study, which included the cases investigated by Urquhart *et al* (chapter 30), yielded no significant associations (chapter 39). Kinlen has also recently published data on 11 cases of leukaemia and non-Hodgkin's lymphoma diagnosed in residents of Seascale age 0–24 years during 1951–91. He confirmed the excess of these malignancies in Seascale, noting that it stemmed not only from the six cases born in Seascale but also from the five born outside Seascale. He further argued that paternal preconceptual exposure to ionising radiation was unlikely to explain the increased incidence of these cancers in the area, as the association was less evident in the five case children born outside Seascale than in the six born in Seascale (chapter 40). The forthcoming report by Parker and her colleagues also concludes that fathers' occupational exposure to ionising radiation is unlikely to explain the excess in Seascale.[5]

In a study in Ontario, Canada, the characteristics of 112 children born to mothers residing in the vicinity of five nuclear facilities who died of, or were diagnosed as having, leukaemia between 1950 and 1988, were compared with 890 age and residence matched control children. No evidence of an association with paternal preconceptual dose was found (chapter 55).

By contrast, two other studies have reported an increased risk associated with fathers' exposure at work to ionising radiation and cancer in their children, but because they were based on self reported information the findings are difficult to interpret.[6 7]

SUMMARY

In depth, locally based, studies of leukaemia in children and young adults who have lived near nuclear establishments have yielded some unexpected findings. Few have engendered such intense scientific and public debate as the findings of the Gardner report. The principal point of contention was that men who were exposed at work to relatively high doses of ionising radiation from external sources might have children who were at an increased risk of leukaemia. The findings from other studies have been less clear and as yet there seems to be little consistency in their results or coherent interpretation of them. The relative importance of parental occupation, child's place of birth, and child's place of residence at diagnosis are still not clear. More studies are under way, and it is too early to draw firm conclusions on the basis of existing evidence.

Is the increased incidence of childhood leukaemia continuing?

When the cluster of leukaemia in children and young adults living in Seascale was first described a crucial question was whether the increase would continue. Draper and colleagues (chapter 35) have recently reported on the incidence of leukaemia and other cancers in people aged 0–24 years during the seven years subsequent to the Yorkshire Television programme (1984–90). There were two cases of non-Hodgkin's lymphoma and none of leukaemia; the expected number of cases was 0·12. Thus there is some evidence that there continues to be an increased incidence of lymphoid malignancies – but there were some differences from the original observations in that the type of cancer has changed from leukaemia to non-Hodgkin's lymphoma and that one case occurred at the relatively old age of 23, whereas the original "cluster" was in younger people. Additional information on the situation around Dounreay and Aldermaston and Burghfield is awaited.

Other childhood cancers

Although information about other childhood malignancies could aid our interpretation of the findings for leukaemia, no systematic study has yet been concluded. Around Sellafield, no excess has been reported (chapter 35), but COMARE noted a significant excess of all other cancers combined (excluding leukaemia) in children under 5 around Aldermaston and Burghfield (chapter 44).

RETINOBLASTOMA

In 1990 Morris and colleagues reported that they had identified three children with retinoblastoma whose grandfathers had worked at Sellafield and whose mothers had lived in Seascale. Subsequently two further cases came to light in children whose mothers had lived in Seascale but whose grandfathers had not worked at Sellafield, and Morris and colleagues estimated that the incidence of this rare tumour is increased about 20-fold in the children of women who had lived in Seascale (chapters 26, 37). This curious observation is difficult to interpret. Forty percent of retinoblastomas in children are associated with an identifiable germ cell mutation, and research is now under way to establish whether the retinoblastomas in these children were the consequences of susceptibility transmitted to the child by its mother or father, or whether they were of the non-familial type.

Conclusions

Ten years after James Cutler's remarkable observation about the cluster of leukaemia in children and young adults in Seascale, scientific opinion has shifted considerably. When the documentary was screened in November 1983 the response of many experts was that of incredulity – the general view at the time was that the excess had been exaggerated either by the unconventional way that Cutler had identified people with leukaemia or the unusual age and geographical boundaries he had used to describe it, or that the cluster was due to the play of chance. It is now widely accepted that there is a real excess of leukaemia and lymphoma in young people in Seascale – not only was the excess demonstrable over a wide range of age and geographical boundaries, but it seems to have persisted after Cutler's first observations were made (chapters 35, 40). Careful investigations have also confirmed excesses of childhood lymphoid malignancies around Dounreay, and Aldermaston and Burghfield.

Scientific debate has moved from questioning whether these excesses are real to finding explanations for them. Cutler's allegation that environmental contamination by radioactive materials caused the increases does not at this stage have strong support. According to conventional radiobiological knowledge, the levels of radioactivity in the soil and air appear to be orders of magnitude too low to account for the excesses. Even around Sellafield the levels of contamination are comparable with those found in many areas of the world contaminated by the fallout from atomic bomb tests, where no increases in childhood leukaemia have been observed. The levels are lower near Dounreay (chapter 9)[8] and lower still near Aldermaston and Burghfield.

Childhood cancer is a rare disease and its causes are, for the most part, unknown. In Britain about 1200 children are diagnosed as having cancer each year, about a third of these have leukaemia. This rarity has meant that many of the studies that have set out to investigate the occurrence of cancer in children who live near nuclear establishments have been bedevilled by the small numbers involved. Interpretation has been further hampered by the fact that despite the many suggested hypotheses about the causes of childhood cancer, particularly leukaemia, direct evidence is lacking. At present, the only established external causes of leukaemia in children are exposure to ionising radiation in utero or shortly after birth and chemotherapy.

In 1990 Gardner presented evidence that suggested that father's employment in the nuclear industry was responsible for the excess in Seascale. The fathers of children with leukaemia had received relatively high doses of external radiation before their children were conceived. One curious finding in Gardner's original report was that the association with father's exposure at work was far stronger for children born in Seascale than for children born elsewhere in west Cumbria (table). This has led to criticism of Gardner's work, since if father's exposure to radiation were the sole reason for the excess, then it should be evident in the children of other similarly exposed workers, regardless of where they lived. In the absence of corroboration from other studies, the suggestion that paternal preconceptual exposure to ionising radiation can cause leukaemia or lymphoma in children remains to be proved. A study investigating the occurrence of all cancers, not only leukaemia, and the incidence of other illnesses and conditions that could have a genetic cause among children of workers in the

Numbers (and percentages) of children diagnosed as having leukaemia (cases) and their corresponding controls by place of residence at diagnosis and by their fathers' employment at Sellafield and recorded preconceptual dose of external ionising radiation while working at Sellafield*

Father's employment/radiation group	Resident in Seascale		Resident elsewhere	
	Cases (%)	Controls (%)	Cases (%)	Controls (%)
Not employed at Sellafield	0	4 (20)	37 (88)	227 (89)
Employed at Sellafield				
No dose	0	0	1 (2)	5 (2)
1–49 mSv	0	8 (40)	3 (7)	18 (7)
50–99 mSv	1 (25)	7 (35)	0	4 (2)
⩾100 mSv	3 (75)	1 (5)	1 (2)	2 (1)
Total	4 (100)	20 (100)	42 (100)	256 (100)

* From Gardner *et al* (chapter 19)

nuclear industry is now under way. A study linking a national data on childhood cancer to parental radiation records is also in progress. The findings from these studies should eventually provide reliable information on the incidence of cancer and other conditions in the children of fathers employed in the nuclear industry.

Kinlen has proposed that the excess of leukaemia around Sellafield and Dounreay and Aldermaston and Burghfield might have resulted from unusual patterns of migration and population mixing, affecting the local incidence of an infectious agent that caused leukaemia (chapters 13, 32, 38–40).[9] Though this hypothesis has its attractions, the evidence to date is indirect. The search for an infectious cause of childhood leukaemia has a long history; although research to date has largely been unsuccessful, there is now renewed interest in this topic.[10] Whether infectious agents play an important part in the aetiology of childhood leukaemia is being investigated in a national case-control study. This study, which began in 1992, is the largest and most comprehensive investigation of childhood cancer ever undertaken, and its findings will not be available for several years.

It has taken a decade to establish that there is a real excess of childhood leukaemia in the vicinity of certain nuclear establishments in Britain. The published work that has accrued on this topic is extensive, and in this book emphasis has been given to reports that present original data. Reports of studies conducted in the United Kingdom are reproduced in full in chapters 1–40, extracts of government reports are presented in chapters 41–44, and letters and summaries by authors about investigations conducted elsewhere in the world are listed in chapters 45–55.

At least another decade will pass before the reasons for the increased incidence of childhood cancer around certain nuclear establishments are understood, if they ever will be. Cutler's television programme and the

Gardner report have stimulated the launching of some of the most thorough investigations of childhood cancer ever undertaken. The findings so far and the results of the new studies will undoubtedly expand our knowledge of the causes of childhood cancer, about which so little was known before. Martin Gardner's integrity, wisdom, and clarity of thought will be sadly missed, especially when the results of the new studies become available.

We should particularly like to thank Gerald Draper for his help and advice. We are also grateful to Lucy Carpenter, Sarah Darby, Hazel Inskip, and Leo Kinlen for their comments.

1 Baron JA. Cancer mortality in small areas around nuclear facilities in England and Wales. *Br J Cancer* 1984; **50**: 815–24.
2 Cook-Mozaffari PJ, Ashwood FL, Vincent T, Forman D, Alderson M. *Cancer incidence and mortality in the vicinity of nuclear installations England and Wales 1959–80.* London: HMSO, 1987. (Studies on medical and population subjects, No. 51.)
3 Stiller CA, Bunch KJ. Trends in survival for childhood cancer in Britain diagnosed 1971–85. *Br J Cancer* 1990; **62**, 806–15.
4 Stiller C. Aetiology and epidemiology. In: Ploughman PN, Pinkerton CR, *Paediatric oncology: clinical practise and controversies.* London: Chapman Hall, 1992: 1–24.
5 Parker L, Craft AW, Smith J, Dickinson H, Wakeford R, Binks K, McElvenny D, Scott L, Slovak A. Childhood leukaemia and occupational radiation exposure: the geographical distribution of preconceptional radiation doses associated with fathers employed at the Sellafield nuclear installation, west Cumbria, for births during 1950–1989, *BMJ* (in press).
6 McKinney PA, Alexander FE, Cartwright RA, Parker L. Parental occupations of children with leukaemia in west Cumbria, north Humberside, and Gateshead. *BMJ* 1991;**302**:681–7.
7 Sorahan T, Roberts PJ. Childhood cancer and parental exposure to ionising radiation: preliminary findings from the Oxford survey of childhood cancers. *Am J Ind Med* 1993; **23**:343–54.
8 Darby SC, Olsen JH, Doll R, Thakrar B, Nully Brown P, Storm HH, *et al.* Trends in childhood leukaemia in the Nordic countries in relation to fallout from atmospheric nuclear weapons testing. *BMJ* 1992; **304**: 1005–9.
9 Kinlen LJ, Clarke K, Hudson C. Evidence from population mixing in British new towns 1946–85 of an infective basis for childhood leukaemia. *Lancet* 1990; **336**, 577–82.
10 Greaves MF, Alexander FE. An infectious etiology for common acute lymphoblastic leukemia in childhood? *Leukemia* 1993; 7: 349–60.

1: Mortality in Cumberland during 1959–78 with reference to cancer in young people around Windscale

Letter to the *Lancet*

M J GARDNER, P D WINTER

In a Yorkshire Television programme on 1 November 1983, concern was expressed that the incidence of cancer, and of leukaemia in young people especially, might be raised in Cumbria and that this could be related to radiation exposure from the Sellafield (formerly Windscale) nuclear reprocessing plant. The issue is the subject of a Government inquiry, chaired by Sir Douglas Black. We present here information that we have readily available on death rates in the surrounding areas for the years 1959–78, though we accept that statistics on cancer incidence might be more pertinent. Craft and Birch's data from two childhood cancer registries in 1968–82 showed that the subdistrict of Cumbria containing Windscale had some of the higher incidence rates for leukaemia and all cancer under the age of 15.[1] However, there was no suggestion, on the large scale of area used, of an excess as large as that reported in the television programme for one village near the reprocessing plant.

From abstracts of records for deaths on computer tape, giving year of death, age, sex, underlying cause of death, and local authority area of residence at time of death (but no personal identification), we have compiled an atlas of cancer mortality covering 1968–78,[2] the period when the eighth revision of the International Classification of Diseases (ICD 8) was in operation. We also have computerised mortality data for 1959–67 (ICD 7).

The former county of Cumberland (in Cumbria since 1974) and its subdivisions were used in the analysis reported here. Deaths are compared with numbers expected from age-sex specific death rates for England and

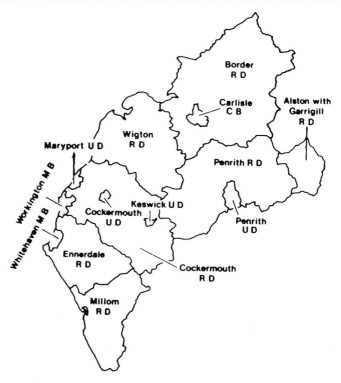

Local authority areas of Cumberland (before reorganisation in 1974). (CB = county borough, MB = municipal borough, RD = rural district, UD = urban district.)

Wales. Population figures are taken from the 1961 and 1971 censuses. We have more extensive results for 1968–78 because of the analyses done for the cancer atlas.[2] We do not yet have post-1978 mortality data in comparable form.

The British Nuclear Fuels Ltd plant at Sellafield is at the southern coastal extreme of Ennerdale rural district, and the village of Seascale (the focus of the television programme) is at the northern coastal tip of Millom rural district (see map).

In Cumberland during 1968–78 there was a 6% excess death rate for both men and women (table I), but for cancer deaths there were deficits of 6% for men and 2% for women and there were slightly fewer leukaemia deaths than expected. Among other types of cancer, there were significant excesses (10–15%) for stomach, large intestine, and pancreas. The excess mortality from non-cancer causes is largely a result of high death rates from ischaemic heart disease, for which there was an excess of 26% in 1969–73. During 1959–63 the overall excess death rate in Cumberland was 7%, whereas there was a deficit in cancer deaths of 4% for 1959–67.

TABLE I—*Mortality by cause of death and sex in Cumberland during 1968–78*

	Men			Women		
Causes	Observed (O)	Expected (E)	SMR (100 × (O/E))	Observed (O)	Expected (E)	SMR (100 × (O/E))
All	20 904	19 801	106*	19 755	18 570	106*
Non-cancer	16 811	15 464	109*	16 213	14 961	108*
Cancer	4 093	4 338	94*	3 542	3 608	98
Leukaemia	104	113·2	92	96	93·5	103

E = expected number of deaths at age, sex, and cause specific rates in England and Wales during 1968–78; SMR = standardised mortality ratio; ICD eighth revision codes 140–209 for cancer, 204–207 for leukaemia.
* Significantly different from 100 at p < 0·01.

In the data for Ennerdale and Millom rural districts (table II) men and women have been combined. The two districts had death rates at all ages similar to those for Cumberland as a whole during 1968–78, except for a raised leukaemia rate in Millom rural district. At young ages (under 25) there were apparent raised cancer death rates in both areas during 1968–78, but not during 1959–67. For Millom rural district the high rate was largely accounted for by the leukaemia figures, but this was not so for the statistically non-significant excess in Ennerdale rural district. In Millom rural district three of the six leukaemia deaths were in men and three in women (0·82 and 0·56 expected, respectively); three of the deaths were at under the age of 15 and three between the ages of 15 and 24 (0·95 and 0·43, respectively); two of the deaths were due to acute lymphatic leukaemia

TABLE II—*Mortality by cause of death and age in Ennerdale and Millom rural districts*

		Ennerdale rural district			Millom rural district		
Cause	Period	Observed	Expected	SMR	Observed	Expected	SMR
		All ages					
All causes	1959–67						
	1968–78	3897	3684	106*	1785	1737	103
Cancer (140–207)	1959–67	564	648·5	103	234	266·9	88†
(140–209)	1968–78	726	765·6	95	330	359·7	92
Leukaemia (204)	1959–67	15	15·6	96	6	7·6	79
(204–207)	1968–78	16	20·6	78	13	9·5	137
		Ages 0–24					
All causes	1959–67						
	1968–78	167	145·8	115	63	60·5	104
Cancer (140–207)	1959–67	7	9·1	77	3	4·5	67
(140–209)	1968–78	14	9·3	150	10	4·0	253†
Leukaemia (204)	1959–67	3	3·3	91	1	1·6	63
(204–207)	1968–78	4	3·3	121	6	1·4	435*

All causes figures not calculated for 1959–67; ICD 7th revision (1959–67) and 8th revision codes in parentheses (1968–78).
Significantly different from 100 at *p < 0·01. †p < 0·05.

TABLE III—*Mortality from leukaemia under age of 25 in Cumberland*

Local authority area	1959–67			1968–78		
	Observed	Expected	SMR	Observed	Expected	SMR
Carlisle county borough	13	6·7	195†	6	7·0	86
Cockermouth urban district	0	0·6	0	0	0·6	0
Keswick urban district	0	0·4	0	0	0·4	0
Maryport urban district	0	1·1	0	0	1·2	0
Penrith urban district	1	1·0	100	0	1·2	0
Whitehaven municipal borough	3	3·0	101	2	2·9	69
Workington municipal borough	2	2·8	70	1	2·8	36
Alston with Garrigill rural district	0	0·2	0	0	0·2	0
Border rural district	0	2·9	0	2	2·7	74
Cockermouth rural district	0	2·0	0	0	1·9	0
Ennerdale rural district	3	3·3	91	4	3·3	121
Millom rural district	1	1·6	63	6	1·4	435*
Penrith rural district	0	1·1	0	0	1·1	0
Wigton rural district	6	2·1	282†	1	2·2	45
Cumberland	29	28·9	100	22	28·8	76

Significantly different from 100 at *p<0·01. †p<0·05.

(0·77), three to acute myeloid leukaemia (0·37), and one to chronic lymphatic leukaemia (0·01). Over the age of 25 there were no excess leukaemia deaths.

Table III summarises the findings in relation to leukaemia mortality in Cumberland under the age of 25. The standardised mortality ratio for leukaemia fell from 100 during 1959–67 to 76 during 1968–78. There is no other individual area with a raised figure comparable with Millom's for the latest 11-year period. During the earlier period two areas, Carlisle county borough and Wigton rural district, stand out: in Wigton rural district the six deaths were all among children under the age of 15 (1·6 expected).

The results for leukaemia among people aged under 25 show that there appears to have been an excess during 1968–78 in the areas around Windscale. However, from the mortality data—even though the upper 95% confidence limit for the standardised mortality ratio at Millom rural district during these 11 years was equivalent to a 9·5 times raised risk—the excess appears to be lower than the tenfold excess suggested in Yorkshire Television's *Windscale: the Nuclear Laundry.* However, the television programme looked at cases of cancer not deaths and focused on a small locality, Seascale, within Millom rural district. Our findings at least confirm the need for further investigation.

A more extensive analysis of mortality data would be most useful, and this is being done by Dr P Cook-Mozaffari and her colleagues in Oxford. They are investigating death rates for selected cancers by distance from nuclear installations in Britain with other neighbouring areas as controls. Cancer incidence is being studied at the Office of Population Censuses and Surveys, using information from the National Cancer Registration

Scheme. For a condition such as leukaemia, survival from which by young patients is now so much better than it was in former years, it is important to collect information on all cases, not just deaths.

Studies of this sort will inevitably yield some excesses (and deficits) as a result of statistical fluctuation alone, and both the high rates near Windscale and the raised mortality levels in Carlisle county borough and Wigton rural district during 1959–67 could have happened in this way. However, if the excess of leukaemia in young people in Millom rural district is substantiated, a more detailed study will be needed with inquiry into, for example, the validity of the certified causes of death, the place of residence at birth, during life, and at death, whether or not they drank potentially radiation-contaminated milk, and whether or not they were exposed to radiation in utero.

1 Craft AW, Birch JM. Childhood cancer in Cumbria. *Lancet* 1983;**ii**:1299.
2 Gardner MJ, Winter PD, Taylor CP, Acheson ED. *Atlas of cancer mortality for England and Wales, 1968–78*. Chichester: Wiley, 1983.

2: Cancer in Cumbria: the Windscale connection

Letter to the *Lancet*

JOHN URQUHART, MICHAEL PALMER,
JAMES CUTLER

Craft and Birch conclude that there have been no significant increases in the incidence of childhood cancer in Cumbria, the county in which the British Nuclear Fuels Ltd plant at Sellafield (Windscale) is situated.[1] However, they fail to consider smaller areas within Cumbria which show abnormal patterns, and they ignore cancers in young persons aged 15 or more. In the areas closest to the BNFL plant and coastal areas where high levels of radioactivity have been found there is a significant excess of deaths from malignancy and leukaemia in the 0–24 age group. The data in table I are from Office of Population Censuses and Surveys sources (SD 25s, DH 2s, and earlier series). The seven deaths in the age group 0–24 from all malignancies, the four from leukaemia recorded for Seascale and coastal villages, and the eight from leukaemia in Millom rural district are all significantly more than expected for England and Wales as a whole ($p < 0.02$, $p < 0.02$, $p < 0.01$, respectively).

Craft and Birch's contention that clusters can occur by chance fails to meet the point that a cluster of cases may also be a sign that some specific cause is at work. However, the six cases of leukaemia diagnosed in children under the age of 15 and living at Seascale (the ones mentioned in the Yorkshire Television programme) are not a "cluster" in that sense. They are more an "excess". Details of these six children are: (a) F, aged 8 years, died 1956; (b) M, 2, died 1960; (c) 1967, M, 10, recovered; (d) M, 6, died 1970; (e) F, 2, died 1971; (f) 1979, F, 4, recovered. Five were aged under 10 (expected 0.45, $p < 0.0002$).

There is no sign that the excess childhood malignancies near Windscale are decreasing. The cases in the under 15 age group found by the Yorkshire Television research team are shown in table II.

It has been suggested that excess cancers may be linked to the radioactive discharges from Windscale, so data for Maryport were also analysed.

TABLE I—*Deaths per 100 000 person years 1963–82 (and numbers of deaths in parentheses) for England and Wales and for selected parts of Cumbria*

Age (years)	England and Wales	Copeland	Millom rural district*†	Seascale and coastal villages*
		All malignancies		
0–14	6·7	6·2 (22)	7·7 (6)	19·7 (4)
15–24	7·9	12·3 (27)	20·9 (9)	27·5 (3)
0–24	7·2	8·5 (49)	12·4 (15)	22·4 (7)
		All leukaemias		
0–14	2·8	2·8 (10)	3·8 (3)	9·7 (2)
15–24	2·1	3·2 (7)	11·6 (5)	18·3 (2)
0–24	2·5	3·0 (17)	6·6 (8)	12·7 (4)

* The population of Millom rural district is about 20% that of Copeland. The coastal villages and Seascale are all the coastal parishes in Millom rural district nearest Windscale and consist of Seascale itself, Drigg and Carleton, Bootle, Waberthwaite, and Muncaster. The population is about 5% of that of Copeland.
† There were 50 non-cancer deaths in Millom rural district in children aged under 15 and 20 in those aged 15–24, the non-cancer death rates are similar to those for England and Wales.

Maryport has the most contaminated river estuary on the Cumbrian coast after Ravenglass.[2] There has been a significant increase in deaths from malignant disease in the 15–24 age group both for Maryport ($p < 0.02$) and for Millom rural district ($p < 0.01$) when 1963–72 data are contrasted with 1973–82 (table III).

We suggest that Craft and Birch analyse their registry data again, looking at smaller areas in Cumbria, particularly those near the coast or on river

TABLE II—*Malignancy cases 1968–83: rates per 100 000 person years (totals in parentheses) in children aged under 15*

Years	England and Wales*	Copeland†	Millom rural district‡	Seascale and coastal villages‡
1968–72	10·8	15·8 (15)	18 (4)	55 (3) ($p < 0.05$)
1973–77	11·5	10·6 (9)	13 (2)	44 (2)
1978–83	11·0	10·5 (8)	20 (4)	90 (4) ($p < 0.004$)
1968–83	11·1	11·6 (32)	17 (10)	62 (9) ($p < 0.0001$)

* Source: OPCS cancer statistics registration series MB 1 and earlier series (1978–83 is estimated).
† These rates are given by Craft and Birch and are for 1968–82.
‡ Cases compiled from death certificates and interviews, and confirmed by local general practitioner.

TABLE III—*Malignancy deaths rates per 100 000 person years (totals in parentheses) in people aged 15–24*

Years	England and Wales	Copeland	Millom rural district	Allerdale*	Maryport†
1963–72	8·4	12 (11)	10 (2)	—	0 (0)
1973–82	7·4	14 (16)	32 (7)	6 (7)	29 (5)

* 1974–81 only.
† Maryport is a small part of Allerdale.

estuaries, and that they extend their studies to include non-lymphoblastic leukaemias and malignancy data in the 15–24 year age group.

1 Craft AW, Birch JM. Childhood cancer in Cumbria. *Lancet* 1983;**ii**:1299.
2 Hunt GJ. *Aquatic environment monitoring report no 8*. London: Ministry of Agriculture, Fisheries and Food, 1982.

3: New estimates of radioactive discharges from Sellafield

Letter to the *British Medical Journal*

DEREK JAKEMAN

I would like to add a few points to the note on this subject (*BMJ*, 2 August 1986, p 340). My estimates of discharges in the 1950s and the possible effects of these are contained in a report which has recently been published for me by the United Kingdom Atomic Energy Authority.[1]

The release of radioactivity in the early 1950s was substantial, consisting of thousands of millions of highly radioactive particles, which were deposited within a few kilometres of the Windscale nuclear reactor chimneys from which they were discharged. In contrast with the Windscale fire, the release was predominantly of long lived fission products. The total release was about 259 TBq (7000 Ci). Large numbers of radioactive particles were found in gardens and homes, including the larders, in Seascale. In 1955, when the particles were first found, only recently deposited activity was measured. No attempt was made to trace the full extent of the radioactivity within the local environment or the transfer to the food chain; consequently, there are large uncertainties in estimates of the effects of the release. A decision to monitor milk was not taken until July 1957, some three years after the particles were believed to have been released.[2]

Since I drew attention to these releases two years ago, it has been recognised that levels of the radioactivity in milk and other foods in the mid-1950s would have been extremely high at Seascale. They may have averaged more than 10 times the maximum permissible levels in milk for one or two years. Farms nearer to Sellafield would have had even higher levels.

Very young children who were living at Seascale at the time of the release were at highest risk. In my report I explain why I believe the cumulative dose received by these children could have been in the region of 50 mSv.

Although there is some uncertainty in this figure, it probably represents the worst known example of exposure to radiation for members of the public in the United Kingdom from operations of nuclear power plant. Most of this dose would have been received within the first four years of life. You quote the National Radiological Protection Board's conclusion that two thirds of the total risk from all sources came from background and only 16% from Sellafield discharges. These figures refer to the cumulative effect between 1950 and 1980 and include children born in Seascale during the whole of this period. For children born after 1956 the risk arising from the particles released in the early 1950s was quite small. Furthermore, comparing cumulative doses over long periods of time may have little relevance in relation to childhood leukaemia, which on average is contracted before the age of 4. The dose received in the first four years of life may be more important in relation to the development of leukaemia in children. For the group of children born in the 1950s, this dose could have exceeded that from natural background by a factor of 10. The mechanisms that give rise to leukaemia in young children are not well understood and possibly this large increase relative to the background could be more important than is assumed at present.

If, however, the National Radiological Protection Board's methods of risk analysis are correct, then 1 death is to be expected per 5000 children who have received a dose of 50 mSv. This can be compared with the highest risk of 1 in 100 000 from Sellafield discharges reported to the Black inquiry. As the population of children under 5 living in Seascale in 1955 was about 250 the probability of a death resulting from these releases is estimated to be small although the uncertainties in the analysis are large. No deaths from leukaemia have been reported in children who were born before 1956 in Seascale and who continued to live there until death. Some cases were reported to the Black inquiry of leukaemia and other cancers in children who were living in Seascale in the early 1950s although, as they either were not born there or did not die there, they were not included as part of the epidemiological data considered by the Committee on Medical Aspects of Radiation in the Environment. Although no clear and indisputable link between leukaemia and the Sellafield discharges has been established, uncertainty remains.

1 Jakeman D. *Notes on the level of radioactive contamination in the Sellafield area arising from discharges in the early 1950s.* London: HMSO, 1986. (AEEW R 2104).
2 Anonymous. Strontium-90 at Windscale. *BMJ* 1960;ii:658–9.

4: Childhood leukaemia in west Berkshire

Letter to the *Lancet*

CAROL J BARTON, EVE ROMAN,
HILARY M RYDER, ANN WATSON

Since the establishment of a paediatric oncology/haematology clinic at the Royal Berkshire Hospital, Reading, in 1971[1] we have been concerned that we were seeing more children with acute leukaemia than might be expected in a population the size of our health district's. After the investigation of the incidence of childhood leukaemia near the nuclear complex at Sellafield,[2] and because the west Berkshire health district contains two nuclear establishments—namely, the Atomic Weapons Research Establishment at Aldermaston and the Royal Ordnance Factory at Burghfield—and has two others as near neighbours, we decided to collate our figures. While doing so we learned that Yorkshire Television plans to show a documentary about childhood cancer in this area. We have not discussed our data with the media, but want to publish our preliminary findings before the programme is shown.

For the years 1972–84, 49 children aged 0–9 years were newly diagnosed at the paediatric oncology/haematology clinic as having acute leukaemia; 45 were residents of west Berkshire at the time of diagnosis. The population of children at risk in west Berkshire during 1972–84 was estimated from age-specific mid-year population figures obtained from the population estimates department, Office of Population Censuses and Surveys (OPCS). The average annual incidence rate of leukaemia among children in west Berkshire (1972-84) is compared with that in England and Wales (1972–81) in the accompanying table.

The apparent significance of the excess in children under 5 years old must be interpreted with caution because we were already suspicious that there was an excess in children and this was the reason for the analysis. Moreover, there are problems with using incidence data for England and Wales as the basis for calculating expected cases.[2] For example, registration

Incidence of leukaemia among children aged 0–9 years in west Berkshire 1972–84* and England and Wales 1972–81†

Age (yr)	Average annual rate (per 100 000)		No of cases in west Berkshire	
	E & W†	W Berks	Observed	Expected‡
0–4	5·6	9·3	34	20·6 (p < 0·01)
5–9	3·1	2·7	11	12·7
0–9	4·3	5·8	45	33·3 (p = 0·06)

* ICD codes: 1972–78 8th revision codes 204–207; 1979–84 9th revision codes 204–208.
† Source: 1972–81 OPCS series MBI (numerator) and PP1 (denominator). Data for 1982–84 not yet available.
‡ E & W rate × total person-years at risk in west Berkshire 1972–84. p Values are two tailed.

of leukaemia may be more efficient in some parts of the country and there may be variations in leukaemia incidence due to factors such as socioeconomic class. Both factors could, if they operate in this district, artificially inflate the observed/expected difference. We have excluded non-resident cases; on the other hand, we know of some west Berkshire children with leukaemia who are being treated outside the district.

The study is still in progress. Information about other time periods and age groups, the geographical and temporal distributions, and the incidence of other childhood cancers are being collected.

1 Neil VS, Weindling AM, Ryder HM, Barton CJ, Newman Cl. Approach to the management of children with malignant disease in one district general hospital. *BMJ* 1981;**283**:366–67.
2 Black D for the Independent Advisory Group. *Investigation of the possible increased incidence of cancer in West Cumbria.* London: HMSO, 1984. (Black report.)

5: Childhood leukaemia in northern Scotland

Letter to the *Lancet*

M A HEASMAN, I W KEMP, J D URQUHART,
R BLACK

In preparation for the public inquiry to be held later in 1986 on the planning application for a nuclear reprocessing plant at Dounreay on the north coast of the Scottish mainland we were asked to examine cancer registration and other data from that area. Our primary concern here is to report findings for lymphatic and haematopoietic neoplasms (ICD ninth revision; codes 200–208) in people aged 0–24 years during the period 1968–84. The places of residence of the patients at the time of registration have all been postcoded and grouped into five groups: mainland enumeration districts whose centroids fall within 12·5 km or within 25 km of the existing Dounreay installation, the remaining mainland districts falling within the KW postal area (KW relates also to Kirkwall, Orkney) and within 25–75 km of Dounreay, and places of residence on the islands of Orkney (range 35–120 km) and Shetland (range 160–300 km). Expected figures are based on all-Scotland cancer registration rates. Population data were extracted from the 1971 and 1981 censuses.

The table shows the observed and expected registrations for the periods 1968–73, 1974–78, and 1979–84. The cell in this table that gives cause for concern is that for leukaemia (ICD 9: 204–208) during 1979–84, less than 12·5 km from Dounreay ($p < 0·001$, one tailed test). In this group four of the five patients with leukaemia lived in Thurso, the only appreciable centre of population within 12·5 km of Dounreay, and the fifth lived about 3 km from Dounreay. Four patients were aged under 15 at registration. Four were originally registered as having acute lymphoid, and one acute myeloid leukaemia, but subsequent validation has changed the diagnosis of one lymphoid case to myeloid.

The importance of this finding is difficult to evaluate. The choice of radii and periods is arbitrary and, although there is an excess of cases over the whole period 1968–84, no cases at all were registered within 25 km in the

13

Registrations for lymphatic and haematopoietic neoplasms in defined areas in northern Scotland: age group 0–24

Area and period	Leukaemia (ICD 9, 204–208)		Other lymphatic and haematopoietic neoplasms (ICD 9, 200–203)	
	Observed	Expected	Observed	Expected
1968–73				
< 12·5 km from Dounreay	0	0·169	1	0·185
12·5 to < 25 km from Dounreay	0	0·171	0	0·188
Other mainland*	2	0·413	1	0·453
Orkney	1	0·321	2	0·352
Shetland	1	0·336	0	0·169
1974–78				
< 12·5 km from Dounreay	0	0·498	0	0·369
12·5 to < 25 km from Dounreay	0	0·443	0	0·309
Other mainland*	0	1·123	1	0·766
Orkney	1	1·102	0	0·724
Shetland	0	1·496	2	0·974
1979–84				
< 12·5 km from Dounreay	5	0·513	0	0·529
12·5 to < 25 km from Dounreay	1	0·453	2	0·453
Other mainland*	1	1·151	1	1·098
Orkney	0	1·130	1	1·031
Shetland	3	1·534	0	1·386

* Remainder of KW postcode area on mainland.

period 1968–78. On the other hand, the facts that all reported cases within 25 km occurred within a five year period, five were in children under 15, and five occurred within 12·5 km of Dounreay may increase its potential importance. Similar findings have been reported from near other United Kingdom nuclear installations (for example, Sellafield,[1] Hunterston,[2] and Aldermaston and West Burghfield[3]).

Preliminary examination of all other cancers in childhood and of leukaemia and selected sites of cancer in adults, and of the occurrence of congenital malformations, showed no significantly raised figures in the area around Dounreay.

These findings will be reported to the Committee on Medical Aspects of Radiation in the Environment. A further report will deal with the validation of all cases of leukaemia in people aged 0–24 in Scotland for the period 1968–81. It is hoped also to report on any other clusters throughout Scotland and to update findings to 1983.

1 Black D for the Independent Advisory Group. *Investigation of the possible incidence of cancer in west Cumbria 1984.* London: HMSO, 1984. (Black report.)

2 Heasman MA, Kemp IW, MacLaren Anne-Marie, Trotter P, Gillis CR, Hole DJ. Incidence of leukaemia in young persons in west of Scotland. *Lancet* 1984;**i**:1188–9.
3 Barton CJ, Roman E, Ryder HM, Watson A. Childhood leukaemia in west Berkshire. *Lancet* 1985;**ii**:1248–9.

Correction

M A HEASMAN, I W KEMP, J D URQUHART, R BLACK

We regret that in our letter (Feb 1, p 266) the expected figures for registration 1968–73 were incorrect. The correct figures (see table) do not alter the comment in our letter.

Area and period	Leukaemia (ICD 204–208)		Other lymphatic and haematopoietic neoplasms (ICD 200–203)	
	Observed	Expected	Observed	Expected
1968–73				
< 12·5 km from Dounreay	0	0·554	1	0·411
12·5 to < 25 km from Dounreay	0	0·547	0	0·445
Other mainland*	2	1·316	1	1·104
Orkney	1	1·043	2	0·881
Shetland	1	1·097	0	0·993

* Remainder of KW postcode area on mainland.

6: Leukaemia and lymphatic cancer in young people near nuclear installations

Letter to the *Lancet*

JOHN URQUHART, JAMES CUTLER,
MICHAEL BURKE

Dr Barton and her colleagues (*Lancet* 30 November, p 1248) described a significant excess of leukaemia in the age group 0–4 years in the West Berkshire Health District, which contains the Aldermaston and Burghfield nuclear weapons establishments. A Yorkshire Television documentary (*Inside Britain's Bomb*, 3 December 1985) drew attention to leukaemia and lymphatic cancer in young people in areas very close to the Berkshire nuclear weapons installations.

The area examined consisted of the nine rural wards in the Newbury and Basingstoke county districts contiguous with and including the two electoral wards containing the establishments. These wards formed two "circles" of roughly 4 km ($2\frac{1}{2}$ miles) radius around each plant. Populations for the wards with age and sex breakdowns were supplied by Berkshire and Hampshire county councils for the years 1971 and 1981. Cases of cancer in the under 25 year age group were ascertained by a Yorkshire Television researcher and confirmed by death certificate or by confidential inquiries to local general practitioners. They were assigned to the study area on the basis of residence at time of diagnosis or death.

Table I gives details of 15 cases of leukaemia or lymphatic malignancy (ICD 8, 200–08) identified in the nine wards.

The total population of the nine wards in the age group 0–24 was 10 314 in 1971 and 9967 in 1981.

The expected registration rate was taken as the average rate for England and Wales for 1976–81. This was 6·6 per 100 000 for age 0–4, 4·3 for age 5–14, and 6·2 for age 15–24. For deaths the comparison was made with the national rates for the year in which the death occurred. Table II shows the

TABLE I—*Details of 15 children with leukaemia or lymphatic cancer (ICD 8, 200–208) aged under 25 years, Berkshire, 1971–85*

Year*	Diagnosis	Sex	Age†	Year*	Diagnosis	Sex	Age†
1971	Hodgkin's	M	7	1978	Leukaemia	M	4 (†1979)
1972	Hodgkin's	F	17	1982	Hodgkin's	M	16
1972	Leukaemia	F	16 (†1973)	1982	Hodgkin's	F	3
1972	Leukaemia	M	4 (†1973)	1982	Hodgkin's	F	19
1972	Leukaemia	F	9 (†1978)	1983	Leukaemia	M	2 (†1984)
1973	Leukaemia	F	6 (†1976)	1983	Hodgkin's	F	21 (†1985)
1976	Hodgkin's	F	22 (†1977)	1985	Non-Hodgkin's		
1977	Leukaemia	F	14 (†1978)		lymphoma	F	3

* Year of diagnosis († and of death).

TABLE II—*Rates per 100 000 person years, 1971–85, of leukaemia or lymphatic cancer at age under 25 years in the Aldermaston and Burghfield areas*

Area	Age 0–4	Age 0–14	Age 0–24
Aldermaston and Burghfield circles	25·2 (7)	9·7 (9)	9·9* (15)
Burghfield circle	43·6 (5)	15·6 (6)	12·8 (8)
Burghfield parish†	65·6 (3)	20·5 (3)	16·5 (4)
England and Wales	6·6	5·0	5·5

Figures in parentheses are observed cases (ages related to diagnosis). *All rates in this table are significantly different from the rate for England and Wales at the 5% level at least. For all three ages and for both circles combined $p < 0.025$.

rates for the Aldermaston and Burghfield "circles" for leukaemia and lymphatic cancer cases (ICD 8, 200–08) under age 25 per 100 000 person years for 1971–85.

Only four cases of solid tumour (three brain, one testis) were found in the area in under 25 year olds. This high ratio of leukaemia or lymphatic cancer cases to other cancers is similar to the pattern found near Sellafield.[1]

Radioactivity is discharged from the Aldermaston and Burghfield sites,[2,3] and the possibility of a causal association between the high rates of leukaemia and the lymphatic cancers and radioactive discharges requires further investigation.

1 Black D for the Independent Advisory Group. *Investigation of the possible increased incidence of cancer in west Cumbria*. London: HMSO, 1984.
2 *Aquatic environment monitoring reports*. Lowestoft: Ministry of Agriculture, Fisheries, and Food.
3 *Digest of environmental pollution and water statistics: No 6, radioactivity*. London: Department of the Environment, 1983.

7: Childhood leukaemia in the west of Scotland

Letter to the *Lancet*

D J HOLE, C R GILLIS

Public attention to cases of leukaemia in areas close to nuclear installations has created concern that exposure to low dose ionising radiation may be a major risk factor in the local incidence of leukaemia. Four publications relating to areas around nuclear installations have recorded higher rates of leukaemia in children and young adults living in these areas than occur nationally.[1-4] To interpret these observations we need to ask whether the differences reported are greater than those observed in areas of similar sizes containing no nuclear installations and whether these publications are representative of populations around all nuclear installations.

Data for the West of Scotland Cancer Registry region, which consists of 26 local government districts and contains four nuclear installations, may be helpful. They relate to children aged 0–14, to avoid problems of diagnosis and ascertainment. The variation in rates of childhood leukaemia has been ascertained by using data relating to the 26 districts, thus avoiding any selective bias in choice of study areas as local government boundaries are fixed for administrative not scientific purposes. The choice of boundaries around the four nuclear installations is less clear. For Hunterston, the immediate postcode sectors do not contain the nearby conurbation of Ardrossan, Saltcoats, and Stevenston, so we have defined two sets of boundaries corresponding to Hunterston inner and outer areas (see table II). For Holy Loch (Dunoon), Faslane, and Chapelcross, the postcode sectors immediately adjacent to the installations contain all the immediate resident population.

Table I shows average annual incidence rates ranging from 7·3 to 1·3 per 100 000 in local government districts that do not contain nuclear installations, a range of rates precisely representative of Scotland as a whole.[5] The three local government districts that contain nuclear installations, Cunninghame (Hunterston), Argyll and Bute (Holy Loch, Faslane), and Annandale and Eskdale (Chapelcross) rank 11th, 14th, and 23rd, respectively,

TABLE I—*Incidence of leukaemia in children aged 0–14 years in local government districts in west of Scotland, 1974–85*

Rank	District	Rate*	Rank	District	Rate*
1	Stewartry	7·28 (4)	14†	Argyll and Bute	3·39 (6)
2	Bearsden and Milngavie	6·60 (7)	15	Kyle and Carrick	3·08 (9)
3	Strathkelvin	6·60 (17)	16	Kilmarnock and Loudoun	2·88 (7)
4	Cumnock and Doon Valley	6·02 (8)	17	Hamilton	2·74 (9)
5	Cumbernauld and Kilsyth	5·40 (11)	18	Falkirk	2·74 (11)
6	Nithsdale	5·35 (8)	19	Eastwood	2·72 (4)
7	Wigtown	4·94 (4)	20	East Kilbride	2·72 (7)
8	Dumbarton	4·92 (12)	21	Motherwell	2·53 (11)
9	Clackmannan	4·77 (7)	22	Stirling	2·28 (5)
10	Renfrew	4·23 (25)	23†	Annandale and Eskdale	2·22 (2)
11†	Cunninghame	4·20 (17)	24	Monklands	2·03 (7)
12	Clydesdale	3·78 (6)	25	Inverclyde	1·79 (5)
13	Glasgow City	3·48 (73)	26	Clydebank	1·31 (2)
				West of Scotland	3·56 (285)

* Age standardised rates have been calculated by applying the age (in 5 year age groups), sex, and time period (1974–78, 1979–85) specific rates for each of the local government districts to the west of Scotland 1981 population. Number of cases in parentheses.
† Local government districts that contain a nuclear installation.

TABLE II—*Observed and expected numbers of cases of leukaemia in children aged 0–14 years in postcode areas close to nuclear installations in west of Scotland for 1964–85*

Location (date)	Postcodes used	No of leukaemias		Rate	p Value
		Observed	Expected		
Holy Loch (1961)	PA23	4	2·1	6·8	0·16
Faslane (1963)	G84	5	4·2	4·3	0·41
Chapelcross (1962)	DG12	3	2·3	4·6	0·40
Hunterston (1963) inner	KA23, KA29, KA28	1	1·1	3·2	0·67
Hunterston (1963) outer	KA20, KA21, KA22, KA24, KA25, KA30, KA13, KA14	18	14·6	4·4	0·22
Total		31	24·3	4·6	0·11

Expected numbers have been calculated using west of Scotland age (in 5 year age groups), sex, and time period (1964–68, 1969–73, 1974–78, 1979–85) specific rates of childhood leukaemia applied to the populations aged 0–14 resident in the appropriate postcodes as defined in the 1981 census and the 1971 census reconstituted to provide comparable denominations for the postcode areas as currently defined. Hunterston (inner area) includes the villages of West Kilbride, Seamill, Fairlie, and Millport. Hunterston (outer area) includes Ardrossan, Saltcoats, Stevenston, Kilwinning, Dalry, Kilbirnie, and Largs.

19

producing an overall rate of 3·7 per 100 000, which is similar to the west of Scotland as a whole. As stated previously, coastal areas of the west of Scotland show no observed rates that are consistently higher than inland areas.[6]

Examination of the observed and expected numbers of childhood leukaemias in the postcode sectors adjacent to the four nuclear installations (table II) indicates that over a 22 year period, two additional cases have occurred in Dunoon, one extra case each has occurred near Faslane and Chapelcross, and three extra cases have occurred in Hunterston outer area.

The low level of occurrence together with the small excess of cases makes it impossible to comment precisely on whether such an increase can be attributed to exposure to low dose ionising radiation. Thus, in the absence of direct evidence as to whether any increased exposure to low dose ionising radiation has occurred and whether an increased risk due to living near a nuclear installation exists, what comments can usefully be made? Firstly, there is a sixfold variation in the rates of childhood leukaemia in the west of Scotland when small areas that have been independently chosen are examined. Secondly, the rates for local government districts that contain nuclear installations and for postcodes immediately adjacent to nuclear installations lie within the variation expected in the west of Scotland. Thirdly, the increases seen in the areas adjacent to the three nuclear installations are small, do not include Hunterston inner area, and could well be explained by random fluctuations ($p = 0·11$). If increases can be produced by choosing different criteria for space and time, these will only be genuine if sustained by examining as many choices of criteria as exist.

We believe these data are evidence that ionising radiation is not a major risk factor in the areas concerned. Whether it is a minor risk factor acting alone, with viruses, chemicals, or any other environmental factor is not known. Mere statistical studies of these data will not help; combined epidemiological and biological approaches will. Further studies must include careful categorisation of life events from conception to diagnosis, but what is the best protocol?

1 Black D for the Independent Advisory Group. *Investigation of the possible increased incidence of cancer in west Cumbria.* London: HMSO, 1984. (Black report.)
2 Heasman MA, Kemp IW, MacLaren AM, Trotter P, Gillis CR, Hole DJ. Incidence of leukaemia in young persons in west of Scotland. *Lancet* 1984;1:1188–9.
3 Barton CJ, Roman E, Ryder HM, Watson A. Childhood leukaemia in west Berkshire. *Lancet* 1985;ii:1248–9.
4 Heasman MA, Kemp IW, Urquhart JD, Black R. Childhood leukaemia in northern Scotland. *Lancet* 1986;i:266.
5 Kemp I, Boyle P, Smans M, Muir C, eds. *Atlas of cancer in Scotland, 1975–1980: (incidence and epidemiological perspective).* Lyon: International Agency for Research on Cancer, 1985. (IARC Scientific Publication No 72.)
6 Gillis CR, Hole DJ. Childhood leukaemia in coastal areas of west Scotland 1969–83. *Lancet* 1984;ii:872.

8: Childhood leukaemia in the West Berkshire and the Basingstoke and North Hampshire District Health Authorities in relation to nuclear establishments in the vicinity

EVE ROMAN, VALERIE BERAL, LUCY CARPENTER, ANN WATSON, CAROL BARTON, HILARY RYDER, D LYNN ASTON

During the years 1972–85, 89 children aged 0–14 were registered as having leukaemia in the West Berkshire and the Basingstoke and North Hampshire District Health Authorities. Two nuclear establishments are located within the two district health authorities, and a third is situated nearby. Fifty of the 143 electoral wards in the two district health authorities lie wholly within, or have at least half their area lying within, a circle of radius 10 km around the establishments. In those 50 electoral wards 41 children aged 0–14 were registered as having leukaemia, 28·6 registrations being expected on the basis of leukaemia registration rates in England and Wales (incidence ratio = 1·4, $p < 0·05$). This excess was confined to children aged 0–4, among whom there were 29 registrations of leukaemia, 14·4 being expected (incidence ratio = 2·0, $p < 0·001$). In the remaining 93 electoral wards there was a small and non-significant increase in the number of registrations of leukaemia at age 0–14 (48 observed, 40·8 expected; incidence ratio = 1·2). There was no obvious trend in the incidence of childhood leukaemia over the 14 years and the overall occurrence of the malignancy in the 143 electoral wards was consistent with a random distribution. In the surrounding Oxford and Wessex Regional Health Authorities the number of registrations of leukaemia at age 0–14 was virtually identical with that expected on the basis of registration rates in England and Wales (362 observed, 372·5 expected; incidence ratio = 1·0).

These data indicate that in the two district health authorities studied there was an excess incidence of childhood leukaemia during 1972–85 in the vicinity of the nuclear establishments. In the West Berkshire and the Basingstoke and North Hampshire District Health Authorities an average of 60 000 children aged 0–14 lived within a 10 km radius of a nuclear establishment each year. The normal expectation of leukaemia in these children was two cases a year, whereas the recorded incidence was three cases a year, representing one extra case of leukaemia each year among these 60 000 children.

Introduction

The incidence of childhood leukaemia around nuclear establishments has been a topic of public concern and scientific investigation, especially since the reported cluster of cases near the Sellafield plant in west Cumbria.[1-6] The West Berkshire District Health Authority contains two nuclear establishments: the Atomic Weapons Research Establishment at Aldermaston and the Royal Ordnance Factory at Burghfield. Both establishments lie in the south of the West Berkshire District Health Authority, close to its border with the Basingstoke and North Hampshire District Health Authority (see fig 1). The United Kingdom Atomic Energy Authority's establishment at Harwell lies less than 2 km to the north of the West Berkshire District Health Authority.

In 1985 we reported a preliminary analysis of the incidence of leukaemia for the years 1972–84 in children aged 0–9 living in the West Berkshire District Health Authority, noting that the incidence among the 0–4 year olds was increased by 63% (p < 0·01).[2] At that time complete information was not available for children who, although resident in the West Berkshire

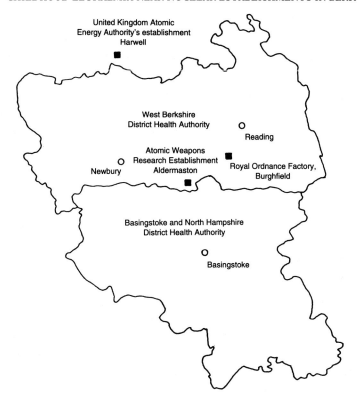

FIG 1—*Map of the West Berkshire and the Basingstoke and North Hampshire District Health Authorities, showing main towns (○) and nuclear establishments (■) in the area.*

District Health Authority, were referred elsewhere for diagnosis and treatment. In addition, we could not examine the incidence of childhood leukaemia in the immediate area surrounding the nuclear installations, as data from the neighbouring Basingstoke and North Hampshire District Health Authority had not been compiled, nor could we assess whether the excess incidence of childhood leukaemia was specific to the West Berkshire District Health Authority or characteristic of the general area in which the West Berkshire District Health Authority is situated. The preliminary data have now been extended to include children from the neighbouring health authority of Basingstoke and North Hampshire, children diagnosed as having leukaemia in 1985, those aged 10–14 years, and residents in the district health authorities who were referred elsewhere for diagnosis and treatment. The places of residence of the children with leukaemia have been investigated with specific reference to their proximity to the nuclear establishments in the vicinity.

23

Subjects and methods

The West Berkshire District Health Authority forms part of the Oxford Regional Health Authority, constituting about one sixth of its population. The Royal Berkshire Hospital is situated in Reading, and a paediatric oncology and haematology clinic was established there in 1971.[7] The Basingstoke and North Hampshire District Health Authority forms part of the Wessex Regional Health Authority, constituting almost one tenth of its population. The Basingstoke District Hospital serves this district health authority. The hospital was opened in 1972 and lies on the outskirts of Basingstoke. Figure 1 shows a map of the two district health authorities and the position of the main towns and the three nuclear establishments in the vicinity.

SUBJECTS

Children aged under 15 years who were first diagnosed as having leukaemia in 1972–85 and who were then living in either the West Berkshire District Health Authority or the Basingstoke and North Hampshire District Health Authority were identified. Fifty eight patients were first diagnosed at the Royal Berkshire Hospital, 56 being residents of the West Berkshire District Health Authority and two of the Basingstoke and North Hampshire District Health Authority. Twenty seven patients were first diagnosed at the Basingstoke District Hospital, 25 being residents of the Basingstoke and North Hampshire District Health Authority and two of the West Berkshire District Health Authority. All diagnoses were confirmed histologically and were supported by documentary evidence in hospital records. Reliable hospital records were not available before 1972, because the oncology and haematology clinic at the Royal Berkshire Hospital was not fully operational until 1972 and the Basingstoke District Hospital was not opened until 1972. To ensure that ascertainment of cases for 1972–85 was as complete as possible consultants from hospitals in the surrounding district health authorities and staff of the Childhood Cancer Research Group in Oxford were approached for information that might identify additional subjects. As a result of these inquiries a further eight cases, six from West Berkshire and two from North Hampshire, were identified. All eight had been referred for diagnosis and treatment outside the district health authority in which they lived.

The completeness of registration of children with leukaemia was checked against national cancer registry data. This could be done only for the years up to 1982, as data were not complete beyond that year. All 48 patients identified by us as living in the West Berkshire District Health Authority and diagnosed as having leukaemia between 1972 and 1982 were also registered in the national scheme. For the Basingstoke and North Hampshire District Health Authority 24 of the 28 patients diagnosed between

1972 and 1982 were also registered in the national scheme. One of those not registered was a 6 year old boy, diagnosed as having lymphoblastic lymphoma in early 1979, who later that year developed acute lymphatic leukaemia. He was registered in the national scheme as having lymphoma but not leukaemia. The three other children who were not registered were aged 2, 3, and 8, respectively, and were all diagnosed as having leukaemia at the Basingstoke District Hospital in 1972. These children probably escaped registration in the reorganisation after the opening of the Basingstoke District Hospital in 1972 and the separation of the Wessex cancer registry from the South Thames registry in early 1973.[8]

METHODS

Yearly mid-year population estimates were provided for the 14 years 1972–1985 for the West Berkshire District Health Authority, the Basingstoke and North Hampshire District Health Authority, the Oxford Regional Health Authority, and the Wessex Regional Health Authority by the population estimates department of the Office of Population Censuses and Surveys. Populations, by five year age groups, are available from the 1981 census for each of the 85 electoral wards in the West Berkshire District Health Authority and the 58 wards in the Basingstoke and North Hampshire District Health Authority. Population estimates for the electoral wards are not made yearly by the Office of Population Censuses and Surveys, and we estimated these by applying the 1981 ward proportions of the district health authority population to the yearly mid-year district health authority population figures supplied by the Office of Population Censuses and Surveys.

The address of each child when leukaemia was diagnosed was allocated to the appropriate electoral ward, using the ward boundaries that existed at the time of the 1981 census. The expected numbers of registrations of leukaemia (International Classification of Diseases (ICD) 8th revision codes 204–207, 9th revision 204–208[9 10]) were estimated by applying the yearly age specific leukaemia registration rates for England and Wales for 1972–82 to the population estimates.[11] National incidence data were not available beyond 1982. As there was no significant trend in national registration rates for childhood leukaemia over the 11 years 1972–82, the mean age specific rates for 1972–82 were applied to 1983–5. Confidence intervals and tests of significance for the ratio of observed to expected cases (incidence ratio) were obtained from the tables based on the Poisson distribution.[12] All tests of significance were two sided.

For each age group we compared the distribution of the incidence ratios for the 143 wards in the two district health authorities with the distribution that would have been expected, assuming that the observed numbers of cases in each ward followed a separate Poisson distribution. For these calculations the age specific incidence in the two health authorities was used as a standard. The expected number of cases in each ward was calculated as a fraction of the total cases observed, this fraction being the proportion of the total population that was contained in the respective ward in 1981. The probability distributions for the incidence ratio of each ward were summed to give a predicted distribution, assuming a random distribution of cases across the wards. Two additional methods were also used to examine for non-uniformity of leukaemia risk across the wards.[13 14]

To study the relation between residence near a nuclear establishment and leukaemia risk, we divided the electoral wards according to whether half or more of their area lay within circles of specified radii from the three nuclear plants in the vicinity. A 10 km radius was chosen for the analyses before the geographical distribution of leukaemia was examined. In view of the findings obtained when the 10 km radius was used, we made further divisions at 5 km and 15 km for subsidiary analyses. Incidence ratios were calculated separately for each category, and, where appropriate, linear tests for trend were carried out using a standard method.[15]

Results

Ninety three children aged 0–14 living in the West Berkshire District Health Authority or the Basingstoke and North Hampshire District Health Authority were identified as having had leukaemia first diagnosed in the years 1972–85. Of these, 49 were boys and 44 girls and 5 (5%) also had Down's syndrome. Seventy eight children (84%) had acute lymphatic leukaemia, but complete information on the different subtypes was not available, as cell marker studies were not routinely performed until 1976. Four of the 93 children were not registered in the national cancer registration scheme (see methods) and were excluded from all analyses presented here. Table I shows the numbers of children registered as having leukaemia in each district health authority, by age. The numbers of cases expected were based on leukaemia registration rates in England and Wales. Overall, there was a significant excess in the numbers of registrations of leukaemia in 0–14 year olds ($p < 0.05$), due almost entirely to the excess among 0–4 year olds ($p < 0.01$). The findings were similar in the West Berkshire District Health Authority and the Basingstoke and North Hampshire District Health Authority, but the incidence ratios were larger in West Berkshire and significant only in that health authority. The data were examined for evidence of a trend in incidence of leukaemia over time. Although this examination was limited by the small number of patients diagnosed each year, there was little suggestion of either an increase or a decrease in incidence over the 14 years 1972–85.

Table II contrasts the childhood leukaemia registration ratios in the West Berkshire and the Basingstoke and North Hampshire District Health

TABLE I—*Incidence of childhood leukaemia in the West Berkshire and the Basingstoke and North Hampshire District Health Authorities 1972–85, by age. (Expected numbers are based on leukaemia registration rates in England and Wales)*

Age (years)	West Berkshire			Basingstoke and North Hampshire			Total		
	No of children with leukaemia		Incidence ratio* (95% confidence interval)	No of children with leukaemia		Incidence ratio* (95% confidence interval)	No of children with leukaemia		Incidence ratio* (95% confidence interval)
	Observed	Expected		Observed†	Expected		Observed†	Expected	
0–4	38	22·3	1·7 (1·2 to 2·3)	15	11·7	1·3 (0·7 to 2·1)	53	34·0	1·6 (1·2 to 2·0)
5–9	15	13·6	1·1 (0·6 to 1·8)	6	7·1	0·8 (0·3 to 1·8)	21	20·7	1·0 (0·6 to 1·6)
10–14	11	9·7	1·1 (0·6 to 2·0)	4	4·9	0·8 (0·2 to 2·1)	15	14·6	1·0 (0·6 to 1·7)
Total	64	45·6	1·4 (1·1 to 1·8)	25	23·7	1·1 (0·7 to 1·6)	89	69·3	1·3 (1·0 to 1·6)

* Ratio of observed to expected number of registrations.
† Excludes four children (aged 3, 4, 6, and 8, respectively) who were not registered in the national cancer registration scheme.

TABLE II—*Incidence ratios (observed to expected registrations) for childhood leukaemia in the West Berkshire and the Basingstoke and North Hampshire District Health Authorities compared with the rest of the Oxford and Wessex Regional Health Authorities 1972–82, by age. (Expected numbers are based on leukaemia registration rates in England and Wales)*

Age (years)	West Berkshire and Basingstoke and North Hampshire District Health Authorities	Oxford and Wessex Regional Health Authorities (excluding West Berkshire and Basingstoke and North Hampshire District Health Authorities)	Total
0–4	1·7** (45/26·9)	1·0 (174/179·6)	1·1 (219/206·5)
5–9	0·8 (13/17·0)	1·0 (115/112·5)	1·0 (128/129·5)
10–14	1·2 (14/11·6)	0·9 (73/80·4)	0·9 (87/92·0)
Total	1·3* (72/55·5)	1·0 (362/372·5)	1·0 (434/428·0)

*$p < 0.05$.
**$p < 0.01$.

Authorities with those in the surrounding Oxford and Wessex Regional Health Authorities. The data relate to 1972–82 because registration data beyond 1982 were not available for the regional health authorities. The expected numbers of cancer registrations are based on registration rates for leukaemia in England and Wales. There was a significant excess in leukaemia registrations in these two district health authorities in the 11 years 1972–82. In contrast, childhood leukaemia rates in the surrounding areas were virtually identical with those in England and Wales in general. The incidence ratio at age 0–14 was 1·0 in the Oxford Regional Health Authority after the data for the West Berkshire District Health Authority were excluded. In the Wessex Regional Health Authority it was also 1·0 after the data for the Basingstoke and North Hampshire District Health Authority were excluded. Because the rates of childhood leukaemia in the remainder of the Oxford and Wessex regional health authorities were so similar to national rates, the expected numbers of registrations of leukaemia estimated for subsequent analyses were based on age specific rates in England and Wales as a whole.

Figures 2 and 3 show the distribution of childhood leukaemia in the 143 electoral wards making up the West Berkshire and the Basingstoke and North Hampshire District Health Authorities for 1972–85. Figure 2 gives data for those aged 0–14 and figure 3 for those aged 0–4. Electoral wards with incidence ratios greater than one are shaded; the striped areas indicate wards with incidence ratios not significantly greater than one and the darker areas indicate wards with incidence ratios significantly greater than one ($p < 0.05$). The distribution of observed incidence ratios within each ward was compared with that predicted when a random distribution of cases across wards was assumed (table III). For each five year age group the

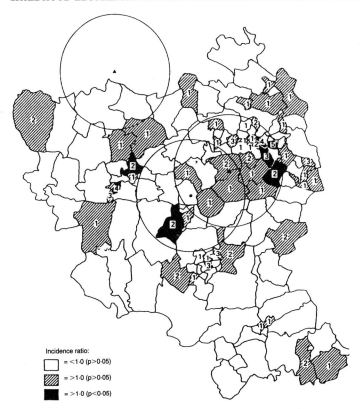

Incidence ratio:
▢ = <1·0 (p>0·05)
▨ = >1·0 (p>0·05)
■ = >1·0 (p<0·05)

FIG 2—*Map showing distribution of leukaemia incidence ratios at ages 0–14 in 143 electoral wards in the West Berkshire and the Basingstoke and North Hampshire District Health Authorities. Figures are numbers of cases. Circles of radius 10 km are drawn around each nuclear establishment (● = Atomic Weapons Research Establishment, Aldermaston, ■ = Royal Ordnance Factory, Burghfield, and ▲ = United Kingdom Atomic Energy Authority's establishment, Harwell).*

observed and predicted distributions of incidence ratios were comparable. Although the data are not shown here, two other methods used to examine for non-uniformity of risk across the wards also suggested that the overall geographical distribution of the cases was not significantly different from that expected by chance.[13][14]

Fifty of the 143 electoral wards had half or more of their area lying within 10 km of one of the three nuclear establishments at Aldermaston, Burghfield, and Harwell (see figs 2 and 3). There was a significantly increased incidence of leukaemia in these 50 electoral wards at ages 0–4 (p < 0·001) and 0–14 (p < 0·05), but not at ages 5–9 or 10–14 (table IV). The excess numbers of registrations at ages 0–14 may be attributed entirely to the excess in the under 5 group. In wards further than 10 km from a nuclear

29

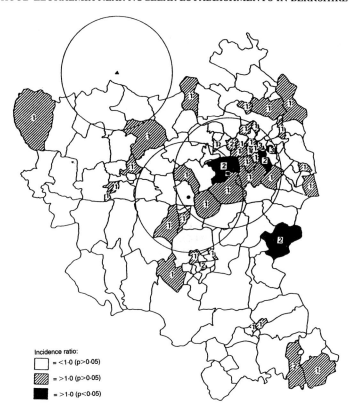

Incidence ratio:
☐ = <1·0 (p>0·05)
▨ = >1·0 (p>0·05)
■ = >1·0 (p<0·05)

FIG 3—*Map showing distribution of leukaemia incidence ratios at ages 0–4 in 143 electoral wards in the West Berkshire and the Basingstoke and North Hampshire District Health Authorities. Figures are numbers of cases. Circles of radius 10 km are drawn around each nuclear establishment (● = Atomic Weapons Research Establishment, Aldermaston, ■ = Royal Ordnance Factory, Burghfield, and ▲ = United Kingdom Atomic Energy Authority's establishment, Harwell).*

establishment the incidence at ages 0–4 and 0–14 was still slightly higher than the national figures, but this excess was not significant at the 5% level. The incidence of leukaemia at ages 0–4 and 0–14 was examined further by dividing the electoral wards into those with at least half of their area lying within 5 km, 6–10 km, 11–15 km, and more than 15 km from a nuclear establishment (table V). At age 0–4 the incidence ratio in the 15 electoral wards lying within 5 km of these establishments was 2·3, significantly greater than the number of registrations expected (p < 0·05); but at age 0–14 the excess was not significant at the 5% level. For electoral wards located 5–10 km from the establishments the incidence ratio was significantly increased both at age 0–4 and at 0–14. Two sided tests for linear trend

TABLE III—*Observed and predicted distributions of childhood leukaemia incidence ratios in the 143 electoral wards of the West Berkshire and the Basingstoke and North Hampshire District Health Authorities 1972–85, by age*

| | Age (years) | | | | | |
| | 0–4 | | 5–9 | | 10–14 | |
Incidence ratio*	Observed No of wards	Predicted No of wards	Observed No of wards	Predicted No of wards	Observed No of wards	Predicted No of wards
0	100	102·3	125	124·1	130	129·1
−2·5	21	20·4	1	1·2	0	0·3
−5·0	12	12·3	8	7·2	2	2·3
>5·0	10	8·0	9	10·6	11	11·3
Total	143	143·0	143	143·0	143	143·0

* Ratio of observed to expected number of registrations.

TABLE IV—*Incidence of childhood leukaemia in the West Berkshire and the Basingstoke and North Hampshire District Health Authorities 1972–85, by age and distance of the electoral ward of residence from a nuclear establishment. (Expected numbers are based on leukaemia registration rates in England and Wales)*

| | Electoral wards within 10 km of a nuclear establishment | | | Electoral wards more than 10 km from a nuclear establishment | | |
| | No of children with leukaemia | | Incidence ratio* (95% confidence interval) | No of children with leukaemia | | Incidence ratio* (95% confidence interval) |
Age (years)	Observed	Expected		Observed	Expected	
0–4	29	14·42	2·0 (1·3 to 2·9)	24	19·58	1·2 (0·8 to 1·8)
5–9	9	8·25	1·1 (0·5 to 2·1)	12	12·48	1·0 (0·5 to 1·7)
10–14	3	5·91	0·5 (0·1 to 1·5)	12	8·70	1·4 (0·7 to 2·4)
Total	41	28·58	1·4 (1·0 to 1·9)	48	40·76	1·2 (0·9 to 1·6)

* Ratio of observed to expected number of registrations.

across the four divisions of distance given in table V were not significant ($\chi^2 = 2\cdot19$, p = 0·14 for age 0–4; $\chi^2 = 1\cdot10$, p = 0·29 for age 0–14).

Table VI shows the incidence ratios and the observed and expected numbers of registrations of childhood leukaemia separately for each of the three nuclear establishments in the vicinity. The numbers are small, but broadly similar incidence ratios are found around both the Atomic Weapons Research Establishment at Aldermaston and the Royal Ordnance Factory, Burghfield. Nine electoral wards lie within 10 km of both of these

31

TABLE V—*Incidence of childhood leukaemia in the West Berkshire and the Basingstoke and North Hampshire District Health Authorities 1972–85, by age and 5 km distances of the electoral ward of residence from a nuclear establishment. (Expected numbers are based on leukaemia registration rates in England and Wales)*

Distance of the electoral ward of residence from from nuclear establishment	Age (years)					
	0–4			0–14		
	No of children with leukaemia		Incidence ratio* (95% confidence interval)	No of children with leukaemia		Incidence ratio* (95% confidence interval)
	Observed	Expected		Observed	Expected	
≤5 km	9	3·85	2·3 (1·1 to 4·4)	10	7·68	1·3 (0·6 to 2·4)
−10 km	20	10·56	1·9 (1·2 to 2·9)	31	20·89	1·5 (1·0 to 2·1)
−15 km	14	12·96	1·1 (0·6 to 1·8)	35	27·07	1·3 (0·9 to 1·8)
>15 km	10	6·63	1·5 (0·7 to 2·8)	13	13·69	0·9 (0·5 to 1·6)
Total	53	34	1·6 (1·2 to 2·0)	89	69·33	1·3 (1·0 to 1·6)

* Ratio of observed to expected number of registrations.

TABLE VI—*Incidence ratios (observed/expected registrations) of childhood leukaemia in electoral wards lying within 5 km and 10 km, respectively, for each of the three nuclear establishments in the vicinity of the West Berkshire and the Basingstoke and North Hampshire District Health Authorities 1972–85, by age. (Expected numbers are based on leukaemia registration rates in England and Wales)*

Age (years)	Distance from nuclear establishment	Atomic Weapons Research Establishment, Aldermaston†	Royal Ordnance Factory, Burghfield†	United Kingdom Atomic Energy Authority's establishment, Harwell
0–4	≤5 km	2·8 (3/1·08)	2·2 (6/2·77)	No data available
	≤10 km	2·2 (7/3·13)	2·2* (27/12·19)	0 (0/0·18)
0–14	≤5 km	1·4 (3/2·15)	1·3 (7/5·46)	No data
	≤10 km	1·2 (8/6·41)	1·6* (38/23·86)	0 (0/0·39)

* p < 0·05.
† Includes data for nine electoral wards that lie within 10 km of both the establishment at Aldermaston and that at Burghfield where five registrations were observed at age 0–4, with 1·08 expected and five registrations were observed at age 0–14, with 2·38 expected.

establishments, and thus there is some overlap between the separate figures. In those nine overlapping electoral wards there was a significant excess in the number of children aged 0–4 years registered as having leukaemia (five registrations observed, 1·08 expected; incidence ratio = 4·6, p < 0·05). Information for the area surrounding the United Kingdom Atomic Energy Authority's establishment at Harwell is incomplete, no data having been examined for the district health authority in which Harwell is located. None of the electoral wards in the West Berkshire District Health Authority had half or more of their area contained within a 5 km circle around this establishment, and in the two West Berkshire wards within 10 km no cases of leukaemia were observed at age 0–14 and 0·39 were expected.

Discussion

These data confirm our preliminary finding of an increased incidence of leukaemia in children aged 0–4 in the West Berkshire District Health Authority.[2] In the adjacent district health authority of Basingstoke and North Hampshire, registrations of leukaemia at age 0–4 were also increased, but not significantly so. When the data for the two authorities were combined there was a significant increase in registrations of leukaemia in the 0–14 age group (89 registrations observed, 69·3 expected), which was almost entirely due to the excess registrations in the 0–4 age group (53 registrations observed, 34·0 expected). The incidence of childhood leuk- aemia in the surrounding regional health authorities, after the two district health authorities under investigation had been excluded, was virtually identical with national figures (incidence ratio = 1·0) suggesting that the increased incidence is specific for the two district health authorities of interest and not characteristic of the region as a whole.

The classification of electoral wards according to whether all or at least half of their area lay within a circle of radius 10 km around the three nuclear establishments in the vicinity indicated that at ages 0–4 and 0–14 the number of children registered with leukaemia was significantly greater than that expected, based on the rates in England and Wales. The 42% excess at age 0–14 (41 cases observed, 28·6 expected, $p < 0.05$) was entirely due to the 101% excess at ages 0–4 (29 cases observed, 14·4 expected, $p < 0.001$). Although fairly few people live within a 5 km radius of the establishments, a significant excess of leukaemia was also found in the 0–4 age group (nine cases observed, 3·85 expected, $p < 0.05$). This area corresponds roughly with that investigated by the Yorkshire Television researchers, who, although examining data for a different period, reported a significantly increased incidence of leukaemia and lymphoma in 0–25 year olds.[3] In areas further than 10 km from the establishments the number of cases observed was slightly greater than that expected, but the excess was not significant (48 observed, 40·8 expected at age 0–14). The 10 km boundary was selected for analysis before the registration data were examined. If a 5 km or 15 km boundary had been selected instead the incidence ratios at ages 0–4 and 0–14 would all have been greater than one and significant at the 5% level, except at 5 km for the 0–14 year olds.

Although the incidence ratios within the 10 km circle were significantly greater than those expected on the basis of rates in England and Wales (table IV), the incidence rates in children living within the 10 km boundary were not significantly different from those in children living outside the 10 km boundary. The statistical power of comparisons of leukaemia rates in two small areas is, however, low: data would have had to be collected for more than 40 years before the almost twofold difference in incidence noted here at age 0–4 between those inside and outside the 10 km boundary would have been significant at the 5% level. That the pattern of childhood leukaemia in the two district health authorities is consistent with a random distribution partly reflects the low statistical power of such methods when applied to small populations. It is also consistent with the findings from systematic analyses of the geographical distribution of childhood leukaemia, which have indicated that there is no strong evidence why this malignancy should cluster geographically.[16] That the overall pattern of leukaemia was compatible with a random distribution might be thought to conflict with the observed excess incidence around the nuclear establishments, but the methods used to assess variation in the spatial incidence of disease were non-specific and not necessarily sensitive for the detection of a raised incidence of disease around a defined point source.

The calculation of the expected numbers of cases of leukaemia necessitated certain assumptions, but none of these is likely to result in major errors in the estimates. Leukaemia registration rates for England and Wales were not available for the years 1983–5 and were assumed to be the average for the years 1972–82. As there was no significant increasing or decreasing trend in national childhood leukaemia registration rates during that period, this assumption seems reasonable. Moreover, even when data for 1983–5 were excluded there were still significantly more registrations of childhood leukaemia than expected in the West Berkshire and the Basingstoke and North Hampshire District Health Authorities (table II). There were also significantly more leukaemia registrations than expected in children living within 10 km of the establishments for the years 1972–82 alone (25 observed, 11·6 expected at ages 0–4, $p < 0.001$; 34 observed, 23·2 expected at 0–14, $p < 0.05$). The use of national rather than local rates to calculate expected registrations is unlikely to have biased the findings, as the registration rates in the surrounding Oxford and Wessex Regional Health Authorities were almost identical with national rates (table II). Four children (5%) were not registered, which is comparable with reported figures on the completeness of cancer registration elsewhere in England and Wales.[8] These four were excluded to permit valid comparisons with national rates. Their inclusion would not have altered the conclusions. Two of the children were aged under 5; one lived outside the 10 km circle and the other lived within 10 km of both the Atomic Weapons Research Establishment at Aldermaston and the Royal Ordnance Factory at Burghfield. The two other children were aged 6 and 8 years, respectively, and both lived outside the 10 km circle.

Could the finding of the increased incidence of leukaemia in 0–4 year olds living within 10 km of the nuclear establishments be explained by other factors? The characteristics of the children with leukaemia—the type of leukaemia, the sex of the children, and the percentage with Down's syndrome—are similar to those described elsewhere,[17-19] and there were no obvious differences in the characteristics of those who lived close to or far from the nuclear establishments in the vicinity. All diagnoses were confirmed histologically. The whole of the Oxford and Wessex Regional Health Authorities, including the West Berkshire and the Basingstoke and North Hampshire District Health Authorities, are areas of fairly high social class compared with the rest of England and Wales, and it has been suggested that the incidence of leukaemia is increased in children whose parents are in the upper social classes. If such a gradient exists, however, it is weak,[19 20] and social class differences are unlikely to account for the almost twofold increase in risk noted for the 0–4 year olds living within 10 km of the establishments. There have also been suggestions that the incidence of childhood leukaemia may be greater in urban than rural areas.[18 19] It is unlikely that our findings could be explained by such variation in incidence of disease. The incidence ratios among 0–4 year olds were significantly increased within both the 5 km and the 10 km circles, yet the 5 km circles included predominantly rural areas, whereas the 10 km circles included the urban centre, Reading. Infection, birth order, and certain parental occupations have also been linked with childhood leukaemia,[18-20] but it is impossible to assess their roles or that of other environmental influences here. To investigate these findings further, and in particular to study the possible contribution of other factors, a case-control study of childhood cancer in the area is planned.

Could the excess registration of leukaemia in the electoral wards lying within 10 km of the nuclear establishments be due to chance? The probability of the excess in the 0–4 age group occurring by chance is less than 0·001 and in the 0–14 year olds 0·05, based on a stringent two sided statistical test. Moreover, this investigation is now one of a series examining the incidence of childhood leukaemia around nuclear establishments.[1-6] Table VII summarises the findings from the published reports. Although the years included and the age groups studied differed, the incidence ratio for leukaemia was greater than 1·0 for each establishment but not always significant at the 5% level. When all the data are added together a total of 96 cases of leukaemia are observed, compared with the expected total of 65 ($p < 0.001$). As the suspicion of an increased occurrence of childhood leukaemia in a village near the Sellafield plant prompted many of the other investigations, the Sellafield data should be viewed as generating, rather than testing, the hypothesis that the incidence of childhood cancers is increased around nuclear establishments. If the Sellafield data are excluded from the totals 77 cases of leukaemia are observed and 54·5 expected. The

TABLE VII—*Summary of the reported findings on the incidence of childhood leukaemia in the vicinity of nuclear establishments in the United Kingdom*

Nuclear establishment	Start up (approx)	Area included in the analysis	Childhood leukaemia incidence				
			Time period	Age group (years)	Observed No of cases	Expected No of cases	Incidence ratio (95% confidence interval)*
Sellafield[1]	1947	Copeland district	1961–80	0–14	19	10·5	1·8 (1·1 to 2·8)
Dounreay[4,5]	1954	Enumeration districts whose centres fell within 12·5 km of the establishment	1968–84	0–24	5	1·6	3·2 (1·0 to 7·3)
Holy Loch[6]	1961	Postcode sectors immediately adjacent to the installations	1964–85	0–14	4	2·1	1·9 (0·5 to 4·9)
Faslane[6]	1963		1964–85	0–14	5	4·2	1·2 (0·4 to 2·8)
Chapel Cross[6]	1962		1964–85	0–14	3	2·3	1·3 (0·3 to 3·8)
Hunterston[6]	1963		1964–85	0–14	19	15·7	1·2 (0·7 to 1·9)
AWRE, Aldermaston, ROF, Burghfield, and small part of UK AEAE, Harwell	1952 1962 1946	Electoral wards with at least half their area within 10 km of the establishments	1972–85	0–14	41	28·6	1·4 (1·0 to 2·0)

* Incidence ratio (95% confidence interval) = 1·5 (1·2 to 1·8) and for all establishments excluding Sellafield = 1·4 (1·1 to 1·8). For Hunterston inner and outer postcode sectors are included.
AWRE = Atomic Weapons Research Establishment; ROF = Royal Ordnance Factory; UK AEAE = United Kingdom Atomic Energy Authority's Establishment.

probability of such an excess occurring by chance is less than 0·01. Our data dominate the figures, as, unlike many nuclear establishments, those we studied are situated near areas of fairly high population density. Almost all the excesses described here were attributable to children aged 0–4. Other analyses of childhood leukaemia near nuclear establishments have not presented data for 0–4 year olds separately. The difficulty in accounting for the observed excesses of childhood leukaemia in terms of known emissions from nuclear establishments is a complex issue, which has been discussed in detail only for the Sellafield data.[1]

The data repoorted so far do not cover all nuclear establishments in the country, and our data include only a small part of the area around the United Kingdom Atomic Energy Authority's establishment at Harwell. There were no cases at all in the two West Berkshire electoral wards with at least half of their area included in the 10 km circle around Harwell, and only 0·38 cases were expected at ages 0–14. Other research groups are studying the incidence of childhood leukaemia around Harwell, and it is hoped that their findings will be available soon. The data described here are essentially confined to the area around the Atomic Weapons Research Establishment, Aldermaston, and the Royal Ordnance Factory, Burgh-field, and all the excess registrations of childhood leukaemia described occurred there. The incidence ratios were similar around each of the two establishments, although significant only around the Royal Ordnance Factory, which lies near areas of high population density. The reports so far may have selected establishments that happen to be located near areas with an increased rate of childhood leukaemia. The analyses for Dounreay were prompted by the impending local inquiry,[4 5] as were those relating to Holy Loch, Faslane, Chapel Cross, and Hunterston, which were reported as showing no evidence of an increase in childhood leukaemia.[6] Staff at the Royal Berkshire and Basingstoke District Hospitals have had a longstanding clinical impression, dating from the 1970s, that more children were attending their hospitals with leukaemia than might be expected but did not suggest that the excess incidence was confined to an area within 10 km radius of the local nuclear establishments.

Despite the significance of our findings the actual risk of leukaemia to children living in the West Berkshire and the Basingstoke and North Hampshire District Health Authorities and within a 10 km radius of the nuclear establishments is not great. About 60 000 children aged 0–14 were living at any one time within a 10 km radius of the nuclear establishments. About two of these children would normally be expected to develop leukaemia each year, but three have been registered, representing one extra case of leukaemia among these 60 000 each year.

We thank the consultants in the surrounding district health authorities for providing additional data about the children in the area with leukaemia. Charles

Stiller and his colleagues at the Childhood Cancer Research Group kindly provided data on childhood leukaemia in the Oxford and Wessex Regional Health Authorities, based on cancer registrations provided by the Office of Population Censuses and Surveys, and checked whether the children identified by us were also registered in the national scheme. Anna Brown and Jayne Hartnell kindly helped with the analyses, and Abe Adelstein and Peter Smith made helpful comments on the manuscript. The Office of Population Censuses and Surveys produced population estimates for the district and regional health authorities. Helen Edwards and Nina Saroi typed the manuscript. ER and LC are supported by the Medical Research Council.

1 Black D for the Independent Advisory Group. *Investigation of the possible increased incidence of cancer in west Cumbria.* London: HMSO, 1984. (Black report.)
2 Barton CJ, Roman E, Ryder HM, Watson A. Childhood leukaemia in west Berkshire. *Lancet* 1985;**ii**:1248–9.
3 Urquhart J, Cutler J, Burke M. Leukaemia and lymphatic cancer in young people near nuclear installations. *Lancet* 1986;**i**:384.
4 Heasman MA, Kemp IW, Urquhart JD, Black R. Childhood leukaemia in northern Scotland. *Lancet* 1986;**i**:266.
5 Heasman MA, Kemp IW, Urquhart JD, Black R. Leukaemia and lymphatic cancer in young people near nuclear installations. *Lancet* 1986;**i**:384.
6 Hole DJ, Gillis CR. Childhood leukaemia in the west of Scotland. *Lancet* 1986;**ii**:524.
7 Neil VS, Weindling AM, Ryder HM, Barton CJ, Newman CL. Approach to the management of children with malignant disease in one district general hospital. *BMJ* 1981;**283**:366–7.
8 Swerdlow AJ. Cancer registration in England and Wales: some aspects relevant to interpretation of the data. *Journal of the Royal Statistical Society* 1986;**149**:146–60.
9 World Health Organisation. *International classification of diseases. 8th revision, 1965.* Geneva: WHO, 1967.
10 World Health Organisation. *International classification of diseases. 9th revision, 1975.* Geneva: WHO, 1978.
11 Office of Population Censuses and Surveys. *Cancer statistics. Registrations.* Series MB1. London: HMSO, 1979–85. (Nos 2–14).
12 Bailar JC. Significance factors for the ratio of a Poisson variable to its expectation. *Biometrics* 1964;**20**:639–43.
13 Walter SD. On the detection of household aggregation of disease. *Biometrics* 1974;**30**:525–38.
14 Ohno Y, Aoki K, Aoki N. A test of significance for geographic clusters of disease. *Int J Epidemiol* 1979;**8**:273–81.
15 Breslow NE, Lubin JH, Marek P, Langholz B. Multiplicative models and cohort analysis. *Journal of the American Statistical Association* 1983;**78**:1–12.
16 Smith P. Spatial and temporal clustering. In: Schottenfeld D, Fraumeni JF, eds. *Cancer epidemiology and prevention.* Philadelphia: WB Saunders, 1982:391–407.
17 Knox G. Epidemiology of childhood leukaemia in Northumberland and Durham. *British Journal of Preventive and Social Medicine* 1964;**18**:17–24.
18 Alderson M. The epidemiology of leukaemia. *Adv Cancer Res* 1980;**31**:1–76.
19 Linnet MS. The leukaemias: epidemiologic aspects. *Monographs in epidemiology and biostatistics.* Vol 6. Oxford, New York: Oxford University Press, 1985.
20 McWhirter WR. The relationship of incidence of childhood lymphoblastic leukaemia to social class. *Br J Cancer* 1982;**46**:640–5.

9: Fallout, radiation doses near Dounreay, and childhood leukaemia

SARAH C DARBY, RICHARD DOLL

Possible explanations for the recently reported increased incidence of childhood leukaemia around Dounreay were examined in the light of changes in the national incidence of leukaemia that occurred during the period of exposure to fallout from international testing of nuclear weapons in the atmosphere. It was concluded that the increase could not be accounted for by an underestimate of the risk of leukaemia per unit dose of radiation at low doses and low dose rates, nor by an underestimate of the relative biological efficiency of high as compared with low linear energy transfer radiation. One possible explanation was underestimation of doses to the red bone marrow due to the discharges at Dounreay relative to the dose from fallout, though investigation of ways in which this might have occurred did not suggest anything definite. Other possible explanations included a misconception of the site of origin of childhood leukaemia, outbreaks of an infectious disease, and exposure to some other, unidentified environmental agent.

These findings weigh heavily against the hypothesis that the recent increase in childhood leukaemia near Dounreay might be accounted for by radioactive discharges from nuclear plants, unless the doses to the stem cells from which childhood leukaemia originates have been grossly underestimated.

TABLE I—*Mortality from leukaemia at aged 0–24 years in vicinity of Sellafield.*† *(Data derived from Gardner and Winter[1])*

	Ennerdale rural district			Millom rural district		
	Observed	Expected‡	O:E	Observed	Expected‡	O:E
1959–67	3	3·3	0·91	1	1·6	0·63
1968–78	4	3·3	1·21	6**	1·4	4·35
1959–78	7	6·6	1·06	7*	3·0	2·33

† Sellafield plant is at the southern coastal extreme of Ennerdale rural district. Millom rural district lies immediately to the south.
‡ Based on England and Wales national mortality rates.
* $p < 0.05$, ** $p < 0.01$ (one tailed tests).

TABLE II—*Incidence of leukaemia at ages 0–24 years in vicinity of Dounreay. (Data derived from Heasman et al[2])*

	< 12·5 km from Dounreay			12·5 to < 25 km from Dounreay		
	Observed	Expected†	O:E	Observed	Expected†	O:E
1968–78	0	1·1	0	0	0·99	0
1979–84	5***	0·5	9·75	1	0·45	2·21
1968–84	5*	1·6	3·19	1	1·44	0·69

† Based on all Scotland cancer registration rates.
* $p < 0.05$, *** $p < 0.001$ (one tailed tests).

Introduction

An increased incidence of childhood leukaemia has recently been reported in the vicinity of two nuclear installations in the United Kingdom[1][2]—namely, that at Sellafield, where spent nuclear fuel from nuclear power stations is reprocessed, and that at Dounreay, where a prototype fast breeder reactor has been developed and where there is also a reprocessing operation that deals with fuel from various reactors. Tables I and II summarise the evidence.

The National Radiological Protection Board has published calculations of the estimated radiation doses due to discharges from Sellafield and the risk of leukaemia that might be expected in children living in the nearby village of Seascale.[3][4] Similar calculations have also been published for Thurso, the town nearest Dounreay.[5] These calculations are based on assumptions that have generally been accepted by radiobiologists and those concerned with radiological protection, and they lead to the conclusion that the doses received by the children are insufficient to have caused anything like the increase in leukaemia that has been recorded in the vicinity of either installation. It is disturbing, however, that an increased incidence should have been found near two separate installations—and especially near the only two in Britain reprocessing substantial amounts of spent fuel—and this demands further investigation. Increases have also been suggested near several other nuclear installations but it is difficult to know what attention should be paid to these until a full study of all installations is available.

The possibility that the increased incidence of leukaemia near these two special installations might be due to chance is too unlikely to be acceptable unless all other explanations are ruled out, and we need to find an explanation that will account for both findings. We have therefore examined the evidence relating to the amount of irradiation received by children near Dounreay as a possible cause of leukaemia and viewed the findings in the light of the known effects of the worldwide fallout from the testing of nuclear weapons in the atmosphere. We considered that a hypothesis that failed to explain the increased incidence in one area could not be regarded as a satisfactory explanation in the other.

Radiation exposures to children in Thurso

Children living in Thurso are exposed to radiation from several sources, the most important of which are naturally occurring radiation, fallout from weapons testing, medical x rays, discharges into the sea and to the atmosphere from Dounreay, and discharges into the sea from Sellafield that have spread northwards round the coast. Throughout this chapter discharges into the sea from Dounreay include those from the adjoining reactor site (Vulcan Naval Reactor Test Establishment) operated by the Ministry of Defence.[67] There is clear evidence that leukaemia can be caused by exposure to radiation and it is widely assumed that even very low doses will cause a small increase in risk of the disease. If this is true, then all the sources of radiation listed above will contribute to the risk of radiation induced leukaemia in children in Thurso. In the National Radiological Protection Board's study of radiation doses to these children Dionian *et al* have estimated the absorbed dose to the red bone marrow from each source up to 1985 for children living in Thurso, the types of radiation being separated into low linear energy transfer radiation, such as x rays and γ rays, and high linear energy transfer radiation, chiefly α particles.[5] Detailed figures have been published for the cohort born in 1960 (table III). Three quarters of the estimated dose from low linear energy transfer radiation and 93% of the estimated dose from high linear energy transfer is attributable to natural sources. Given the conventional assumption that high linear energy transfer radiation is 20 times as harmful as low linear energy

TABLE III—*Average dose to red bone marrow integrated to 1985 for person born in 1960 and living in Thurso by source of radiation and radiation type. (Data derived from Dionian et al[5])*

Source of radiation	Absorbed dose to red bone marrow (μGy)		Dose equivalent to red bone marrow	
	Low linear energy transfer* (includes x rays, γ rays)	High linear energy transfer (chiefly α particles)	μSv*	%
Natural radiation	$2 \cdot 4 \times 10^4$	$1 \cdot 3 \times 10^2$	$2 \cdot 7 \times 10^4$	76·8
Fallout	$4 \cdot 6 \times 10^3$	3·0	$4 \cdot 7 \times 10^3$	13·4
Medical exposure	$2 \cdot 9 \times 10^3$		$2 \cdot 9 \times 10^3$	8·3
Dounreay discharges	$3 \cdot 6 \times 10^2$	4·0	$4 \cdot 4 \times 10^2$	1·3
Sellafield discharges	$1 \cdot 2 \times 10^2$	$9 \cdot 0 \times 10^{-2}$	$1 \cdot 2 \times 10^2$	0·3
Total	$3 \cdot 2 \times 10^4$	$1 \cdot 4 \times 10^2$	$3 \cdot 5 \times 10^4$	100·0

* Calculated assuming that relative biological efficiency of high linear energy transfer radiation is 20.

transfer radiation per unit of absorbed dose, just over three quarters of the dose equivalent to the red marrow is attributable to natural radiation; 13% is estimated to have been due to fallout and very much smaller proportions to discharges from Dounreay (1·3%) and Sellafield (0·3%)

For comparison of the effects produced by different sources of radiation with those possibly produced by the discharges, fallout has several advantages. The three recognised pathways of exposure for the discharges are (a) external exposure from radionuclides deposited on the beach or on soil or from the radioactive cloud, (b) internal exposure from inhalation of radionuclides in the air or in resuspended beach sands and sea spray, and (c) internal exposure from ingestion of radionuclides in marine foods, especially shellfish, and terrestrial foods and the inadvertent ingestion of beach sands and soil. These three pathways of exposure are also thought to operate for fallout—that is, external exposure from radionuclides deposited on the ground, both by dry deposition and in rainfall, and internal exposure from inhalation of radionuclides in the air and from terrestrial foods in which radionuclides have been incorporated.

Fallout, moreover, has several radionuclides in common with the discharges. Many of these are capable of irradiating the red bone marrow, which is assumed to be the tissue in which leukaemia is induced. Those that contributed appreciably to the dose to the red marrow in children born in Thurso in 1960 were listed by Dionian et al in two groups according to the type of radiation produced (low or high linear energy transfer) for each source (table IV).[5] External low linear energy transfer radiation, six radionuclides producing low linear transfer radiation, and two radionuclides producing high linear energy transfer were common to all three

TABLE IV—*Radionuclides occurring in fallout or in discharges from Dounreay or Sellafield and contributing to radiation dose to red bone marrow of child born in Thurso in 1960. (Data derived from Dionian et al[5])*

	Radionuclides	
Sources of radiation	Low linear energy transfer	High linear energy transfer
Fallout, Dounreay discharges* and Sellafield discharges†	Strontium-90, ruthenium-106, caesium-137, cerium-144, plutonium-239, plutonium-238‡ external radiation	Plutonium-229, plutonium-238‡
Fallout and Dounreay discharges*	Strontium-89, iodine-131	
Dounreay* and Sellafield† discharges only	Zirconium-95, niobium-95, caesium-134, plutonium-241,§ americium-241§	Plutonium-241,§ americium-241§
Fallout only	Carbon-14‖	

* Discharges to sea and atmosphere.
† Discharges to sea.
‡ Plutonium-238 not listed explicitly by Dionian *et al* as occurring in discharges from Dounreay and Sellafield.[5] Nevertheless, small amount does occur and was taken into account by Dionian *et al* in their calculations (J Dionian, personal communication).
§ Plutonium-241 and americium-241 are produced in fallout but contribution to dose is very small by comparison with other radionuclides.
‖ Carbon-14 is present in Dounreay discharges but in only small quantities compared with other radionuclides.

sources, and two further radionuclides producing low linear energy transfer radiation were common to both fallout and to the discharges at Dounreay. This contrasts sharply with the picture for the other two main sources of exposure—namely, medical and natural irradiation. The estimated dose to the red bone marrow in children due to medical irradiation is almost entirely from external x rays, whereas the dose due to natural irradiation is from low linear energy transfer external radiation and from the radionuclides potassium-40, polonium-210, lead-210, radium-226, radon-220, and radon-222, none of which occurs in substantial quantities in liquid discharges from Sellafield or in liquid or atmospheric discharges from Dounreay.

Lastly, fallout has the advantage for our analysis that the resulting exposure to radiation has varied greatly over time. Figure 1 shows the number of nuclear explosions in the atmosphere by calendar year. The first nuclear weapon test in the atmosphere took place at Alamagordo in 1945, before the bombings of Hiroshima and Nagasaki. Atmospheric testing increased after the war and reached a peak in the late 1950s and early 1960s. After the 1962 test ban treaty the level of atmospheric testing fell and has remained low, only France and China continuing to test.

Discharges from the Dounreay site began in 1958[7] and from Sellafield

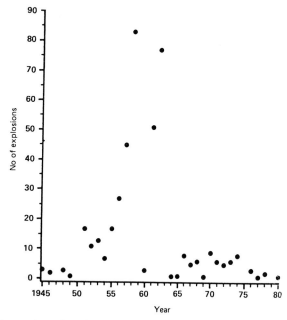

FIG 1—*Yearly number of nuclear explosions in atmosphere during 1945–80. (Data derived from United Nations Scientific Committee on the Effects of Atomic Radiation.[8])*

around 1950.[4] Estimates of the average yearly absorbed doses from low and high linear energy transfer radiation received in the bone marrow by children born in Thurso in 1960 from these two sources and from fallout have been published by Dionian *et al.*[5] Figure 2 shows the contributions from Dounreay and fallout; the maximum yearly contributions from Sellafield for both high and low linear energy transfer radiation were very small by comparison with the maximum contributions from either fallout or Dounreay and are omitted. The contributions from medical exposure and natural radiation are also omitted from figure 2. They will have been roughly the same each year—namely, from medical radiation (low linear energy transfer only) 270 µGy to the fetus and between about 40 µGy and 160 µGy a year after birth, depending on age; and from natural radiation (low linear energy transfer) 690 µGy to the fetus and 950 µGy a year after birth and (high linear energy transfer) about 0·2 µGy to the fetus and between 4·4 µGy and 6·0 µGy a year after birth, depending on age.

Figure 2 shows that the standard yearly dose from low linear energy transfer radiation due to fallout rose to a maximum a few years after the period of peak testing activity and then declined. In every year, however, the estimated dose due to fallout was greater (and sometimes much greater)

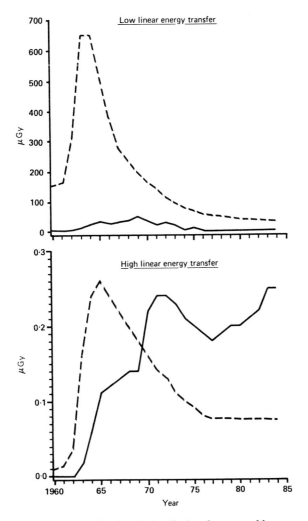

FIG 2—*Estimated average yearly absorbed radiation doses to red bone marrow resulting from fallout (----) and Dounreay dischages (——) for high and low linear energy transfer radiation for person born in 1960 in Thurso. (Fetal doses not included but estimated as follows—low linear energy transfer: fallout 86 µGy, Dounreay 8·4 µGy; high linear energy transfer: fallout $6·4 \times 10^{-4}$ µGy, Dounreay $7·3 \times 10^{-5}$ µGy.) (Data derived from Dionian et al.[5])*

than that due to the discharges from Dounreay. The estimated dose from high linear energy transfer fallout also reached a peak in the mid-1960s and then declined. By the late 1970s the decline had halted and the estimated yearly dose subsequently remained roughly constant. This constant dose was due to inhaled plutonium-239, which is thought to have a long retention time on bone surfaces and to irradiate the red bone marrow continuously. The estimated yearly high linear energy transfer dose from the discharges at Dounreay tended to increase throughout the period, and from about 1970 it exceeded that from fallout. The maximum estimated yearly high linear energy transfer dose due to the discharges at Dounreay occurred in the early 1980s and was comparable with the estimated dose due to fallout in the mid-1960s.

Possible explanations for increased incidence of leukaemia near Dounreay

Four explanations for the increased incidence of leukaemia near Dounreay seem possible—namely, (a) that some leukaemias were caused by the discharges from Dounreay, in which case others will have been caused by fallout from weapon tests; (b) that estimates of the relative magnitude of the average doses to the red marrow due to fallout and the discharges are wrong; (c) that the dose to the red bone marrow is irrelevant for childhood leukaemia; and (d) that the leukaemias have been caused by some agent other than radiation exposure from the discharges. These four explanations are examined below.

SOME LEUKAEMIAS NEAR DOUNREAY CAUSED BY DISCHARGES AND SOME CAUSED BY FALLOUT FROM WEAPON TESTS

One explanation is that most of the leukaemias near Dounreay are, in fact, caused directly by the discharges. If this is true it follows that doses from fallout must also have been large enough to cause a material increase in the risk of childhood leukaemia, unless explanation (b) or (c) is also true. Fallout, however, is not specific to the area around Dounreay, which enables the effect of fallout to be tested. Airborne material transferred from the stratosphere is widely dispersed in the northern hemisphere. There is some variation with latitude, but this effect is small for the geographical regions considered in this paper. Thus doses from inhaling fallout material from weapons testing may be considered to be independent of geographical location. Deposition of some radionuclides depends on rainfall, and transfer of the deposited material through food chains may depend on local agriculture. Thus doses from ingesting radionuclides in food may vary geographically. For high linear energy transfer radiation most of the dose is thought to arise from inhaled plutonium in the air; thus the high linear energy transfer plutonium dose from fallout in England and Wales, and also throughout Scotland, is estimated to be similar to that in the vicinity of Thurso and to have occurred with a similar temporal pattern. For low linear energy transfer radiation the dose is chiefly due to radionuclides deposited on the ground in rainfall and subsequent uptake through food

TABLE V—*Proportion of leukaemic children surviving five years or more after diagnosis by calendar period. (Manchester data derived from Draper et al[9]; data for Britain derived from C Stiller (personal communication))*

	Year of diagnosis	Percentage of children surviving five years or more
All leukaemias (Manchester)	1954–8	0
	1959–63	3
	1964–8	5
	1969–73	26
	1971–3	36
Acute lymphatic leukaemia (Britain)	1974–6	47
	1977–9	52

chains; hence it varies in magnitude from place to place, though the temporal pattern will still be broadly similar. It follows that the average dose from low linear energy transfer radiation in England and Wales as a whole is lower than that in Thurso, where the rainfall is above average for the United Kingdom, though the amount is thought not to differ by more than a factor of two. For Scotland as a whole the estimated doses from low linear energy transfer radiation lie between those for England and Wales and those for Thurso.

Death rates, which were commonly used as a surrogate for the incidence of leukaemia when the disease was almost uniformly fatal, became no longer usable for the study of trends around 1960, when improvements in the treatment of leukaemia in children began to be reflected in a falling mortality (see table V). Incidence rates depend on the efficiency of registration and, though this began in some areas before the second world war, it was not extended nationally until the 1950s; even then it was grossly incomplete in some parts of Britain owing to poor administrative support. In England and Wales registration remained lower than the death rates until 1969 and did not exceed the average level of mortality in the 1950s until 1971 (fig 3). After 1971 there was an increase of around 10%, which persisted until 1979, when the recorded incidence fell to the level of the mortality in the 1950s. The data for Scotland show a similar pattern (fig 3). Published data for childhood cancer are reportedly inflated by some 10% owing to duplicate registrations and the failure to deregister incorrectly diagnosed cases.[9] This, however, does not account for the observed temporal pattern, as the data obtained by the Childhood Cancer Research Group, in which these errors have been corrected, show the same pattern (C Stiller, personal communication). We are therefore left with the possibility of a small increase in incidence in the early 1970s, which is proportionally two orders of magnitude less than that observed in Doun-

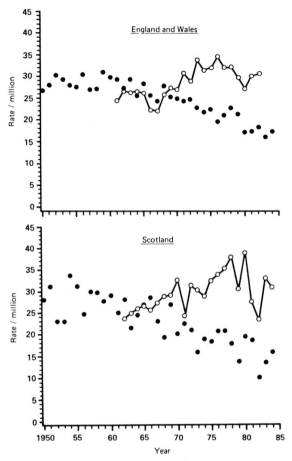

FIG 3—*Leukaemia mortality (●) and registration (○) rates in patients aged 0–24 years in England and Wales and in Scotland during 1950–84 directly standardised to world standard populaton.[11] (Data derived from reports published by Office of Population Censuses and Surveys and Registrar General, Scotland, and unpublished data supplied by Scottish Health Service Common Services Agency.)*

reay and, on the basis of studies of radiation induced leukaemia, some five years later in time than would have been expected had it been due to fallout.

If the leukaemia trends in Britain in the 1970s were due to fallout we should expect similar trends to have been recorded in Denmark and Norway, where national cancer registries have long been established and where the same temporal trend in fallout was observed. For high linear energy transfer radiaiton the estimated doses in those two countries are similar to those in Britain. For low linear energy transfer radiation the

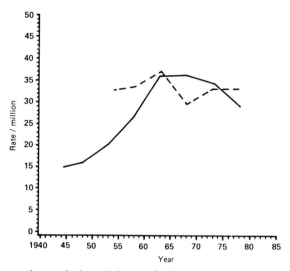

FIG 4—*Incidence of acute leukaemia in population aged 0–24 years in Norway during 1953–80 (———) and Denmark during 1943–80 (———) directly standardised to world standard population.[11] (Data derived from Hakulinen et al.[10])*

estimated doses are higher than in the United Kingdom, especially in Norway because of its high rainfall. Measured concentrations of caesium-137 in Norwegian milk have been about six times those in the United Kingdom and measured concentrations of strontium-90 about three times the United Kingdom values, whereas concentrations in Denmark have been intermediate between those for Norway and the the United Kingdom for ^{90}Sr and similar to the United Kingdom values for ^{137}Cs.

Data on the incidence of acute leukaemia (which would include almost all childhood leukaemia) are available from 1943 for Denmark and from 1953 for Norway.[10] Figure 4 shows these for ages 0–24 years standardised for age.[11] In neither country was there a peak in incidence in the early 1970s or late 1960s. The increasing trend in Denmark before 1960 is thought to have been at least partly artificial and due to an increase in the proportion of children with leukaemia who were diagnosed correctly.[12]

Thus, though the rates of childhood leukaemia have varied in each of the three countries, there is no convincing evidence of an increase in incidence that could be attributed to fallout, let alone any comparable with that found around Dounreay.

The arguments presented in this chapter make the conventional assumption that risk per unit dose is roughly uniform throughout the range of doses that have been received by children living in Thurso. It has sometimes been suggested, however, that for low linear energy transfer radiation the risk per unit dose varies within the low dose range, resulting in a higher risk per unit of absorbed dose for those at the upper end of the range and making the average dose an inappropriate measure. Nevertheless, that the average yearly dose due to fallout from weapons testing have varied up to well over 10 times the maximum yearly dose resulting from discharge means that if this were so an even greater effect of fallout in comparison with the discharges would be expected. For high linear energy transfer radiation radiobiological work does not, on the whole, suggest a departure from a uniform risk per unit of absorbed dose, even in the low dose range.

ESTIMATES OF RELATIVE MAGNITUDE OF AVERAGE DOSES TO RED MARROW DUE TO FALLOUT AND DISCHARGES WRONG

A second possible explanation of the findings is that the true dose to the red marrow due to the discharges when averaged over all subjects is much higher than that due to fallout. A popular explanation postulates the existence of a small subgroup of people who have received very high doses due to the discharges and who have been omitted from the calculations. We have discounted this as accounting for the findings for the following reasons. Even if a very small proportion of the children had received very high doses and had not been taken into account in the calculations this would have a negligible effect on the overall average dose; for example, if 1% of children had in fact received 10 times the estimated average dose and been omitted, then altering the calculations to take them into account would increase the average by only 10%. Thus to explain the findings it is necessary to postulate that the proportion of children receiving extraordinarily high doses is substantial. The mechanisms by which this might occur—for example, living on the beach, eating a diet of pure shellfish, or deliberately ingesting large quantities of beach sands—are such that it is not plausible that they would apply to a substantial proportion of children. There are, however, several ways in which it might theoretically be possible for a large discrepancy in the estimates of the relative magnitude of doses from fallout and from the discharges to have occurred.

Firstly, the amounts of radioactive materials assumed to be present in the environment may be wrong. Those from fallout are based on environmental measurements and are therefore unlikely to be grossly in error. Those from the discharges are based primarily on mathematical models, as this approach permits a more comprehensive assessment than would be possible on the basis of environmental measurements alone.[7] The results obtained by comparing the model predictions with such environmental measurements as have been made in Thurso and the surrounding area suggested that the predicted doses are unlikely to be far out. Indeed, the doses predicted by the models appear to overestimate the concentrations of radionuclides in the environmental materials that are thought to be the most important causes of exposure by a factor of two or three.[7]

Secondly, assumptions regarding individual behaviour, such as the amount of time spent on the beach, quantities of various different types of food eaten, etc, may be wrong; and, thirdly, the metabolic models relating the dose in an individual organ or tissue to an intake of radionuclide may be wrong. As it is impossible to measure the body content of plutonium in vivo at the levels of interest, it is not possible to test all the assumptions directly. Nevertheless, in two studies comparing measured and predicted concentrations of ^{137}Cs in the body the models tended to overestimate dose.[13 14] In Germany measurements of the concentration of plutonium due to fallout from weapons testing have also been made at necropsy for several organs and good agreement has been shown between measured and predicted values.[15] We emphasise that the same metabolic models are used for both discharges and fallout and so cannot distort the relative magnitude of the dose from the two sources in so far as the same radionuclides and methods of intake are concerned. For low linear energy transfer radiation the estimated doses from external radiation are much the same from the discharges and fallout and much additional low linear energy transfer internal radiation was received only from fallout. For high linear energy transfer radiation most of the dose from both fallout and the discharges is due to ^{239}Pu. For fallout, however, the dose is received mainly from inhalation, whereas for the discharges it is received mainly from ingestion. Substantial differences might therefore be produced if the assumed proportion of plutonium transferred from the lung into the bloodstream is much too high or the assumed proportion transferred from the digestive tract is much too low.

DOSE TO RED BONE MARROW IRRELEVANT FOR CHILDHOOD LEUKAEMIA

The target cells for adult myeloid leukaemia are located in the bone marrow, and there is now evidence that a substantial proportion of childhood leukaemias also arise in the bone marrow, a small proportion of cases arising in the fetal liver or thymus. The question, however, is not completely resolved (M Greaves, personal communication).

We do not know where in the bone marrow the target cells lie, but even if they are restricted to a small region of the marrow it seems unlikely that the ratio of fallout dose to discharge dose for that region would differ substantially from that for the marrow as a whole.

LEUKAEMIAS CAUSED BY SOME AGENT OTHER THAN RADIATION EXPOSURE FROM DISCHARGES

The fourth possible explanation is that these leukaemias are caused not by radiation exposure from the discharges at Dounreay but by some other environmental agent. It is not easy, however, to suggest what such an agent might be. The only agents other than ionising radiations that are known to have caused leukaemia are benzene, some of the alkylating agents and other drugs used for cancer, and two viruses (human T cell lymphotropic viruses types 1 and 2), and none of these has caused the typical acute lymphoblastic leukaemia of childhood.

Viral infection has often been suspected as the most likely principal cause; but no direct evidence of such a cause has been obtained, unless it is thought to have been provided by the occurrence of leukaemia in the donor's marrow cells after the treatment of leukaemia in a child by whole body irradiation and marrow transplantation.[16] Reports of clusters of cases have recurred frequently in the past 50 years and the evidence that clusters may occur more often than would be expected by chance alone is not conclusive.[17] If an infective agent is responsible for the disease it is possible that mini epidemics would be particularly likely to occur under the conditions that have brought together a young workforce in a comparatively isolated area.

Many other environmental agents have been suspected as possible causes from time to time (for example, electromagnetic fields[18] and parental occupation, particularly paternal exposure to chlorinated solvents, pesticides, and incense (J Peters, personal communication)). None has yet been substantiated and there is no obvious reason, other than parental occupation in a nuclear installation, why such factors should have caused an increased number of cases specifically around Dounreay and Sellafield.

Conclusions

The available data weigh heavily against the hypothesis that the recent increase in childhood leukaemia near Dounreay might be accounted for by exposure to radiation due to discharges from the Dounreay and Sellafield plants, unless the doses to the red marrow from the discharges are grossly underestimated by comparison with the doses received from fallout. In particular, the possibility that an underestimate either of the risk of leukaemia per unit of absorbed dose to the bone marrow at low doses and low dose rates or of the relative biological efficiency of high linear energy transfer as compared with low linear energy transfer radiation is ruled out by the lack of any consistent increase in childhood leukaemia after the period of peak fallout. Investigation of the various ways in which underestimates of dose might have occurred does not suggest any ready explanation, but there remains the possibility that childhood leukaemia does not arise from the red marrow and that the radioactive nuclides are disproportionately concentrated in the relevant tissue. Alternatively the increase might be the result of a cluster of cases brought out by an infective agent or perhaps by some other environmental agent. Which, if any, of these explanations is correct can be decided only by further research.

We thank Miss F A Fry, Professor M Greaves, Dr L Kinlen, Dr M C Pike, Mr L Salmon, and Dr A D Wrixon for helpful discussions during the preparation of this paper; Mr C Stiller for providing data from the Childhood Cancer Research Group registry, based on the national cancer registration scheme; and the information services division of the Scottish Health Service Common Services Agency for supplying leukaemia registrations for Scotland. Thanks are also due to Mrs I Stratton for help with computing, Mrs V Weare for clerical work, and Mrs C Harwood for preparing the manuscript.

1 Gardner MJ, Winter PD. Mortality in Cumberland during 1959–79 with reference to cancer in young people around Windscale. *Lancet* 1984;i:216–7.

2 Heasman MA, Kemp IW, Urquhart JD, Black R. Childhood leukaemia in northern Scotland. *Lancet* 1986;i:266, 385.

3 Stather JW, Wrixon AD, Simmonds JR. *The risks of leukaemia and other cancers in Seascale from radiation exposure.* London: HMSO, 1984. (NRPB report R171.)

4 Stather JW, Dionian J, Brown J, Fell TP, Muirhead CR. *The risks of leukaemia and other cancers in Seascale from radiation exposure.* London: HMSO, 1986. (Addendum to NRPB report R171.)

5 Dionian J, Muirhead CR, Wan SL, Wrixon AD. *The risks of leukaemia and other cancers in Thurso from radiation exposure.* London: HMSO, 1986. (NRPB report R196.)

6 Hunt GJ. *Aquatic environment monitoring report.* Lowestoft: Ministry of Agriculture, Fisheries, and Food, 1986.

7 Hill MD, Cooper JR. *Radiation doses to members of the population of Thurso.* London: HMSO, 1986. (NRPB report R195.)

8 United Nations Scientific Committee on the Effects of Atomic Radiation. *Ionizing radiation: sources and biological effects.* New York: United Nations, 1982.

9 Draper GJ, Birch JM, Bithell JF, *et al. Childhood cancer in Britain.* London HMSO, 1982. (OPCS studies on medical and population subjects, No 37.)

10 Hakulinen T, Anderson AH, Malker B, Pukkala E, Schon G, Tulinius H. Trends in cancer incidence in the Nordic countries. *Acta Pathol Microbiol Immunol Scand [A]* 1986;94(suppl 288):1–151.

11 Waterhouse J, Muir C, Shanmugaratnam K, Powell J. *Cancer incidence in five continents.* Vol 4. Lyon: International Agency for Research on Cancer, 1982.

12 Hansen NE, Karle H, Jensen OM. Trends in the incidence of leukaemia in Denmark, 1943–77. *Journal of the National Cancer Institute* 1983;71:697–701.

13 Fry FA, Sumerling TJ. *Measurements of caesium-137 in residents of Seascale and its environs.* London: HMSO, 1984. (NRPB report R172.)

14 Fry FA. *Comparison of measured and predicted body contents of ^{137}Cs in adults resident near Sellafield.* London: HMSO, 1986. (Appendix D of addendum to NRPB report R171.)

15 Bunzl K, Henrichs, K, Kracke W. Distribution of fallout ^{241}Pu, $^{239+240}Pu$ and ^{238}Pu in persons of different ages from the Federal Republic of Germany. In: *Assessment of radioactive contamination in man 1984.* Vienna: International Atomic Energy Agency, 1985;541–53.

16 Smith JL, Heerema NA, Provisor AJ. Leukaemic transformation of engrafted bone marrow cells. *Br J Haematol* 1985;60:415–22.

17 Smith PG. Spatial and temporal clustering. In: Schottenfeld D, Fraumeni JF Jr, eds. *Cancer epidemiology and prevention.* Philadelphia: Saunders, 1982.

18 Wertheimer N, Leeper E. Electrical wiring configurations and childhood cancer. *Am J Epidemiol* 1980;109:273–84.

10: Follow up study of children born elsewhere but attending schools in Seascale, west Cumbria (schools cohort)

M J GARDNER, A J HALL, S DOWNES, J D TERRELL

Records on 1546 children who were identified as having attended schools in Seascale up to November 1984 and were born since 1950 but not in the civil parish were studied. These children lived in or near Seascale for a period of time while they were attending one or more of three local schools and are an additional group to the 1068 children who were identified as born to mothers resident in Seascale in the next chapter. Even though some of the schoolchildren apparently remained in the village for only a short period, all but 7% were followed up through the National Health Service central register. Mortality among these children to 30 June 1986 is comparable to that expected at national rates. From all causes there were 10 observed deaths compared with 12·69 expected—a ratio of 0·79 (95% confidence interval 0·38 to 1·45)—and from cancer one observed death compared with 2·04 expected—a ratio of 0·49 (95% confidence interval 0·01 to 2·73). No deaths from leukaemia or lymphoma were reported, but only 0·83 was expected. Since 1971 (the year when cases of cancer were first notified to the NHS central register) three non-fatal cases of cancer were reported, including two lymphomas, compared with 2·04 expected and two cases of carcinoma in situ of the cervix compared with 1·79 expected. In addition, there was a case of leukaemia among the schoolchildren which was known previously and had been diagnosed in 1968.

There is an interesting difference between the results of this study and the results of the study of children born to mothers who were resident in Seascale. In the latter study there was an excess of leukaemia and of other cancers, but a similar finding is not apparent among children who spent some time at schools in Seascale but were born elsewhere. This raises the question of whether one or more aetiological factors in childhood cancer were acting on a locality specific basis before birth or early in life. This cannot be answered from these cohort studies, but it is hoped that the case-control study that is under way in west Cumbria will provide relevant information.

Introduction

The Black report made recommendations for four epidemiological studies related to childhood cancer in west Cumbria and the village of Seascale, which is close to the Sellafield nuclear fuel reprocessing site.[1] Some of the rationale for these is given in the next chapter, which reports the results of one of the investigations—namely, the follow up of children born since 1950 to mothers resident in Seascale at the time of birth (recommendation 2).

The third recommendation was that "a study should be considered of the records of schoolchildren who have attended schools in the area." After due consideration the records were found to be suitable to proceed, and this chapter reports the methodology and the findings on mortality and cancer registration of this second follow up study.

Methods

We were made aware of four schools in Seascale which had taken pupils for all or some of the period from 1950. With the cooperation of the local education department, headmasters, and headmistresses we examined the school registers to find out whether the information in them was sufficiently detailed to identify uniquely the children who had attended. For three of the schools the recorded details were of suitable quality for follow up. The fourth school was a preparatory boarding school for boys which closed during 1972 but had taken some 150 pupils since 1950, of whom about half came from outside Cumbria. Although for each boy the year of

TABLE I—*Numbers of children in Seascale birth cohort and schools cohort by register of first identification*

Cohort	Register of first identification	Later identified in school register		
		Singing Surf	Local authority	Calder Girls
Birth cohort	1068	44	565	1
Schools cohort:				
Singing Surf School	124	—	54	1
Local authority school	1311	—	—	1
Calder Girls School	111	—	—	—

birth was recorded, the full date of birth was not and hence follow up through the National Health Service central register was not feasible. This school had, therefore, to be omitted.

Children who had attended the other three schools and who were born after 1 January 1950, as in the Seascale birth cohort, were included in the study. But any schoolchildren who were also born to mothers resident in Seascale civil parish at the time of birth, and so were already members of the birth cohort, were left out of this study.

Singing Surf School—This was a small coeducational school in Seascale that was open from 1949 to 1968 and mainly took children at preschool ages. Only 168 children born since 1950 were recorded as having attended. Among these were 44 who were already included in the Seascale birth cohort, and thus 124 children were identified for follow up.

Seascale local authority school—This is the main local village school. A total of 1930 pupils who were born after 1 January 1950 and entered the school up to November 1984 were recorded in the school register. Of these children, 565 (29%) had already been identified in the Seascale birth cohort, and a further 54 (3%) had previously attended Singing Surf School. The remaining 1311 (68%) children, who must have moved into Seascale since birth or lived nearby, were included in the follow up.

Calder Girls School—This was a boarding school for girls that was open from 1950 to 1967. Altogether 114 girls born from 1950 onwards were recorded in the school register as having attended, many of whom came from far away, some from abroad. Only one of the 114 girls was in the Seascale birth cohort, one other had earlier attended Singing Surf School, and a further one the local authority school. The remaining 111 girls were thus included in the follow up.

The allocation of children to birth and schools cohorts in the way described was carried out to avoid duplication in counting children and events such as cancer registration and death. Table I gives the numbers of children in the various cohorts and their interrelationships. A total of 2614 children were followed up (given by summing the figures in the first column of the table), of which 1068 (41%) are in the birth cohort and the remaining 1546 (59%) in the schools cohort.

The birth and schools cohorts do not include all children who were born after 1950 and lived in Seascale for some period of time. In addition to boys who were pupils only at the excluded preparatory school, any child who, for example, moved to the village after birth but left before school age or went to boarding school elsewhere cannot be identified by the means we have used. The studies, however, will have included most of the Seascale children.

Suitable details of identification for all of these schoolchildren, except those already in the birth cohort, were forwarded to the NHS central register, which then provided us with information on deaths, cancer registrations, and emigrations. We were also notified by the central register of all family practitioner committee areas, together with dates, in which the children had been recorded as registered with general practitioners. We also obtained dates of starting and leaving school from the registers where available. These details give two indications of dates and duration of residence in or near Seascale. Again, as for births to mothers in Seascale, neither the children nor their parents were approached direct.

In this chapter mortality among the children from the time they started school in Seascale until 30 June 1986 is analysed and compared with that expected at national rates. As for the birth cohort, although some of the follow up and deaths in the study are among individuals who have strictly passed childhood, the term children is used throughout the chapter to refer to the members of the schools cohort. The person years method of analysis was used, incorporating calendar period, cause, sex, and age specific death rates for England and Wales. Confidence intervals were calculated using standard methods based on the Poisson distribution.

Results

Table II gives the numbers of children in the schools cohort by school and year of entry to school. An average of under 10 children a year entered Singing Surf School from 1955 to the date of its closure. Entry to the local authority school of children not included in the birth cohort peaked at about 70 children a year during the early 1960s, with a subsequent fall and secondary peak in the late 1970s. For Calder Girls School the maximal years of entry were 1960–4, averaging about 15 girls a year.

Table II also shows the numbers of children by age at entry to the three schools, indicating the first age at which they are known to have attended school—and possibly lived—in Seascale. Most children who attended Singing Surf School entered before 5 years of age. The most frequent ages of entry to the local authority school were 4 and 5 years, even though the

TABLE II—*Numbers of children by year of entry and age at entry to each school*

	School		
	Singing Surf (n = 124)	Local authority (n = 1311)	Calder Girls (n = 111)
Years of entry to school:			
1950–4	2	1	0
1955–9	38	202	6
1960–4	42	338	79
1965–9	42	251	25
1970–4	0	187	0
1975–9	0	204	0
1980–4	0	128	0
Unknown	0	0	1
Age (years) at starting school:			
2	6	0	0
3	44	0	0
4	58	529	0
5	10	281	0
6	3	119	0
7	1	98	1
8	2	97	6
9	0	80	13
10	0	51	19
11	0	55	39
12	0	1	17
13	0	0	12
14	0	0	2
15	0	0	1
Unknown	0	0	1

565 children who were born in Seascale and later attended this school are excluded. The numbers who joined the school at older ages indicate the degree of movement of families into the area. An indication of movement out is given by the proportion of children, 545 out of 1173 (46%) with recorded dates of leaving school, who left before the usual age of 11 years. For Calder Girls School starting ages were older and mainly between 9 and 13 years. The median length of time at school in Seascale for all the children was nearly four years, and about 30% stayed over six years.

Table III summarises the follow up information received from the central register for children in the schools cohort by school. Up to 30 June 1986 no deaths were reported among the Singing Surf and Calder Girls schoolchildren but there were 10 among the local authority schoolchildren. Overall 65 (4%) of the children were reported to have left the country. Of 1546 children in the three schools combined, the records of 1439 (93%) were traced in the central register. Though this is a high percentage, it compares unfavourably with the 100% trace rate in the birth cohort, for which NHS numbers were available.

TABLE III—*Vital statistics of children at 30 June 1986 in each school cohort*

	School		
At 30 June 1986	Singing Surf	Local authority	Calder Girls
Alive	108	1177	79
Dead	0	10	0
Emigrated	3	45	17
No trace	13	79	15
Total	124	1311	111

The deficit is largely among children born before July 1963 for whom the no trace rate was 9% (90 of 1000 births) compared with 3% (17 of 546) for later births. The reason for this is likely to be related to the fact that between February 1952 and July 1963 the central register's alphabetical index was compiled from applications for welfare foods, and about 15% of parents nationally apparently did not complete the application form issued at birth registration. This limits the searching option to the alternative births index which is more difficult without NHS numbers. In addition, there are inevitably some inaccuracies in the information in the school registers that will have contributed to children not being traced. We know of instances where small errors in, for example, the spelling of the name, have none the less not excluded a successful trace.

Table IV gives mortality figures for the children in the schools cohort compared with national rates. For Singing Surf and Calder Girls Schools, with no deaths reported, the expected numbers from all causes are small at 1·45 and 0·82 respectively. For the children in the local authority school the 10 observed deaths are similar to the 10·42 expected at death rates in England and Wales. For the three schools combined there were 10 observed deaths compared with 12·69 expected—a ratio of 0·79 (95% confidence interval 0·38 to 1·45). When examined by cause one of the 10 deaths was certified as due to cancer compared with 2·04 expected—a ratio of 0·49 (95% confidence interval 0·01 to 2·73). The particular diagnosis was "malignant melanoma" in a man aged 33 who had moved away from Seascale. The other nine deaths were all coded under "injury and poisoning" according to the International Classification of Diseases[2] and consisted of four traffic accidents, three poisonings, one asphyxiation, and one drowning. These nine deaths contrasted with 6·13 expected in this category (observed/expected = 1·47, 95% confidence interval 0·67 to 2·79) and included two pairs of siblings. Table V shows that in no age group were the numbers of observed deaths particularly different from those expected, that mortality was similar to expected for both sexes, and that there was no pattern of deaths by calendar year of follow up.

TABLE IV—*Numbers of deaths by cause to 30 June 1986 among children in each school cohort compared with deaths expected at national rates*

Cause of death	No of deaths			95% Confidence interval for O/E
	Observed (O)	Expected (E)	O/E	
Singing Surf School				
Malignant neoplasms (140–208):	0	0·21	0	0 to 17·23
Non-Hodgkin's lymphoma (200, 202)	0	0·02	0	0 to 212·68
Hodgkin's disease (201)	0	0·01	0	0 to 272·68
Leukaemia (204–208)	0	0·06	0	0 to 59·89
Other cancers	0	0·12	0	0 to 30·49
Other causes	0	1·24	0	0 to 2·98
All causes	0	1·45	0	0 to 2·54
Local authority school				
Malignant neoplasms (140–208):	1	1·63	0·61	0·02 to 3·42
Non-Hodgkin's lymphoma (200, 202)	0	0·13	0	0 to 29·08
Hodgkin's disease (201)	0	0·10	0	0 to 35·46
Leukaemia (204–208)	0	0·45	0	0 to 8·13
Other cancers	1	0·94	1·06	0·03 to 5·90
Other causes	9	8·79	1·02	0·47 to 1·94
All causes	10	10·42	0·96	0·46 to 1·77
Calder Girls School				
Malignant neoplasms (140–208):	0	0·20	0	0 to 18·74
Non-Hodgkin's lymphoma (200, 202)	0	0·01	0	0 to 350·94
Hodgkin's disease (201)	0	0·01	0	0 to 302·65
Leukaemia (204–208)	0	0·03	0	0 to 119·05
Other cancers	0	0·14	0	0 to 25·80
Other causes	0	0·62	0	0 to 5·96
All causes	0	0·82	0	0 to 4·52

Figures in parentheses are code numbers in the International Classification of Diseases (9th revision).[2]

In addition to the one cancer death, three further cases of cancer were registered between 1971 and 1984 compared with 2·04 non-fatal cases of cancer expected (observed/expected = 1·47, 95% confidence interval 0·30 to 4·30) using published annual figures for cancer registration by age and sex[3] and subtracting the number of expected deaths during the same period. All three cases occurred among the local authority schoolchildren. One of these three, a patient with non-Hodgkin's lymphoma diagnosed while living in Seascale, was included in the Black report (case 16 of table 2.3[1]). Of the other two, one is a case of Hodgkin's disease diagnosed in a man aged 26 and the second a carcinoma of the lung diagnosed in a 21 year old woman. These two cases were diagnosed after the patients left Seascale, although one was still resident in Cumbria at the time. In addition, from the central register two cases were reported to us of carcinoma in situ of the

TABLE V—*Numbers of deaths by age, sex, and calendar year to 30 June 1986 among children in local authority school cohort compared with deaths expected at national rates*

| Category | No of deaths | | | 95% Confidence interval for O/E |
	Observed (O)	Expected (E)	O/E	
Age (years):				
Under 5	0	0·09	0	0 to 41·37
5–9	0	1·56	0	0 to 2·37
10–14	0	1·51	0	0 to 2·44
15–19	4	2·71	1·47	0·40 to 3·78
20–24	2	2·18	0·92	0·11 to 3·31
25–29	2	1·46	1·37	0·17 to 4·94
30 and over	2	0·90	2·23	0·27 to 8·06
Sex:				
Male	7	6·85	1·02	0·41 to 2·10
Female	3	3·56	0·84	0·17 to 2·46
Calendar year of follow up				
1955–9	0	0·20	0	0 to 18·25
1960–4	0	0·65	0	0 to 5·65
1965–9	2	1·32	1·51	0·18 to 5·46
1970–4	1	1·95	0·51	0·01 to 2·87
1975–9	2	2·46	0·81	0·10 to 2·94
1980–6	5	3·83	1·30	0·42 to 3·04
Total	10	10·42	0·96	0·46 to 1·77

cervix uteri diagnosed outside Cumbria compared with 1·79 expected between 1971 and 1984 at national rates—a ratio of 1·12 (95% confidence interval 0·14 to 4·04). One case was in a 29 year old who had attended Singing Surf School and the other in a 21 year old who had attended the local authority school. Including females in the birth cohort, among whom no cases have been reported, raises the expected number to 2·55—more than the two cases observed.

One further case of cancer, diagnosed as "acute lymphocytic leukaemia" while the patient was resident in Seascale, is known to have occurred among these schoolchildren and was included in the Black report (case 2 of table 2.1[1]). Information from the National Cancer Registration System, however, was not reported to the NHS central register before 1971, and hence we were not notified of this case, which was diagnosed in 1968.

Discussion

This chapter reports a follow up study of children who attended one or more of three schools in Seascale but who were not born there. Because they lived for some period of time in Seascale they will have been part of the population at risk of being included as cases in the earlier geographical studies of cancer incidence mortality. Thus it was important to study the records of these children to get as full a picture of Seascale children as possible. Many of the 1546 children moved into Seascale or the nearby area before the usual age of starting school, whereas the remainder came in at later ages. This large degree of movement into the village matched the large movement out that was found in both this study and that of children born to mothers who were resident in Seascale (see next chapter).

Given the ages at which the excess of leukaemia mainly occurred in the Seascale birth cohort, most children entered the schools cohort after the maximal age of risk had passed among the births cohort as two of the deaths occurred at age 2 years and a third at age 3 years. These are also the most common ages for the diagnosis of childhood leukaemia in Britain.[4] Although in the schools cohort overall the expected number of deaths from leukaemia (0·54) was similar to that in the birth cohort (0·53), no deaths from leukaemia were reported compared with five among the birth cohort. The combined figure is five deaths observed compared with 1·07 expected—a ratio of 4·67 (95% confidence interval 1·52 to 10·90). The apparent limitation of the high leukaemia death rate to children born in Seascale is notable, although the lower 95% confidence limit for the ratio of the rates in the birth cohort to the schools cohort is 0·93. In terms of cases of cancer one case of leukaemia is known among the schoolchildren and diagnosed before 1971 which was the year when the National Cancer Registry first passed on details to the NHS central register. Since then three other cases of cancer have been reported in the follow up of these schoolchildren, which is about one more than the expected number (2·04) of non-fatal cases, plus two cases of carcinoma in situ of the cervix uteri compared with 1·79 expected.

Overall 10 deaths were reported among children in the schools cohort compared with 12·69 expected at national rates—a deficit of about 20%. Apart from the one death from cancer the remaining nine deaths were all certified to "injury and poisoning", which is the largest cause of death nationally for the ages that these children have achieved.

Of some concern in this study is the 93% trace rate of the schoolchildren in the NHS central register. The 7% shortfall may have occurred, for instance, because of inaccuracies in the children's details that were recorded in the three school registers and difficulties in tracing entries in the central register from deficiencies in its construction during the early birth years of this study. It is not known whether these deficiencies, which resulted from parents not applying for welfare foods, come from any specific subgroup of families. For this and other reasons we are continuing to investigate ways of successfully identifying the untraced follow up records.

We thank the registration division of the Office of Population Censuses and Surveys, the former headmistresses of Singing Surf and Calder Girls Schools, the Cumbrian County Council education department, and the headmaster of Seascale School for their cooperation in identifying records on children included in the study. We also thank the National Health Service central register for providing follow up details and many staff of the Medical Research Council environmental epidemiology unit who have helped in various ways, particularly Dr Michael Snee for valuable advice, Mr Paul Barnard for the computer analyses, and Miss Brigid Grimes for preparing the manuscript. Professor M Bobrow, Dr V Beral, and Dr P G Smith kindly commented on an earlier version of the paper. The study was approved by the British Medical Association ethical committee and the west Cumbrian ethics of research committee and was supported partially by a grant from the Department of Health and Social Security.

1 Black D for the Independent Advisory Group. *Investigation of the possible increased incidence of cancer in west Cumbria.* London: HMSO, 1984.
2 World Health Organisation. *International classification of diseases, ninth revision.* Geneva: WHO, 1977.
3 Office of Population Censuses and Surveys. *Cancer statistics, registrations, 1971–83, England and Wales.* London: HMSO, 1979–86. (Series MB1, Nos 1, 2, 4, 5, 7, 8, 10–15.)
4 Draper GJ, Birch JM, Bithell JF, *et al. Childhood cancer in Britain: incidence, survival and mortality.* London: HMSO, 1982. (Office of Population Censuses and Surveys, Studies on Medical and Population Subjects, No 37.)

11: Follow up study of children born to mothers resident in Seascale, west Cumbria (birth cohort)

M J GARDNER, A J HALL, S DOWNES, J D TERRELL

Records on 1068 children who were born to mothers resident in Seascale civil parish during 1950–83 were studied. There was a large degree of mobility among the families, and nearly half of the children did not subsequently attend the main local school. Use of the National Health Service central register, however, enabled us to follow up the children's records regardless of place of residence. The excess of leukaemia among Seascale children first supported from the analysis of geographical areas is confirmed. There were five deaths from leukaemia identified to 30 June 1986 compared with 0·53 expected at national rates—a ratio of 9·36 (95% confidence interval 3·04 to 21·84). One of these deaths occurred after the child had left Seascale. There were four deaths from other cancers compared with 1·06 expected—a ratio of 3·76 (95% confidence interval 1·02 to 9·63). In addition, three further cases of cancer, apart from the deaths, were reported compared with 1·19 expected since 1971—a ratio of 2·53 (95% confidence interval 0·52 to 7·40). For other causes of death, including stillbirths and infant mortality, there was a reported deficit compared with national rates, some of which at least was to be expected on the basis of the social class composition of the population of Seascale.

In view of the importance of this cohort of births, continued follow up is planned (with the possibility of extending it to include births since 1983) and the methods available for this type of study will be examined further.

Introduction

In November 1983 a Yorkshire Television programme (*Windscale: the Nuclear Laundry*) suggested that there was an excess incidence of childhood leukaemia in the village of Seascale, which is close to the Sellafield nuclear fuel reprocessing site on the coast of Cumbria. The results of various studies supported this observation and led to the Black inquiry recommending further epidemiological investigations.[1]

Part of the rationale behind the recommendations was that studies of mortality or incidence of disease on a geographical basis suffer from two potential weaknesses. Firstly, they rely on population figures from decennial censuses for the denominators used in the calculation of area rates, whereas the deaths or cases of cancer that form the numerator typically are those that occur in the area over several years before and after a census. Thus no account can be taken of variations in population size from births, deaths, and migrations that will have taken place during these years. Secondly, any deaths or cases of cancer among children who live for some period of time in an area that occur after they have left will not be included in the numerator of the local rate. Such features are of special concern in an area like Seascale where the population, employed largely at Sellafield, is reported to be particularly mobile.[1]

Among four recommendations in the Black report for further epidemiological studies, the second was that "a study should be carried out of the records on all children born since 1950 to mothers resident in Seascale at the time of birth." This chapter reports the methodology and the findings on mortality and cancer of this follow up study.

Methods

Information on each birth registered since 1 January 1950 to a mother whose residential address in her child's birth entry mentioned "Seascale" was abstracted by the registration division of the Office of Population Censuses and Surveys. This required an extensive clerical search through microfilm records of births in several registration districts to the end of 1983, which was the latest possible date at the time of searching. In an attempt to ensure the inclusion of all hospital as well as home births the search included other areas in addition to the main local registration district of Whitehaven. Table I lists the districts in which it was considered possible that births to mothers who were resident in Seascale might have

TABLE I—*Registration districts for which the Office of Population Censuses and Surveys microfilm records were searched to identify births to mothers who were resident in Seascale by calendar period and numbers included in the study*

Calendar period	Registration district	No in birth cohort*
January 1950–March 1974	Alston	0
	Barrow-in-Furness	2
	Border	0
	Carlisle	39
	Cockermouth†	24
	Millom	0
	Penrith	0
	Whitehaven	808
	Wigton	0
April 1974–December 1983	Appleby	0
	Barrow-in-Furness	0
	Carlisle	0
	Cockermouth†	0
	Kendal	0
	Millom	0
	Penrith	0
	Ulverston	0
	Whitehaven	191
	Wigton	0

* Other potential members of the Seascale birth cohort were found but then eliminated as mentioned in the text (see also table II). Four "transferable" births (see text) were identified as registered outside the districts in the table—three in the Liverpool area and one in Northumberland.
† Cockermouth registration district included Workington and Maryport.

taken place and for which registers were searched before and after local authority boundary reorganisation during 1974. The home addresses given in the birth entries were examined against maps of and lists of addresses inside Seascale civil parish. Only births where the mother's residential address was inside the civil parish boundary, as opposed to having Seascale as a descriptive postal address, were included.

A search was also made in the register of births held locally by the West Cumbria District Health Authority at Flatt Walks Clinic and the West Cumberland Hospital in Whitehaven for immunisation and child welfare purposes. This register contains less identifying information on each child so that, for example, forenames were not always recorded, but details on any possible Seascale births found in this way were abstracted. The two differently obtained sets of births were then checked by computer against each other using the recorded information on surname and date of birth. For children on the west Cumbria list who were not on the Office of Population Censuses and Surveys list a further search was made in the Office of Population Censuses and Surveys microfilm records at the appropriate date, and information on birth entries was abstracted where found.

For all eligible births thus identified details were sent to the National Health Service central register in Southport with a request for vital status data, including information on deaths, cancer registrations, and emigrations. In addition, we were notified by the NHS central register of all family practitioner committee areas in which the children had been recorded since birth as registered with general practitioners and dates, which allowed estimates to be made of durations of residence in Cumbria. This information was supplemented both by a search for the parents' names in the annual Seascale electoral registers (the electoral ward and civil parish boundaries are the same) and by information from the Seascale local authority school register about attendance and dates to obtain estimates of length of residence in Seascale for each child. The West Cumbria District Health Authority register was also searched for recorded information on deaths or cases of cancer among the Seascale births. None of the children or their parents have been approached personally for information.

In this chapter mortality up to 30 June 1986 among the children identified as born to mothers who were resident in Seascale is analysed and compared with that expected at national rates. Some of the follow up information and deaths in the study are of people who have passed childhood, such as those born before 1970, but the term children is used throughout the chapter to refer to the members of the birth cohort. The person years method of analysis was used, incorporating calendar period, cause, sex, and age specific death rates for England and Wales. Confidence intervals were calculated using standard methods based on the Poisson distribution.

Results

SEASCALE BIRTH COHORT

Table II gives details of how the "Seascale birth cohort" was assmbled. The original Office of Population Censuses and Surveys search identified 1202 birth entries with Seascale home addresses, of which 211 were later found to be outside the civil parish boundary and one a duplicate birth registration (a reregistration after the subsequent marriage of the child's parents).

Among the 1056 Seascale births found in the west Cumbria register 92 did not apparently match with any from the 1202 children identified by the Office of Population Censuses and Surveys using the information available. Of these 92 births, five children with addresses outside Seascale civil parish were excluded. A second search was made at the Office of Population Censuses and Surveys for the remaining 87, during which 80 birth entries were identified; three could not be traced and four were found to be

TABLE II—*Births identified during 1950–83 to mothers who were resident in Seascale by source of information*

Source of identification and outcome		No
First OPCS birth register search (n = 1202):		
Included in birth cohort		990
Address outside Seascale civil parish	211	
Duplicate registration	1	
First west Cumbria register search:		
Possible "Seascale" births not found at OPCS (n = 92):		
Address outside Seascale civil parish	5	
Birth entry found at second OPCS search	80	
Included in birth cohort		61
Address outside Seascale civil parish	16	
Duplicate entry (among original 1202):	3	
No trace at OPCS	3	
Stillbirths (no live birth entry)	4*	
"Transferable" births (n = 22)		
Birth entry found at second OPCS search:	18	
Included in birth cohort		16
Address outside Seascale civil parish	2	
Born in Scotland	4	
Second west Cumbria register search:		
Included in birth cohort		1
Total included in birth cohort (relevant livebirths)		1068

OPCS = Office of Population Censuses and Surveys.
* A further five stillbirths were identified both by OPCS and in the west Cumbria register.

stillbirths (stillbirth entries are kept on separate microfilms). Among the 80 birth entries traced three were duplicates of births found in the original Office of Population Censuses and Surveys search for which the matching had not been clear previously, 16 had addresses outside Seascale civil parish, and 61 were extra births to be included in the study. In addition to the four stillbirths mentioned above, searches at the Office of Population Censuses and Surveys and at west Cumbria each identified five further stillbirths during 1950–83.

In addition to entries for births that took place locally, the West Cumbria District Health Authority register has a separate section with details of births registered outside the area which are subsequently "transferred in" and recorded for, for instance, health visiting and immunisation. Details of a further 22 potential Seascale births were abstracted from this section and sent to the Office of Population Censuses and Surveys for further searching. Consequently, four were found to have been born in Scotland and two others had addresses outside Seascale civil parish. Thus 16 more births were added to the birth cohort.

Subsequently, during a search in the west Cumbria register for deaths among children born to Seascale mothers a further eligible birth was identified and included in the study. Thus the count of live births from 1950 to 1983 to mothers with a residential address in Seascale civil parish was $990 + 61 + 16 + 1 = 1068$ births. The distribution of registration districts in which the birth entries were found (table I) shows that the Office of Population Censuses and Surveys search covered a wider area than that in which most Seascale births were actually registered. In fact since 1971 all entries were in Whitehaven following the wide use of the maternity unit opened during 1964 at the West Cumberland Hospital. Including the nine stillbirths the final total in the Seascale birth cohort is 1077 births.

Table III gives the numbers of live births and stillbirths to mothers who were resident in Seascale by calendar year from 1950 to 1983. The numbers of live births by year differ slightly from those given in figure 2.1 of the Black report, which was based on an earlier search of the West Cumbria District Health Authority register.[1] The annual number averaged about 30 over the period, with a peak in the early 1960s and somewhat lower numbers since the middle 1970s. This time trend is similar to figures for births in England and Wales overall, although the recent decrease in Seascale is more pronounced. The ratio of male to female births during the 34 year period was 1·07, similar to the national ratio of 1·06 during these years, with no evidence of any time trend.

The nine stillbirths occurred mainly in the earlier years, as would be expected from national trends in stillbirth rates, which declined from roughly 25 per 1000 births in the early 1950s to about six per 1000 births in the early 1980s. Overall the stillbirth rate—9 of 1077 or 8·4 per 1000 births—is low compared with the period average of 15 per 1000 for England and Wales. The trend, however, in stillbirth mortality according to social class—for example, from 8·8 per 1000 births in social class I to 17·5 per 1000 births in social class V during 1970–2[2]—may partly explain the low rate among the births in the village, most of whose population worked at Sellafield. The percentages of the economically active male population in Seascale in social class I in recent censuses were far higher than national figures—that is, 43% in Seascale for 1961 compared with 4% nationally, 47% for 1971 compared with 5%, and 28% for 1981 compared with 6% (Office of Population Censuses and Surveys, unpublished data). These differences for social class I are extreme, but the general distribution by social class is indicated, for example, in the 1981 census where the percentages were: social class I (professional occupations) 28% in Seascale, 6% in England and Wales; social class II (intermediate) 13%, 22%; social class III (skilled) 42%, 46%; social class IV (partly skilled) 14%, 16%; social class V (unskilled) 0%, 6%; and "unclassified" 3%, 5%.

DURATION OF RESIDENCE IN SEASCALE AND CUMBRIA

In the three different ways outlined earlier, table IV gives figures on

TABLE III—*Live births by sex and stillbirths during 1950–83 to mothers who were resident in Seascale civil parish*

Year of birth	No of live births			Sex ratio M/F	Stillbirths
	Males	Females	Total		
1950	12	15	27	0·80	1
1951	10	15	25	0·67	2
1952	18	22	40	0·82	1
1953	27	19	46	1·42	
1954	20	18	38	1·11	1
1955	13	14	27	0·93	1
1956	14	21	35	0·67	
1957	19	24	43	0·79	
1958	25	16	41	1·56	1
1959	20	16	36	1·25	
1960	25	21	46	1·19	
1961	25	18	43	1·39	
1962	21	15	36	1·40	
1963	32	21	53	1·52	
1964	21	23	44	0·91	1
1965	17	23	40	1·74	
1966	24	10	34	2·40	
1967	14	12	26	1·17	
1968	15	15	30	1·00	
1969	22	17	39	1·29	
1970	16	14	30	1·14	
1971	16	21	37	0·76	
1972	11	13	24	0·85	1
1973	12	15	27	0·80	
1974	12	10	22	1·20	
1975	9	11	20	0·82	
1976	7	15	22	0·47	
1977	7	6	13	1·17	
1978	8	16	24	0·50	
1979	8	2	10	4·00	
1980	9	11	20	0·82	
1981	15	6	21	2·50	
1982	18	14	32	1·29	
1983	10	7	17	1·43	
1950–83	552	516	1068	1·07	9

rough length of residence in Seascale and Cumbria for the 1068 live births in the birth cohort. Table IV(a) gives the numbers of children who had become pupils at the main school in Seascale by November 1984. (For a description of the Seascale schools see the preceding chapter.) If the final four years 1980–3 are excluded then 556 out of the 978 (57%) children attended the school. The remaining 422 (43%) were not found on the school register and can be presumed to have moved out of Seascale between birth and school age. This percentage varied little over the 30 years. Forty four (4·5%), however, are known to have attended a school for preschool

TABLE IV—*Approximate length of residence in Seascale or Cumbria of children born during 1950–83 to mothers who were resident in Seascale civil parish*

(a) *According to Seascale local authority school register up to November 1984*

| Years of birth | Name on register | | Total |
	No	Yes	
1950–4	84	92	176
1955–9	72	110	182
1960–4	101	121	222
1965–9	60	109	169
1970–4	67	73	140
1975–9	38	51	89
(1980–3)*	(81)	(9)	(90)
1950–83	503	565	1068

* Children born during these years had mainly not reached school age by November 1984.

(b) *According to parents' entry on local Seascale electoral registers from 1950 to 1985*

| Years of birth | Years from birth to parents leaving electoral register | | | | | Parents on 1985 electoral register | Parents not found on electoral register | Total |
	<0	0–4	5–9	10–14	15+			
1950–4	1	80	28	9	20	28	10	176
1955–9	5	64	32	18	16	39	8	182
1960–4	6	94	38	7	11	52	14	222
1965–9	9	59	26	6	3	63	3	169
1970–4	3	65	14	7	—	44	7	140
1975–9	4	37	6	—	—	39	3	89
1980–3	0	24	—	—	—	65	1	90
1950–83	28	423	144	47	50	330	46	1068

(c) *According to registrations with a general practitioner in the Cumbria Family Practitioner Committee (FPC) area up to December 1984*

| Years of birth | Years from birth to non-registration with Cumbria FPC | | | | | Still with Cumbria FPC | Unknown | Total |
	0–4	5–9	10–14	15–19	20+			
1950–4	72	27	6	35	15	17	4	176
1955–9	56	24	7	50	12	31	2	182
1960–4	65	11	12	42	11	77	4	222
1965–9	32	8	3	25	—	100	1	169
1970–4	34	5	5	—	—	94	2	140
1975–9	16	3	—	—	—	70	0	89
1980–3	16	—	—	—	—	74	0	90
1950–83	291	78	33	152	38	463	13	1068

age children in Seascale which was open between 1949 and 1968 (see the preceding chapter).

Table IV(b) gives information about the appearance of parents' names on the Seascale electoral register from before the birth of each child up to 10 October 1984, the qualifying date for the 1985 register. Of the 28 births where the parents' names were not on the succeeding electoral register, 23 took place within one year of the date of their qualification for the previous register. Omitting the years 1980–3 as before, 427 out of 933 (46%) identified names had been taken off the electoral register shortly preceding or within five years after the birth. This percentage is comparable to the 43% of children who did not attend the local school. Indeed there is a large overlap between the names of these 427 parents and of the 422 children not on the school register, 360 (85%) of the latter being included in the former, as would be expected and as is suggested by the relevant numbers for the separate quinquennial birth groups in tables IV(a) and (b). Of the 1068 children, 46 parents' names (4%) were not found on the electoral registers, and 330 (31%) were still on in 1985. More and more parents' names were taken off the electoral register over the years since the births, suggesting a continued movement of the children out of Seascale. Among the children who had reached their 15th birthday by the last electoral register examined—that is, born before 1970—532 out of 714 (75%) identified parents were no longer registered. Although such information cannot be equated exactly with children moving out of Seascale, especially at older ages, it is a reasonably good indicator.

Table IV(c) gives the number and duration of registrations of the children with general practitioners in the Cumbria Family Practitioner Committee area, as reported by the NHS central register up to December 1984. This information is less precise than that in tables IV(a) and (b) in relation to residence in Seascale as a change in family practitioner committee registration indicates only a movement out of Cumbria rather than from Seascale. At the end of 1984, excluding the 13 children for whom no family practitioner committee registration was reported, 592 out of 1055 (56%) children had apparently left Cumbria. As might be expected, there was a large increase in non-Cumbria family practitioner committee registrations during the period 15–19 years after birth, corresponding to the children reaching school leaving age. That this movement is largely independent of their parents is indicated by the lack of any similar rise in numbers during these same years in table IV(b).

The general tendency shown in the three parts of table IV concurs with the suggestion of a mobile population in Seascale. Some 40% of children born in Seascale did not stay to attend the local school, a similar percentage of parents came off the electoral register within five years of their child's birth, and over half the children had moved out of Cumbria by the end of 1984.

TABLE V—*Numbers of deaths by cause to 30 June 1986 among children born during 1950–83 to mothers who were resident in Seascale civil parish compared with deaths expected at national rates*

| Cause of death* | No of deaths | | | 95% Confidence interval for O/E |
	Observed (O)	Expected (E)	O/E	
Malignant neoplasms (140–208):	9	1·60	5·63	2·58 to 10·69
Non-Hodgkin's lymphoma (200, 202)	1	0·12	8·45	0·21 to 47·10
Hodgkin's disease (201)	0	0·07	0	0 to 53·71
Leukaemia (204–208)	5	0·53	9·36	3·04 to 21·84
Other cancers	3	0·88	3·42	0·71 to 10·00
Other causes	18	30·70	0·59	0·35 to 0·93
All causes	27	32·30	0·84	0·55 to 1·22

* Figures in parentheses are code numbers in the International Classification of Diseases (9th revision).[3]

MORTALITY AND CANCER FOLLOW UP

Because of the availability of NHS numbers from the birth entries the NHS central register traced all the children's records. Among the 1068 live births in the Seascale birth cohort, 27 deaths and 43 emigrations were reported to us, and the remaining 998 children were thought to be alive.

Table V gives the numbers of deaths by cause among the cohort and the numbers expected according to death rates for England and Wales. As expected from earlier reports[45] there is an excess mortality from leukaemia—five deaths compared with 0·53 expected. Four of these were known to the Black inquiry (cases 3, 4, 5, and 6 of table 2.1[1]), and the fifth was a death from leukaemia that occurred after the child had left Seascale. She was born in 1950, died at age 3 years in 1954, and death was certified as due to "subacute lymphatic leukaemia." She had lived in Seascale to the age of about 3 years according to the electoral registers and family practitioner committee registrations. This is the only death from leukaemia or lymphoma reported among children born in Seascale in addition to those known to the Black inquiry, as the one death from the latter cause, in a child after moving away from Seascale, was listed (case 14 of table 2.3[1]). The other three deaths from cancer, compared with 0·88 expected, include one known previously—certified as "retroperitoneal sarcoma" (case 26 of table 2.4[1])—and two occurring after the children had left Seascale. One of these was certified as "metastatic squamous carcinoma of the tongue" in a 28 year old man, and the other as a "Wilms's tumour of the left kidney" in a girl aged 4.

In contrast with the excess of deaths from cancer in the birth cohort there is a deficit against national figures of some 40% for deaths from other causes—18 compared with 30·70 expected. Table VI shows that this relates

TABLE VI—*Numbers of deaths by age and sex to 30 June 1986 among children born during 1950–83 to mothers who were resident in Seascale civil parish compared with deaths expected at national rates*

Category	No of deaths			95% Confidence interval for O/E
	Observed (O)	Expected (E)	O/E	
Age (years):				
Under 1	12	21·53	0·56	0·29 to 0·97
1–4	6	3·20	1·88	0·69 to 4·09
5–9	1	1·55	0·64	0·02 to 3·59
10–14	0	1·14	0	0 to 3·23
15–19	3	2·04	1·47	0·30 to 4·31
20–24	2	1·53	1·31	0·16 to 4·74
25–29	2	0·87	2·30	0·28 to 8·32
30+	1	0·45	2·24	0·06 to 12·49
Sex:				
Male	15	19·33	0·78	0·43 to 1·28
Female	12	12·97	0·93	0·48 to 1·62
Calendar year of follow up:				
1950–4	3	4·78	0·63	0·13 to 1·83
1955–9	7	4·93	1·42	0·57 to 2·92
1960–4	3	5·94	0·51	0·10 to 1·48
1965–9	3	4·72	0·64	0·13 to 1·86
1970–4	3	4·37	0·69	0·14 to 2·01
1975–9	4	3·38	1·18	0·32 to 3·03
1980–6	4	4·18	0·96	0·26 to 2·45
Calendar year of birth:				
1950–4	8	8·12	0·99	0·43 to 1·94
1955–9	9	6·81	1·32	0·60 to 2·51
1960–4	5	7·22	0·69	0·23 to 1·62
1965–9	4	4·45	0·90	0·25 to 2·30
1970–4	1	3·04	0·33	0·01 to 1·84
1975–9	0	1·49	0	0 to 2·48
1980–3	0	1·17	0	0 to 3·16
Total	27	32·30	0·84	0·55 to 1·22

particularly to infant deaths under 1 year of age—12 deaths were reported compared with 21·53 expected. During the period of this study infant mortality in England and Wales fell from about 30 per 1000 live births around 1950 to about 10 per 1000 live births in the early 1980s, whereas in this birth cohort it was near 11 per 1000 live births. Of these 12 deaths, eight only were originally notified from the NHS central register. Because of this apparently small number a thorough search was made through the West Cumbria District Health Authority register where an additional four deaths before the mid-1960s were identified. There was a potential problem with the recording of deaths in the central register owing to the fact that before 1 April 1969 only age at death, not the date of birth, was reported to the central register, which led to difficulties in linkage in the register, particularly for common names and for births during the period 1952–63 when there was a deficiency of about 15% in their alphabetical index. The ages of the infant deaths, however, show a similar distribution to the national figures for this period—five of the 12 were on the day of birth and four more within the first week of life, which does not suggest that early deaths may be particularly vulnerable to omission.

Infant mortality in the birth cohort fell during the study, with seven infant deaths out of 358 births during the 1950s, five out of 391 births during the 1960s, and none out of the succeeding 319 births. Again, as for stillbirths, the social class composition of Seascale and the trend in infant mortality—for example, from 12 per 1000 live births in social class I to 31 per 1000 live births in social class V during 1970–2[2]—may partly explain the low rate. There is no suggestion that rates are low in general in the locality. Thus for a comparable period of years, 1969–73, infant mortality in the combined rural districts of Cumberland at 20 per 1000 live births was slightly greater than that of 18 per 1000 live births in England and Wales.[6]

Table VI shows that at ages over 1 year there is an excess mortality of 15 observed compared with 10·77 expected (ratio of observed to expected (O/E) = 1·39, 95% confidence interval 0·78 to 2·30) due entirely to the excess of cancer deaths (nine observed, 1·53 expected) particularly leukaemia (five observed, 0·51 expected). The six non-cancer deaths (compared with 9·24 expected) in children over 1 year of age were recorded as being from different causes, including acute pyelitis, congenital heart disease, suicide, bronchopneumonia, myocardial infarction, and a traffic accident.

Also, there is no notable difference between the death rates of boys and girls born in Seascale, nor any suggestion of a time trend by calendar year of follow up. On the other hand, there is an apparent decline in mortality relative to that expected for children born in successive five year periods, which largely reflects the fall in stillbirth and infant mortality discussed earlier. Death rates for young persons in Cumberland, other than infants, are slightly lower than in England and Wales overall, but incorporating an adjustment for this into the expected numbers has no real effect on the interpretation of results in this chapter.

In addition to the nine deaths from cancer in table V three further cases of cancer were notified from the NHS central register. Two of these patients, who lived in Seascale at diagnosis, were included in the Black report (case 7 of table 2.1[1] diagnosed as "acute lymphoblastic leukaemia" and case 17 of table 2.3[1] diagnosed as "non-Hodgkin's lymphoma"). A third case was in a man diagnosed as having a "malignant melanoma" at 28 years of age after having moved away from Seascale.

Table VII gives mortality findings in relation to estimated residence in

TABLE VII—*Number of deaths* by cause to 30 June 1986 among children born during 1950–83 to mothers who were resident in Seascale civil parish compared with deaths expected at national rates by rough length of residence in (a) Seascale or (b) Cumbria*

(a) *According to parents' entry on local Seascale electoral registers from 1950 to 1985*

Cause of death	During parents' residence in Seascale†	No of deaths			95% Confidence interval for O/E
		Observed (O)	Expected (E)	O/E	
Leukaemia	Yes	4	0·24	16·52	4·50 to 42·28
	No	1	0·27	3·75	0·10 to 20·88
Other malignant neoplasms	Yes	1	0·40	2·53	0·06 to 14·07
	No	3	0·62	4·88	1·01 to 14·26
Other causes	Yes	11	22·88	0·48	0·24 to 0·86
	No	5	6·41	0·78	0·25 to 1·82
All causes	Yes	16	23·52	0·68	0·39 to 1·11
	No	9	7·23	1·23	0·56 to 2·34

(b) *According to registrations with a general practitioner in the Cumbria Family Practitioner Committee area up to December 1984*

Cause of death	During Cumbria GP registration‡	No of deaths			95% Confidence interval for O/E
		Observed (O)	Expected (E)	O/E	
Leukaemia	Yes	3	0·32	9·35	1·93 to 27·31
	No	2	0·21	9·57	1·16 to 34·56
Other malignant neoplasms	Yes	2	0·50	4·01	0·49 to 14·48
	No	2	0·56	3·60	0·44 to 12·99
Other causes	Yes	13	25·47	0·51	0·27 to 0·87
	No	5	5·01	1·00	0·32 to 2·33
All causes	Yes	18	26·29	0·69	0·41 to 1·08
	No	9	5·77	1·56	0·71 to 2·96

* Children were excluded from this table if their data on Seascale electoral registers or general practitioner registrations were unknown.
† Person years of follow up during parents' Seascale residence: yes 8711; no 11750.
‡ Person years of follow up during Cumbria registration with general practitioner: yes, 11898; no 9396.

Seascale or Cumbria. In table VII(a) figures are given for observed and expected deaths by cause both during and outside periods when the children's parents were on the Seascale electoral register (see table VI(b)). The observed/expected ratios are greater than unity for leukaemia and for other cancers both during and after Seascale "residence"; although two of the ratios are each based on one death, the other two are statistically significant. In table VII(b) similar information is presented for periods during and after the children's registration with a general practitioner in

Cumbria (see table IV(c)). As would be anticipated the expected numbers of deaths in association with Cumbrian Family Practitioner Committee registrations are larger than those associated with presence on the Seascale electoral register. In this analysis similarly high observed/expected ratios are found for both leukaemia and other cancers in each "residence" category. One of the four deaths from leukaemia where the parents were still on the electoral register in Seascale was of a child whose general practitioner registration had been changed to outside Cumbria. The low level of mortality from other causes during Seascale/Cumbria "residence" shown in tables VII(a) and (b) respectively is largely associated with the low rate of infant deaths described earlier, but it is noticeable in both sections of table VII that overall mortality is higher outside than during Seascale/Cumbria "residence".

Discussion

One of the important purposes of this study was to investigate further the findings of the earlier geographical analyses of the incidence of cancer among young people in Seascale where the main observation had been an excess of leukaemia. We have corroborated that result in reporting five deaths from leukaemia among children born during 1950–83 to mothers who were resident in Seascale compared with 0·53 expected from death rates in England and Wales. Thus by approaching the estimation of the local rate by another method we found a similar estimated level to that originally suggested—that is, about 10-fold higher than expected from national rates. The previous figure of 10-fold referred to children under the age of 10 years,[1] whereas this study reported on births followed up to the ages reached by 30 June 1986. Examination of leukaemia deaths up to age 10 years only in this study, however, produces a similar outcome of four observed compared with 0·32 expected. During the years 1959 to 1978, for which mortality data for the county of Cumberland as a whole are available, the leukaemia death rate was 12% lower than in England and Wales at ages 0–24 years.[7] Using the county figures rather than the national figures for comparison for the Seascale children would raise the observed/expected ratio in table V from 9·36 to 10·59 (95% confidence interval 3·46 to 24·91). We know, however, that a sizable number of the children spent many of the years between 0 and 24 years of age outside Cumbria (table IV(c)). Also these figures exclude the results on Seascale schoolchildren given in the preceding chapter.

There is some evidence that childhood leukaemia rates are highest in social class I and show a declining trend to social classes IV and V.[89] For example, in figures for children aged 0–14 years in England and Wales during 1959–63 the annual leukaemia mortality rates varied from 44 per million in social class I to 37 per million in social class V, with the lowest rate of 31 per million in social class IV.[8] On the other hand, in a report on childhood leukaemia up to the age of 15 years in north west England (which includes Cumbria) during 1954–77 Birch and her colleagues reported that the social class distribution of the cases "did not differ from the population as a whole."[10] It thus seems unlikely that social class factors are sufficient to explain the raised level of leukaemia among the Seascale birth cohort. Clearly there was a lot of movement out of Seascale, as shown in table IV, whether measured by school attendance or by registration on the Seascale electoral roll or with the Cumbria Family Practitioner Committee. By taking account of the mobility of the local population, which caused concern about the use of census figures for calculating death rates, the excess has been confirmed. This finding must remove any doubt that there had previously been an artefact due to the possible underestimation of the appropriate population at risk.

Of the five deaths from leukaemia, four occurred while the children were still resident in Seascale and the other one after the child left the area. The first four deaths were expected to be found in this study as the children were previously known to have been born and had their leukaemia diagnosed in Seascale.[1] If they had not been identified, both in the searches of the Office of Population Censuses and Surveys and west Cumbria birth registers and in the NHS Central Register follow up, this would have cast doubts on the procedures used here. These four and other relevant cases of cancer listed in the Black report, however, were all reported from the central register, the only exception being for case 25 of table 2.4,[1] which is incorrectly given there as born in "Seascale" rather than "Other Millom rural district.' The one death from leukaemia after the child moved from Seascale was reported in a girl aged 3 years who was one of the earliest births in the study. She would have lived some 3 years in Seascale during the early period of operation of the Sellafield site.

As well as the excess of leukaemia deaths in the Seascale birth cohort there is an increase of deaths from other cancers, though also based on small numbers. Compared with an expected number of deaths on national rates of 1·06 there have been four deaths reported, a ratio of 3·76 (95% confidence interval 1·02 to 9·63). These are from various cancers as identified earlier, but include one case of non-Hodgkin's lymphoma. Three of these deaths occurred after the children left Seascale.

For other causes of death there has been a deficit in the reported mortality rates among the Seascale birth cohort related particularly to infant mortality. Extensive searches were made in available records to assess whether this deficit was due to missing deaths that should have been reported. Four infant deaths not identified in the NHS central register were found in the west Cumbria register, and all took place before April 1969 when it was not possible to link successfully all deaths into the central register owing to the insufficient detail supplied. The rate of stillbirths reported is of a similar apparently low level compared with national figures. All nine stillbirths, however, were found independently in both the Office of Population Censuses and Surveys and the west Cumbria registers. The special social class composition of the Seascale population may have contributed importantly to the low rates for stillbirths and infant mortality.

For cancer registrations, rather than deaths, three were reported to us from the NHS central register. The coverage is, however, limited to the years since 1971 when the National Cancer Registration system first notified cases to the central register. Thus only 14 years of the follow up period can be included in the present analysis as notification of cancer cases to the central register has not yet been made by all regional registers beyond 1984. Using published annual figures for cancer registration by age and sex[11] and subtracting the number of expected deaths during the same period, we calculated that 1·19 non-fatal cancers would be expected among the birth cohort from 1971 to 1984 (observed/expected = 2·53, 95% confidence interval 0·52 to 7·40). Although this is a rough calculation, as cancer deaths and registrations occurring in a defined calendar period do not refer to exactly the same cases, it does indicate also a relative, though not statistically significant, excess of living cases of cancer. The case-control study of childhood cancers in west Cumbria that we are carrying out is aimed at obtaining pertinent information on cases in this analysis and on cases diagnosed in other areas of west Cumbria.

The "flagging" of the 1068 birth records in the central register for this study means that follow up can be continued beyond the current date of reporting. In addition, it is possible to include births that have taken place from 1984 onwards to examine the records of children born recently, which is particularly appropriate for childhood leukaemia as most cases are diagnosed in children under 5 years. We will also examine solutions to the difficulties caused in this study and others like it by the lack of complete linkage of birth, death, cancer registration, and other records in the NHS central register. This includes, for example, investigating linkage of the records on children in this study into the national records held by the Childhood Cancer Research Group (G J Draper, personal communication).

We thank the registration division of the Office of Population Censuses and Surveys, the Cumbria County Council education department, and the headmaster of Seascale School for their cooperation in identifying records on children included in this study. We also thank various people at the West Cumberland Hospital and Flatt Walks Clinic in Whitehaven for their help and the National Health Service central register for providing follow up details. Many staff of the Medical Research Council Environmental Epidemiology Unit have helped, particularly Dr Michael Snee, who gave valuable advice; Mr Paul Barnard, who performed the computer analyses; and Miss Brigid Grimes, who prepared the manuscript. Professor M Bobrow, Dr V Beral, and Dr P G Smith kindly commented on an earlier version of the chapter. The study was approved by the British Medical Association Ethical Committee and the West Cumbrian Ethics of Reseearch Committee and was supported partially by a grant from the Department of Health and Social Security.

1 Black D for the Independent Advisory Group. *Investigation of the possible increased incidence of cancer in west Cumbria.* London: HMSO, 1984.
2 Office of Population Censuses and Surveys. *Occupational mortality, decennial supplement, 1970–72, England and Wales.* London: HMSO, 1978. (Series DS, No 1.)
3 World Health Organisation. *International classification of diseases, ninth revision.* Geneva: WHO, 1977.
4 Urquhart J, Palmer M, Cutler J. Cancer in Cumbria: the Windscale connection. *Lancet* 1984;**i**:217–8.
5 Craft AW, Openshaw S, Birch J. Apparent clusters of childhood lymphoid malignancy in northern England. *Lancet* 1984;**ii**:96–7.
6 Office of Population Censuses and Surveys. *Area mortality, decennial supplement, 1969–73, England and Wales.* London, HMSO, 1981. (Series DS, No 4.)
7 Gardner MJ, Winter PD. Mortality in Cumberland during 1959–78 with reference to cancer in young people around Windscale. *Lancet* 1984;**i**:216–7.
8 Adelstein AM, White GC. Causes of children's deaths analysed by social class. In: *Child health—a collection of studies.* London: HMSO, 1976:23–40. (Office of Population Censuses and Surveys, Studies on Medical and Population Subjects, No 31.)
9 Sanders BM, White GC, Draper GJ. Occupations of fathers of children dying from neoplasms. *J Epidemiol Community Health* 1981;**35**:245–50.
10 Birch JM, Swindell R, Marsden HB, Jones PHM. Childhood leukaemia in north west England 1954–1977: epidemiology, incidence and survival. *Br J Cancer* 1981;**43**:324–9.
11 Office of Population Censuses and Surveys. *Cancer statistics, registrations, 1971–83, England and Wales.* London: HMSO, 1979–86. (Series MB1, Nos 1, 2, 4, 5, 7, 8, 10–15.)

12: Cancer near nuclear installations

DAVID FORMAN, PAULA COOK-MOZAFFARI,
SARAH DARBY, GWYNETH DAVEY, IRENE
STRATTON, RICHARD DOLL, MALCOLM PIKE

There has been no general increase in cancer mortality near nuclear installations in England and Wales during the period 1959–80. Leukaemia in young people may be an exception, though the reason remains unclear.

The Office of Population Censuses and Surveys (OPCS) has recently published a report *"Cancer Incidence and Mortality in the Vicinity of Nuclear Installations England and Wales, 1959–80"*.[1] The report is very detailed and difficult to assimilate. We have, therefore, summarised here what we believe to be the principal results and the main conclusions that can be drawn from them.

The OPCS report

The installations included in the report are shown in table I. All pre-1974 local authority areas with at least one third of their population living within 10 miles of any of these installations were included in the analysis. The report provided standardised mortality and registration ratios (SMRs and SRRs) for 25 specific and combined cancer sites for groups of these local authority areas around each installation using appropriate regional rates (age, sex, and year specific rates for the standard region,[2] excluding conurbations, in which the installation was situated) for standardisation. These standard mortality ratios and standardised registration ratios were presented for both sexes combined and essentially for three discrete age groups: 0–24, 25–74, and 75+ years, although the information was also made available for the age group 0–9 years. The report also compared the

TABLE I—*Nuclear installations and summary groupings*

Installation	Summary grouping	Date of first criticality or waste release*
BNFL Sellafield	—	1950
BNFL Springfields		1948
BNFL Capenhurst		1953
Amersham International plc	Pre-1955 (excluding Sellafield)	1946
MoD Aldermaston		1952
UKAEA Harwell		1947
UKAEA Winfrith	—	1964
CEGB Bradwell		1961
Berkeley and Oldbury		1961
Hinkley		1964
Trawsfynydd	CEGB	1964
Dungeness		1965
Sizewell		1965
Wylfa		1971

BNFL = British Nuclear Fuels Ltd; MoD = Ministry of Defence; UKAEA = United Kingdom Atomic Energy Authority; CEGB = Central Electricity Generating Board.
* Referred to as "start up" date in the text.

trends in standardised mortality ratios and standardised registration ratios both over time and with increasing proximity to the installations.

In addition, comparisons were made between the standardised mortality ratios and standardised registration ratios of the grouped local authority areas around each installation and the standardised mortality ratios and standardised registration ratios of groups of control areas. Each group of control local authority areas was constructed by matching each installation area with a non-installation area, selected, where possible, to be in the same standard region[2] and have a similar urban–rural status and population size as its comparison area. For local authority areas that were county boroughs, control selection was also based on comparable social class structure when there was a choice within the above constraints. The rates for the same standard region were used for calculating the standardised mortality ratios and standardised registration ratios for each installation area and for its control.

To focus attention on overall patterns the report provided summed results for the local authority areas in two mutually exclusive combined groups of installations and the respective control areas. These were, firstly, all the installations that started operation before 1955, except Sellafield (the "pre-1955 installations"), and secondly, all the Central Electricity Generating Board (CEGB) installations combined (see table I).

Four distance zones were considered in the report: (1) local authority areas with at least two thirds of their population within six miles of an installation; (2) areas with at least two thirds of their population within eight miles of an installation; (3) areas with at least two thirds of their population within 10 miles of an installation; and (4) areas with at least one third of their population within 10 miles of an installation.

These cumulative zones are referred to as cumulative zones 1, 2, 3, and 4. For some analyses mutually exclusive ("discrete") distance zones were used; these discrete zones were constructed from the cumulative zones by successively excluding inner zones, for example discrete zone 2 = zone 2 minus zone 1, and so on. It should be noted that local authority areas in the vicinity of all installations are not represented in every distance zone. In particular, the innermost distance zone, as defined above, contains no local authority areas that are near to Sellafield, Aldermaston, Berkeley and Oldbury, or Hinkley.

The report provided data for the 22 years 1959–80, a period that commenced several years after the start of operations at Sellafield and at each of the group of pre-1955 installations. The CEGB installations, however, began operations between 1961 and 1971, and Winfrith became operational in 1964. Data for these installations were also available in the report from the year subsequent to start up for some types of cancer.

In addition to the analyses of areas around installations, the report also presented results for a group of coastal local authority areas to the north and south of Sellafield to investigate whether seaborne discharges from Sellafield might be affecting cancer rates. These coastal areas have some overlap with the local authority areas around Sellafield, Springfields, Capenhurst, and Wylfa. Control areas were selected for these coastal areas using the criteria stated above.

Methods

The principal results, in our opinion, are those relating to mortality at ages 0–24 and 25–74 years for combined groupings of installations, categorised by likely environmental impact or similar start up date. Other data are less relevant, for the following three reasons.

Firstly, cancer registration data are of variable quality[1] and the report itself highlighted a number of inconsistencies in the registration information.[14] In particular, the ratio of the number of cancer registrations to the number of cancer deaths was higher in the local authority areas around pre-1955 installations than in the corresponding control areas, which suggests a general registration bias in favour of the installation areas.

Secondly, the mortality results for the 75 year old and over age group are less reliable than those for other ages because diagnostic accuracy on death certificates diminishes with age.[15]

Thirdly, the results for areas around individual installations are based on small numbers and are likely to be less informative than those for groups of similar installations. We have, therefore, mainly used the results for combined installation groupings provided in the report. We have analysed data for local authority areas grouped around the following installation groups.

(i) *The pre-1955 installations excluding Sellafield.* Although the activities carried out in these installations are heterogeneous, the grouping combines all the establishments other than Sellafield which, by 1980, had been operating for more than 25 years and around which any long term effects could most easily be identified.

(ii) *Combined CEGB installations.* All are thought to have a similar impact on their local environment, in terms of their radioactive discharges.[6]

(iii) *Sellafield.* Sellafield first released waste in 1950, but a specific problem had already been identified in relation to it before the OPCS study,[7] and it also needs to be considered separately because the radiobiological impact of the discharges from Sellafield is likely to have been far in excess of that from any other establishment.[7 8]

(iv) *Winfrith.* Winfrith first released waste in 1964, and does not fit into any of the other categories.

(v) *All installations grouped together*, obtained by summing (i) to (iv) above.

We also analysed results for the group of coastal local authority areas to the north and south of that part of mid-Cumbria in which Sellafield is situated. The three areas in mid-Cumbria have been excluded as they are already included in the Sellafield group (group (iii) above), and Liverpool county borough was excluded as it has a very different population density and social class compsition from the remaining coastal local authority areas. The final group consisted of 58 coastal areas.

The 22 "types" of cancer included in the analysis are listed in the box. The standardised mortality ratios given in the report are comparisons with regional standards which make allowance for gross regional and urban–rural variation in cancer rates. However, any remaining difference in the demographic or socioeconomic structure of the local authority areas around an installation compared with that of a region as a whole will result in an effect on the standardised mortality ratio unrelated to the presence of the installation. This type of effect could be expected to be minimised in the comparison between grouped installation local authority areas and grouped control areas, so we have largely restricted attention to such comparisons.

Our approach, therefore, has been to compare death rates in the above installation groupings within each of the four distance zones and in the coastal local authority areas around Sellafield with the rates in their respective control areas. Data for the CEGB installations and Winfrith were considered only subsequent to start up. (In fact, because the OPCS report did not present all the necessary information, it was not possible to divide the data into before and after start up for certain cancer sites. In

---

Sites of cancer, and combined groupings of sites*, which are covered in the OPCS report and are discussed in this chapter

All malignant neoplasms
All leukaemia
   Lymphoid leukaemia†
   Non-lymphoid leukaemia†
     Myeloid leukaemia†
     Monocytic leukaemia†
     Other leukaemia†
     Unspecified leukaemia†
Malignant neoplasm of liver
Malignant neoplasm of lung‡
Malignant neoplasm of bone
Malignant neoplasm of testis
Malignant neoplasm of thyroid
All brain
   Malignant neoplasm of brain
   Benign neoplasms of brain and central nervous system‡
   Unspecified neoplasms of brain and central nervous system‡
All lymphomas
   Hodgkin's disease§
   Other lymphomas§
Multiple myeloma‡
All lymphomas plus leukaemia

---

* Three of the grouped cancer sites examined in the OPCS report (namely, all malignancies minus leukaemia, all malignancies minus leukaemia and lung cancer, and all malignancies minus leukaemia and brain cancer) were included for the sake of completion of specific analyses. We have excluded them from our analyses.
† Information on leukaemia subtypes was only available since 1968.
‡ For these cancer sites, for the age group 0–24 years only, data relating to the grouped CEGB installations have been used since 1966 and not since start up of the installation.
§ For these cancer sites, data relating to the grouped CEGB installations have been used since 1966 and not since start up of the installation for all age groups.

these instances data were used from 1966–80 instead, see box.) The numbers involved in these instances are small and will not affect the overall pattern of occurrence.

For all the 22 types of cancer, the standardised mortality ratios are presented in (or can be calculated from) the OPCS report for each grouping of installation local authority areas that we have considered and for their control areas. We have calculated the ratios of the standardised mortality ratios for the grouped installation areas to the standardised mortality ratios for the grouped control areas and called these ratios "relative risks". For each cumulative distance zone, one sided significance tests have been performed to test the hypothesis that the relative risk for the grouped

85

installation areas is greater (or less) than unity. These tests were performed on the observed numbers of deaths, which we have assumed follow Poisson distributions with means proportional to the number of deaths expected. Tests for trend in the relative risks in the discrete distance zones with increasing proximity to an installation were also carried out using a likelihood ratio test.

Results

All comparisons which lead to the relative risk for the grouped installation local authority areas being significantly greater than unity (one sided, $p < 0.05$) in any of the four cumulative distance zones are shown in table II ("positive" results). Table III corresponds to table II, and shows all comparisons which lead to the relative risk for the grouped installation areas being significantly less than unity ("negative" results). All significant differences between the grouped coastal areas and their control areas, irrespective of whether the relative risks are greater or less than unity, are shown in table IV.

In tables II and III we show all the distance zones in which significant differences are observed between the standardised mortality ratios in the installation and control areas. We also show the observed number of deaths and the standardised mortality ratios for the installation and control local authority areas in the distance zone that shows the most extreme difference in cancer mortality in terms of its statistical significance.

Numerically there are substantially more negative results listed in tables III and IVb than there are positive results listed in tables II and IVa and a greater variety of different cancer types are included in the negative results. In this chapter we are not, however, concerned with the reasons that the risk of death from a number of cancer types is relatively low in the installation areas, except in so far as they help to interpret the opposite findings. We have, therefore, examined further only those types of cancer that had a relatively higher mortality in local authority areas around the installations than in the control areas.

CANCER AT AGES 0–24

Two types of cancer have caused death relatively more often in persons under 25 years of age around some of the installations than in the corresponding control areas: namely, lymphoid leukaemia and all brain tumours. The relative risk for lymphoid leukaemia is significantly raised in cumulative zones 1 and 2 in the local authority areas grouped around the pre-1955 installations. As the populations in the areas around the pre-1955 installations constitute 81% of the entire study population, this results in a significant rise in lymphoid leukaemia, though in zone 1 only, around all

TABLE II—*Comparison of standardised mortality ratios (SMRs) between groupings of installation local authority areas (LAAs) and their controls**

Category of cancer	Installation grouping	Cumulative distance zone† (a)	(b)	Installation LAAs Deaths	SMR	Control LAAs Deaths	SMR	Relative risk‡	p
				People aged 0–24					
Lymphoid leukaemia	Pre-1955 (excl Sellafield)	1	2	42	113·4	20	54·1	2·10	0·004
	All installations	1	—	44	112·1	22	56·1	2·00	0·005
All brain	Sellafield	2	—	5	144·6	0	0·0	∞	0·033
				People aged 25–74					
Liver	All CEGB	2	3, 4	29	189·0	10	62·4	3·03	0·001
	Winfrith	4	—	16	127·0	6	52·0	2·44	0·043
	All installations	4	2, 3	395	100·0	313	81·3	1·23	0·004
Lung	All CEGB	4	3	2 956	95·0	3 134	90·3	1·05	0·025
Hodgkin's disease	Pre-1955 (excl Sellafield)	1	2, 3, 4	141	95·9	104	70·7	1·36	0·011
	All installations	1	2, 3	149	96·7	112	72·4	1·34	0·010
All lymphomas	Pre-1955 (excl Sellafield)	1	—	382	98·5	338	86·2	1·14	0·040
Unspec brain and CNS	Pre-1955 (excl Sellafield)	4	—	357	109·2	302	95·7	1·14	0·049
All malignancies	All CEGB	4	3	10 855	98·4	11 536	94·5	1·04	0·001
	Sellafield	4	2, 3	2 399	97·7	2 491	89·8	1·09	0·002

CEGB = Central Electricity Generating Board; CNS = central nervous system.
* All comparisons where the SMR for the installation LAAs was significantly greater than for the control LAAs (p < 0·05, one sided test) in any of the four cumulative distance zones are indicated. Detailed results are given for the distance zone with the most extreme significance level. Sellafield does not appear on this table for leukaemia in the 0–24 age group because the increase that has been reported was confined to Millom rural district. In this analysis Millom rural district is in distance zone 4 where it is combined with Ennerdale rural district (also in distance zones 2 and 3) and Whitehaven metropolitan borough (also in distance zone 3). No increase in leukaemia mortality was found in these other areas.
† (a) With most extreme significant difference (lowest probability); (b) with significant differences (p < 0·05).
‡ Relative risk = SMR (installation LAAs)/SMR (control LAAs).

87

TABLE III—*Comparison of standardised mortality ratios (SMRs) between groupings of installation local authority areas (LAAs) and their controls**

Category of cancer	Installation grouping	Cumulative distance zone† (a)	(b)	Installation LAAs Deaths	SMR	Control LAAs Deaths	SMR	Relative risk‡	p
				People aged 0–24					
Myeloid leukaemia	Winfrith	4	—	2	55·0	9	234·9	0·23	0·042
Malignant brain	All CEGB	2	—	5	69·6	15	204·0	0·34	0·025
All brain	All CEGB	2	—	6	64·5	16	167·3	0·39	0·032
Malignant brain	All installations	1	—	34	80·2	51	118·1	0·68	0·050
Non-Hodgkin's lymphoma	All CEGB	2	—	0	0·0	5	147·9	0·00	0·034
All lymphomas and leukaemia	Winfrith	4	—	16	94·3	30	168·7	0·56	0·039
All malignancies	All CEGB	2	—	49	97·7	72	138·6	0·70	0·035
				People aged 25–74					
Myeloid leukaemia	Pre-1944 (excl Sellafield)	3	4	473	97·7	522	114·2	0·86	0·008
	All installations	3	4	575	96·7	651	113·2	0·85	0·003
Non-lymphoid leukaemia	Pre-1955 (excl Sellafield)	3	4	576	97·5	621	111·4	0·87	0·011
	All installations	3	4	701	96·8	772	110·3	0·88	0·007
Lymphoid leukaemia	Winfrith	3	4	2	33·4	12	203·8	0·16	0·007
All leukaemia	Winfrith	3	—	21	87·5	36	150·0	0·58	0·032
	All CEGB	1	2, 3	10	50·1	28	118·6	0·42	0·012
	All installations	1	—	379	89·8	437	101·8	0·88	0·040
Malignant brain	Pre-1955 (excl Sellafield)	3	4	1 116	95·0	1 203	107·5	0·88	0·002
	All CEGB	1	—	12	67·6	28	132·8	0·51	0·033
	All installations	3	4	1 333	94·3	1 474	107·2	0·88	<0·001

People aged 25–74

		(a)	(b)	SMR (inst)	Obs (inst)	Obs (ctrl)	SMR (ctrl)	RR	p
Benign brain	Pre-1955 (excl Sellafield)	4	3	88·6	152	185	112·5	0·79	0·016
	All CEGB	1	–	0·0	0	7	324·4	0·00	0·014
	All installations	4	2, 3	88·0	183	221	109·0	0·81	0·018
All brain	Pre-1955 (excl Sellafield)	3	4	96·7	1 523	1 605	107·0	0·90	0·002
	All CEGB	1	–	65·0	15	38	138·7	0·47	0·008
	All installations	3	4	96·1	1 811	1 952	106·6	0·90	<0·001
Lung	Pre-1955 (excl Sellafield)	2	3, 4	96·0	7 500	7 749	103·8	0·93	<0·001
	Winfrith	3	–	101·4	288	330	119·1	0·85	0·025
	All installations	2	3, 4	96·3	8 765	9 059	102·6	0·94	<0·001
Bone	Sellafield	3	2, 4	49·1	4	16	182·0	0·27	0·011
	All CEGB	4	3	88·7	32	54	136·8	0·65	0·032
	All installations	3	4	89·7	231	277	112·8	0·80	0·006
Multiple myeloma	Pre-1955 (excl Sellafield)	1	–	90·3	146	187	113·6	0·80	0·021
	Winfrith	4	–	75·2	25	39	130·0	0·58	0·021
	All installations	1	2	88·5	153	199	112·1	0·79	0·016
Testis	All CEGB	4	–	62·3	18	37	127·0	0·49	0·008
All lymphomas and leukaemia	All CEGB	1	2, 3	65·0	26	55	116·4	0·56	0·009
All malignancies	Pre-1955 (excl Sellafield)	2	1, 3, 4	96·6	25 928	26 074	101·4	0·95	<0·001
	Winfrith	3	–	102·7	1 055	1 142	113·3	0·91	0·011
	All installations	2	1, 3, 4	97·5	30 645	30 835	101·1	0·96	<0·001

* All comparisons where the SMR for the installation LAAs was significantly less than for the control LAAs ($p < 0.05$, one sided test) in any of the four cumulative distance zones are indicated. Detailed results are given for the distance zone with the most extreme significance level.

† (a) With most extreme significant difference (lowest probability); (b) with significant differences ($p < 0.05$).

‡ Relative risk = SMR (installation LAAs)/SMR (control LAAs).

TABLE IV—*Comparison of standardised mortality ratios (SMRs) between the coastal grouping of local authority areas (LAAs)† and the control grouping* in people aged 25–74*

Category of cancer	Coastal LAAs		Control LAA		Relative risk‡	p
	Deaths	SMR	Deaths	SMR		
Coastal LAAs greater than control LAAs						
Multiple myeloma	659	107·0	518	96·6	1·11	0·043
Coastal LAAs less than control LAAs						
Bone	249	89·6	284	114·1	0·79	0·003
All malignancies	68 433	97·1	60 935	98·4	0·99	0·009

* All comparisons where the SMR for the coastal grouping was significantly greater or less than the controls (p < 0·05, one sided test) are included.
† Excluding mid-Cumbria LAAs and Liverpool county borough.
‡ Relative risk = SMR (coastal LAAs)/SMR (control LAAs).

installations combined. These findings are shown in table V in the context of the overall results for leukaemia (lymphoid, non-lymphoid, and all types) in the four discrete distance zones. For lymphoid leukaemia there is a significantly increasing trend in relative risk with increasing proximity to an installation in the pre-1955 group (two sided p = 0·048) and a significantly decreasing trend with increasing proximity to an installation for the grouped CEGB installations (two sided p = 0·015).

The relative risk for all brain cancer (that is, for brain tumours described as malignant, benign, or of unspecified malignancy) is significantly raised in cumulative zone 2 around Sellafield. When data for this type of cancer are examined in the four discrete zones around all the installation groupings, two comparisons show statistically significant trends. One is of an increasing risk with increasing proximity to Sellafield (two sided p = 0·026). The other is of an increasing risk with decreasing proximity to the CEGB installations (two sided p = 0·013).

CANCER AT AGES 25–74

Seven types of cancer have caused death relatively more often in persons aged 25–74 years around some of the installation groupings or in the grouped coastal local authority areas: namely, Hodgkin's disease, all lymphomas, multiple myeloma, liver cancer, lung cancer, tumours of unspecified malignancy of the brain and central nervous system, and all malignancies.

The mortality from Hodgkin's disease is raised in all four cumulative zones in the local authority areas around the pre-1955 installations in comparison with their control areas. This leads to raised relative risks in cumulative zones 1, 2, and 3 for all installations combined. The results for

TABLE V—*Standardised mortality ratios (SMRs) for leukaemia in installation local authority areas (LAAs) and relative risks (RRs) of installation LAAs to control LAAs, 0–24 years age group, discrete distance zones*

Grouping		Discrete distance zone				Trend	
		1	2	3	4	Sign‡	Probability§
Lymphoid leukaemia (1968–80)							
Pre-1955	SMR	113·4	109·1	103·8	91·29		
	RR	2·10**	0·89	0·98	0·94	+	0·048
All CEGB	SMR	102·1	76·8	106·4	162·0		
	RR	1·05	0·34	1·54	2·96*	−	0·015
Winfrith	SMR	0·0	—†	44·8	123·7		
	RR	—‖	—	0·29	1·32	−	0·297
Sellafield	SMR	—†	138·5	53·8	333·7		
	RR	—	1·11	0·28	∞¶	−	0·276
All installations	SMR	112·1	105·5	101·0	113·2		
	RR	2·00**	0·75	0·96	1·30	+	0·425
Non-lymphoid leukaemia (1968–80)							
Pre-1955	SMR	110·0	119·8	86·1	125·8		
	RR	0·97	1·10	0·71	1·40	−	0·786
All CEGB	SMR	0·0	118·0	75·6	151·1		
	RR	0·00	1·00	5·85	1·65	−	0·121
Winfrith	SMR	0·0	—†	110·1	75·4		
	RR	—‖	—	1·17	0·28	+	0·340
Sellafield	SMR	—†	61·0	70·2	565·0**		
	RR	—	1·09	∞¶	4·00	−	0·412
All installations	SMR	107·0	114·9	84·8	137·4		
	RR	0·91	1·08	0·84	1·28	−	0·478
All leukaemia (1959–80)							
Pre-1955	SMR	105·9	109·4	93·5	95·5		
	RR	1·20	0·98	0·80	0·94	+	0·094
All CEGB	SMR	130·5	98·6	104·0	131·7		
	RR	1·10	0·55	1·50	1·59	−	0·054
Winfrith	SMR	0·0	—†	104·7	113·6		
	RR	—‖	—	0·82	0·56	+	0·696
Sellafield	SMR	—†	102·5	83·4	263·2*		
	RR	—	0·68	0·47	3·94	−	0·076
All installations	SMR	106·3	107·1	94·8	106·9		
	RR	1·19	0·86	0·84	1·02	+	0·382

* p < 0·05; ** p < 0·01 (one sided test for increase above 100 (SMR) or unity (RR)).
† No LAAs in this distance zone.
‡ Sign of trend in RR with increasing proximity to installation.
§ Probability of trend arising due to chance (two sided test).
‖ No deaths in installation or control LAAs.
¶ No deaths in control LAAs.
Data for lymphoid and non-lymphoid leukaemia are only separately available since the introduction of the eighth revision of the International Classification of Diseases in 1968. Data for all leukaemia are presented for the entire time period 1959–1980, but are only included since start up of the CEGB installations and since 1966 for Winfrith.

TABLE VI—*Standardised mortality ratios (SMRs) for Hodgkin's disease in installation local authority areas (LAAs) and relative risks (RRs) of installation LAAs to control LAAs, 25–74 years age group, discrete distance zones*

Grouping		Discrete distance zone				Trend	
		1	2	3	4	Sign‡	Probability§
Pre-1955	SMR	95·9	97·9	99·7	103·5		
	RR	1·36*	0·99	1·12	0·96	+	0·102
All CEGB	SMR	63·5	127·4	112·0	79·4		
	RR	0·64	0·96	1·34	0·78	+	0·966
Winfrith	SMR	540·5**	—†	93·3	101·6		
	RR	∞‖	—	1·24	0·56	+	0·002
Sellafield	SMR	—†	77·1	64·3	92·8		
	RR	—	1·05	0·77	0·74	+	0·643
All installations	SMR	96·7	100·5	99·7	99·2		
	RR	1·34*	0·98	1·14	0·89	+	0·040

* $p < 0.05$; ** $p < 0.01$ (one sided test for increase above 100 (SMR) or unity (RR)).
† No LAAs in this distance zone.
‡ Sign of trend in RR with increasing proximity to installation.
§ Probability of trend arising due to chance (two sided test).
‖ No deaths in control LAAs.

the discrete distance zones are given in table VI. Significant trends are seen for an increasing relative risk with increasing proximity to an installation for all installations combined (two sided $p = 0.040$) and for Winfrith (two sided $p = 0.002$). Hodgkin's disease is a major component in the category of all lymphomas, the mortality from which is also raised in distance zone 1 around the pre-1955 installations.

The mortality from multiple myeloma is significantly raised in the coastal local authority areas, but not in any of the areas around the nuclear installations. Because of the finding of an increased risk of myeloma with increasing dose of radiation in the Sellafield[9] and Hanford[10 11] workers, the results are examined in detail for the areas in each of the discrete distance zones around the grouped installation local authority areas in table VII. There is a significant decrease in relative risk with increasing proximity to an installation (two sided $p = 0.017$) for the areas around the pre-1955 installations.

Liver cancer relative risks are raised in cumulative zones 2, 3, and 4 around the grouped CEGB installations and in cumulative zone 4 around Winfrith. These results are reflected in raised relative risks for this cancer in cumulative zones 2, 3, and 4 around all installations combined.

The other positive results around the CEGB installations are those for lung cancer and for all malignancies in cumulative zones 3 and 4. The relative risk for all malignancies is also raised in all three distance zones around Sellafield. However, both of these cancer categories have signific-

TABLE VII—*Standardised mortality ratios (SMRs) for multiple myeloma in installation local authority areas (LAAs) and relative risks (RRs) of installation LAAs to control LAAs, 25–74 years age group, discrete distance zones*

Grouping		Discrete distance zone				Trend	
		1	2	3	4	Sign§	Probability‖
Pre-1955	SMR	90·3	109·7	104·5	108·3		
	RR	0·79	1·14	1·12	1·14	−	0·017
All CEGB	SMR	50·9	90·1	86·4	125·1		
	RR	0·54	0·72	0·87	1·02	−	0·171
Winfrith	SMR	147·3	−‡	90·1	62·5		
	RR	1·77	−	0·71	0·46	+	0·223
Sellafield	SMR	−‡	57·8	92·0	81·2		
	RR	−	0·71	0·78	0·48	+	0·640
All installations	SMR	88·5	100·9	101·5	106·0		
	RR	0·79	0·99	1·06	0·99	−	0·093

‡ No LAAs in this distance zone.
§ Sign of trend in RR with increasing proximity to installation.
‖ Probability of trend arising due to chance (two sided test).

antly lower relative risks around the grouped pre-1955 installations and around all installations combined (table III).

The results for liver cancer, lung cancer, and all malignancies for all four cumulative zones around the CEGB installations are given in table VIII, which also shows separate data for each zone before and after start up of the installations. For liver cancer the excesses in zones 2, 3, and 4 were all present before the opening of the installations as well as after, and the

TABLE VIII—*Standardised mortality ratios (SMRs) for liver cancer, lung cancer, and all malignancies in installation local authority areas (LAAs) and relative risks (RRs) of installation LAAs to control LAAs, 25–74 years age group, all CEGB installations, all cumulative distance zones, before and after start up*

Grouping		Cumulative zone 1		Cumulative zone 2		Cumulative zone 3		Cumulative zone 4	
		Before	Afer	Before	After	Before	After	Before	After
					Liver cancer				
All CEGB	SMR	85·5	163·3	224·6*	189·0**	178·5*	148·8**	162·4*	136·0**
	RR	1·13	1·41	2·21	3·03**	1·91	1·93**	1·59	1·82**
					Lung cancer				
All CEGB	SMR	110·3	107·8	102·4	100·7	96·6	97·2	92·2	95·0
	RR	1·06	1·04	1·03	1·02	1·04	1·06*	1·01	1·05*
					All malignancies				
All CEGB	SMR	109·2	101·4	105·5	103·5†	99·1	99·1	97·9	98·4
	RR	1·05	0·95	1·06	1·02	1·02	1·03*	1·00	1·04**

* p<0·05; ** p<0·01 (one sided test for increase above 100 (SMR) or unity (RR)).

earlier standardised mortality ratios were, in each case, higher than subsequently. For lung cancer and for all malignancies, the relative risks were all close to unity both before and after start up, the highest being 1·06. In cumulative zones 3 and 4, the relative risks and the standardised mortality ratios tended to be higher in the installation local authority areas than in the control areas after the opening of the installations than before, but the reverse was true for cumulative zones 1 and 2.

The remaining positive result is the increased relative risk for tumours of the brain and central nervous system, of unspecified malignancy, in cumulative zone 4 around the pre-1955 installations and around all installations combined. This was more than compensated for by significantly decreased relative risks for the other three brain cancer categories (malignant brain cancer, benign brain cancer, and all brain cancer) in these installation groupings (table III).

Discussion

The comparison of tables II and IVa with tables III and IVb shows that the standardised mortality ratios for local authority areas in the vicinity of nuclear installations or in the 58 selected coastal areas are significantly less than the standardised mortality ratios in their control areas more often than the reverse. This, moreover, remains true if attention is concentrated on those types of cancer that have been particularly associated with exposure to ionising radiation;[12] namely, leukaemia, bone cancer, and multiple myeloma. This provides strong evidence that there is no generalised increase in cancer mortality around nuclear installations in England and Wales either in young persons or in adults.

Although many of these results will be chance findings as so many comparisons were made, the tendency for cancer mortality to be lower near nuclear installations than in the control local authority areas is too strong to be explained solely on these grounds. We do not think that radioactive discharges can protect against the development of cancer and we conclude that there are likely to have been sufficiently large socioeconomic or environmental differences between the installation and the control areas to have had an effect on the pattern of cancer mortality, despite the efforts that were made to choose pairs of local authority areas that were socially similar. It follows that the excesses of mortality from some types of cancer in the installation areas, if they are not due to chance, may also result from these differences. It is, therefore, necessary to consider carefully whether each of the positive results may be due to chance, or to socioeconomic or environmental differences, or to the direct presence of the installations.

We have concentrated initially on the age group 0–24 years, as any effect of the installations on cancer mortality in the general population might be

TABLE IX—*Standardised mortality ratios (SMRs) for lymphoid leukaemia in installation local authority areas (LAAs) and relative risks (RRs) of installation LAAs to control LAAs, individual pre-1955 installations, 0–24 years age group, discrete distance zones*

Grouping		Discrete distance zone				Trend	
		1	2	3	4	Sign‡	Probability§
BNFL Springfields	SMR	134·2	104·8	184·9**	170·9		
	RR	2·35*	1·95	1·82*	1·44	+	0·530
BNFL Capenhurst	SMR	70·5	116·4	58·4	81·7		
	RR	1·12	0·84	0·28	1·09	+	0·811
Amersham International plc	SMR	171·7	85·6	77·4	93·2		
	RR	3·95*	0·87	1·02	0·83	+	0·040
MoD, Aldermaston	SMR	—†	159·1	89·4	46·9		
	RR	—	0·90	0·77	0·52	+	0·701
UKAEA, Harwell	SMR	77·6	67·8	67·1	—†		
	RR	2·54	0·37	0·41	—	+	0·238

* p < 0·05; ** p < 0·01 (one sided test for increase above 100 (SMR) or unity (RR)).
† No LAAs in this distance zone.
‡ Sign of trend in RR with increasing proximity to installation.
§ Probability of trend arising due to chance (two sided test).

expected to be seen first in young people. Studies of the effects of high doses of radiation have shown that children have a greater proportionate increase in risk after a given level of exposure than adults.[13] In addition, for inhaled and ingested radionuclides, children are thought to receive higher doses than adults from similar levels of environmental contamination, under some circumstances.[14]

In the age group 0–24 years there are two results of possible concern, those for lymphoid leukaemia and for all brain cancer. In the period 1968–80, the relative risks for lymphoid leukaemia are raised in the local authority areas around the pre-1955 installations in cumulative zones 1 and 2, and this is reflected in a raised relative risk around all installations combined in cumulative zone 1. The differences observed between the standardised mortality ratios for lymphoid leukaemia in the installation local authority areas and the control areas are the most highly significant of all the differences in this age group.

Several factors argue against the observed excess of lymphoid leukaemia being a chance association. Most of the evidence for the excess comes from the local authority areas around the pre-1955 installations, and any increase in risk would have had the greatest time to accumulate in these areas. For the pre-1955 installations, the increased relative risk is restricted to those areas closest to the installations, that is, in zone 1 (table V); and each of the four individual pre-1955 installations with areas in zone 1 (Springfields, Capenhurst, Amersham, and Harwell) shows a raised relative risk in this zone, although for Capenhurst and Harwell the individual increases do not reach significance (table IX). There is also a suggestion of an increase of lymphoid leukaemia in the coastal areas (relative risk 1·24, one sided p = 0·115). Because the Sellafield discharges are far in excess of those from any other establishment and a substantial proportion of those discharges are made into the sea, these coastal areas could be expected to be the first to experience any widespread effects associated with the discharges from the plant.

Moreover, because of particular interest in the effects of radiation on very young children,[12] we also looked at the lymphoid leukaemia results for the age group 0–9 years, which are available in the OPCS report on microfiche. In this age group all of the above effects were stronger. For the local authority areas in zone 1 around the pre-1955 installations the relative risk for lymphoid leukaemia is 3·95 (one sided p = 0·001) in comparison with 2·10 (one sided p = 0·004) for the age group 0–24 years. There is also a significant positive trend with increasing proximity to the installation (two sided p = 0·035). Finally in the coastal areas there is a significantly raised relative risk of 1·42 (one sided p = 0·038).

It should be noted that the excesses of lymphoid leukaemia in the local authority areas around the pre-1955 installations depend, in large part, on particularly low standardised mortality ratios in the control areas in zone 1. Thus the combined standardised mortality ratios for the age group 0–24 years in the areas in zone 1 around the pre-1955 installations is 113·4, whereas that for the corresponding control areas is 54·1. For the age group 0–9 the corresponding standardised mortality ratios are 113·7 and 28·8. The reason for these low control standardised mortality ratios is not clear, and demonstration of equivalent low standardised mortality ratios in other possible control areas is needed before it can be concluded confidently that the resulting raised relative risks have aetiological importance.

The difference between the results for lymphoid and non-lymphoid leukaemia, seen in table V, means that the combined category of all leukaemia shows no increased risk in the coastal local authority areas and only a slight indication of an increased relative risk in zone 1 around the pre-1955 installations (relative risk = 1·20, one sided p = 0·116). However, the results for lymphoid leukaemia are based on mortality since 1968 (data on leukaemia subtypes were not available before then). The relative risk for all leukaemia in zone 1 since 1968 is 1·46 and is significant (one sided p = 0·029). Therefore, by restricting attention to the more reliable all leukaemia category and to the later period, 1968–80, there is still reasonable evidence of an increased risk in the age group 0–24 years. In the younger age group, 0–9 years, the relative risk is somewhat higher at 1·66, and is of borderline significance (p = 0·051). In the coastal local authority areas the relative risks for all leukaemia in this later period are 1·10 (p = 0·181) at ages 0–24 and 1·26 (p = 0·072) at ages 0–9. Whether or not these increases are particularly associated with lymphoid leukaemia, as our initial results suggest, is open to question and depends on explaining why the standardised mortality ratios in the control local authority areas are especially low for this type of cancer and not for non-lymphoid leukaemia.

The present finding comes after independent reports of a fourfold increase in leukaemia mortality in the age group 0–24 years in Millom rural district, immediately south of Sellafield.[7] Other increases in childhood leukaemia incidence, based on registration data, have also been reported around two nuclear installations in Scotland (Dounreay[15] and Hunterston[16]) and around Aldermaston.[17] However, current assessments of annual radiation doses, in conjunction with estimates of the risk of leukaemia per unit dose, indicate that the estimated doses received by populations living in the vicinity of nuclear installations are not sufficiently high to cause any detectable increase in leukaemia.[6 18] A recent study of the effects of fallout from atmospheric nuclear weapons testing in the 1950s and 1960s provides good evidence that the estimate of the risk of leukaemia per unit dose is not much too low.[19] It follows that either the received doses are grossly underestimated or the excess risk of leukaemia must be due to some other factors that differ between the installation and control local authority areas. Thus, on present knowledge, it is difficult to attribute the leukaemia results found here to ionising radiation, but it is also not clear what the other factors are that distinguish the installation areas from the areas with which they have been compared.

The other positive observation in the age group 0–24 years, that for all brain cancer, seems most likely to be due to chance. The detailed results for this cancer type are contradictory. The increasing risk with proximity to Sellafield contrasts with a decreasing risk with proximity to the CEGB installations. There is no suggestion of a hazard round Winfrith or the pre-1955 installations. The one significantly raised relative risk in discrete zone 2 around Sellafield derives from a comparison between five and no observed deaths, while in discrete zones 3 and 4 the corresponding relative risks are less than unity (0·86 and 0·00 respectively).

Of the positive results in the older age group, 25–74 years, those for Hodgkin's disease present the most consistent evidence for an association with proximity to the installations. There is a tendency for the relative risk to increase with proximity to the installations in areas around the pre-1955 installations, around Sellafield and Winfrith individually, and around all installations combined (table VI). There is no notable trend in either direction around the CEGB installations. It should be noted, however, that the standardised mortality ratios tend to be below or only slightly above the regional standard, except around Winfrith where an exceptionally high standardised mortality ratio was recorded in zone 1 (540·5 based on four cases).

Studies of populations exposed to high doses of radiation have not, so far, shown significant increases of Hodgkin's disease.[12] However, the available data are not inconsistent with a small increase. It is also entirely possible that the present results for Hodgkin's disease could be a consequence of the possible socioeconomic or environmental differences between installation and control local authority areas, especially as there is some evidence that the causes of the disease are influenced by social factors.[20] The positive result for all lymphomas in the innermost distance zone around the pre-1955 installations is accounted for by the result for Hodgkin's disease. If the latter is subtracted out then the remaining "other lymphomas" category shows no increased risk.

Previous observations on mortality from multiple myeloma are perhaps the most suggestive of all the data on adult cancers of a possible hazard associated with nuclear installations. The consistency of the results among workers at both Sellafield[9] and Hanford[10 11] has suggested that there may be a special hazard of myelomatosis associated with these installations. A dose-related increase in this disease has also been documented in Japanese atom bomb survivors.[13] The observation in this study of a small increased relative risk in the local authority areas of the coastal regions to the north and south of Sellafield (relative risk = 1·11, one sided p = 0·043), and the above average value of 107·0 for the standardised mortality ratio in the same coastal areas provides some additional evidence for the association. The hypothesis would, however, seem to be contradicted by the tendency for the relative risks to decrease with increasing proximity to all installations combined (two sided p = 0·093) and particularly with increasing proximity to the pre-1955 installations (two sided p = 0·017) and by the low standardised mortality ratios in the areas immediately adjacent to Sellafield. The latter three local authority areas are all on the coast and could be combined with the other 58 coastal areas. However, because they represent a very small proportion of the population in the group of coastal local authority areas, the overall relative risk in the group is only marginally affected (relative risk = 1·09, one sided p = 0·079).

All of the positive results around the CEGB installations are probably largely explained by the socioeconomic differences between installation and control areas. This is made most apparent by considering the results for lung cancer and all malignancies in tables II and III. Both of these have relative risks which are significantly raised around the CEGB installations and significantly lowered around the pre-1955 installations and all installations combined. As lung cancer is such a major component of all malignancies, the similarity between the two categories is not surprising. Analysis of the results in discrete zones shows highly significant trends in relative risks, which decrease with increasing proximity to the installation for both lung cancer and all malignancies (two sided p = 0·005 and 0·001 respectively around the pre-1955 installations and p = 0·001 and < 0·001 respectively around all installations combined). No significant trends are apparent around the grouped CEGB installations or around Sellafield or Winfrith.

The most likely explanation for these results is that social factors, especially smoking behaviour, have different distributions in the local authority areas around the pre-1955 installations, especially within the inner distance zones, compared with the areas around the CEGB installations. The matching of control areas does not fully allow for this and, as such large numbers of deaths are involved, even moderate differences between installation and control areas produce highly significant results.

A similar explanation can be made in relation to liver cancer which, like lung cancer, is only more prevalent around the CEGB installations. Liver cancer has not, to our knowledge, been associated with radiation exposure at low doses. A large excess of liver tumours has been seen in patients injected with the radioactive contrast medium, thorotrast,[12] and the liver was selected as a specific site for this study because inhaled or ingested plutonium might act in the same way. However, the CEGB installations do not discharge substantial quantities of plutonium,[6] and any effect would have been expected to be more evident in local authority areas around the pre-1955 installations. The diagnosis of liver cancer as a cause of death after about 45 years of age is, moreover, extremely unreliable, and most deaths attributed to this cause are likely to be due to metastases from primary cancers in the lung, stomach, or large bowel. It is, therefore, only to be expected that liver cancer will show a similar relation with vicinity to nuclear installations as is shown by lung cancer and all malignancies.

Further evidence that the significant results around the grouped CEGB installations are not caused by radioactive discharges from the installations is provided by comparing the relative risks in the local authority areas before and after start up (table VIII). This shows very little difference between the two periods in the standardised mortality ratios or the relative risks for liver cancer, lung cancer, or for all malignancies.

The result for "unspecified brain and central nervous system tumours" in the age group 25–74 years is presumably either due to chance or to diagnostic artefacts. The excess is more than compensated for by the deficiency of brain tumours specified as benign or malignant.

Summary

The OPCS report on cancer incidence and mortality in the vicinity of nuclear installations in England and Wales provides a mass of information that is so large that it should be possible to detect quite small changes in disease levels with considerable confidence. The data on cancer mortality are less subject to selective bias than the registration data on which incidence rates are based, and they provide the firmest grounds on which evidence of any effect can be obtained.

These data show conclusively that there has been no general increase in cancer mortality in the vicinity of nuclear installations in a 22 year period beginning several years after the opening of the installations that have released the largest amounts of radionuclides to the environment. On the contrary, the mortality from cancer has tended to be lower in the local authority areas in the vicinity of nuclear installations than in control areas selected for their presumed comparability with the former. This is unlikely to be due to a protective effect of ionising radiation and suggests that, despite the efforts that were made to choose comparable control areas, there were non-installation differences between the populations that are relevant to the risk of dying from one or other type of cancer.

Detailed examination of the few types of cancer that were relatively more common in the installation areas suggests that several of the differences were most likely to be due to chance, diagnostic artefacts, or social factors rather than to any hazard specifically related to the installations. One disease provides a possible exception—namely, leukaemia in the age group 0–24 years. Two other diseases need further investigation, multiple myeloma and Hodgkin's disease in the older age group, 25–74 years. The excess death rates recorded from these cancers were not large, and it has yet to be established that they are not due to general confounding by other environmental or socioeconomic factors.

We thank Miss Cynthia Bates for typing the numerous drafts of this chapter.

1 Cook-Mozaffari PJ, Ashwood FL, Vincent T, Forman D, Alderson M. *Cancer incidence and mortality in the vicinity of nuclear installations, England and Wales, 1950–51.* London: HMSO, 1987. (Studies on Medical and Population Subjects, No 51.)
2 Office of Population Censuses and Surveys. *The registrar general's statistical review of England and Wales for the year 1971.* London: HMSO, 1973.
3 Swerdlow AJ. *Journal of the Royal Statistical Society [Series A]* 1986;**149**:146–60.
4 Cook-Mozaffari P. *Lancet* 1987;**i**:855–6.
5 Office of Population Censuses and Surveys. *Occupational mortality decennial supplement 1970–72, England and Wales.* London: HMSO, 1978.
6 Clark MJ, Kelly GN. *Nuclear Energy* 1982;**21**:275–88.
7 Black D for the Independent Advisory Group. *Investigation of the possible increased incidence of cancer in west Cumbria.* London: HMSO, 1984.
8 Committee on Medical Aspects of Radiation in the Environment (COMARE). *First report.* London: HMSO, 1986.
9 Smith PG, Douglas AJ. *BMJ* 1986;**ii**:845–54.
10 Gilbert ES, Marks S. *Radiat Res* 1979;**79**:122–48.
11 Tolley HD, Marks S, Buchanan JA, Gilbert ES. *Radiat Res* 1983;**95**:211–3.
12 *The effects on populations of exposure to low levels of ionizing radiation.* Washington DC: National Academy of Science, 1980.
13 Kato H, Schull WJ. *Radiat Res* 1982;**90**:395–432.
14 Adams N. *Phys Med Biol* 1981;**26**:1019–34.
15 Heasman MS, Kemp IW, Urquhart JD, Black R. *Lancet* 1986;**i**:266.
16 Heasman MA, Kemp IW, MacLaren A, Trotter P, Gillis CR, Hole DJ. *Lancet* 1986;**i**:1188–9.
17 Roman E, Beral V, Carpenter L, Watson A, Barton C, Ryder H, et al. *BMJ* 1987;**294**:597–602.
18 Hughes JS, Roberts GN. The radiation exposure of the UK population, 1984 Review. London: HMSO, 1984. (NRPB-R173.)
19 Darby SC, Doll R. *BMJ* 1987;**294**:603–7.

20 Grufferman S. In: Schottenfeld D, Fraumeni JF, eds. *Cancer, epidemiology and prevention*. Philadelphia: Saunders, 1982:739–53.

13: Evidence for an infective cause of childhood leukaemia: comparison of a Scottish new town with nuclear reprocessing sites in Britain

LEO KINLEN

Increases of leukaemia in young people that cannot be explained in terms of radiation have been recorded near both of Britain's nuclear reprocessing plants at Dounreay and Sellafield. These were built in unusually isolated places where herd immunity to a postulated widespread virus infection (to which leukaemia is a rare response) would tend to be lower than average. The large influxes of people in the 1950s to those areas might have been conducive to epidemics. The hypothesis has been tested in Scotland in an area identified at the outset as the only other rural area that received a large influx at the same time, when it was much more cut off from the nearest conurbation than at present—the new town of Glenrothes. A significant excess of luekaemia below age 25 was found (10 observed, expected 3·6), with a greater excess below age 5 (7 observed, expected 1·5).

Introduction

The increased incidence of leukaemia in young people near the only

British nuclear power stations that also reprocess spent nuclear fuel (at Sellafield and Dounreay) has been the subject of much public concern and scientific study.[1-10] Three official reports by groups of independent scientists all concluded that the levels of radiation in these areas are far below those necessary on conventional models to account for the excesses.[8-10] Moreover, the risk estimate of leukaemia per unit is unlikely to be much too low, as there was no increase after the fallout from atmospheric nuclear weapons tests in the 1950s and 1960s.[11] The explanation therefore must be either that the radiation levels are very much larger than stated, or that an entirely different factor is involved. As no evidence for any particular alternative explanation has been found,[8-10] there will be continued public suspicion that radiation is responsible: for in which leukaemogenic respect are the areas near Sellafield and Dounreay remarkable except in their associated radiation?

The CRC cancer epidemiology unit, Edinburgh University, has for some time been investigating the possibility that certain distinctive aspects of the Dounreay and Sellafield areas that owe nothing to radiation are relevant to the causation of leukaemia elsewhere. These aspects involve the combination of geographical isolation and population influx. The hypothesis involves three elements: firstly, that influxes of population into rural and isolated areas are conducive to epidemics of certain infections; secondly, that Sellafield and Dounreay are extreme examples of isolation and population influx; and thirdly, that some unidentified virus (or viruses) can cause childhood leukaemia. The last mentioned is itself hypothetical; but it is plausible, and if it is correct the possible relevance of the first two elements obviously deserves careful examination.

The points are discussed in more detail below.

(1) People who live in geographically isolated places represent one of the few groups who may escape appreciable exposure at usual ages to common and widespread infective agents. To such groups "incomers" can introduce infective agents with dramatic consequences.[12-14] The following interrelated factors may be relevant here. A lower level of natural immunisation to the agent may occur either because of the fewer opportunities for person to person transmission than in more urban areas or because the population is not large enough to maintain the disease in endemic form.[14] Age at exposure may also be greater in rural than in urban areas, and this can influence the form of certain viral infections such as maternal rubella and paralytic poliomyelitis. The dose of the agent may also be important, as it is in several animal models of viral oncogenesis, and when there is large scale mixing of susceptible people with infected people or carriers, particularly under circumstances of crowding, the likelihood must be increased of a susceptible person being heavily exposed.

(2) The nuclear power station at Doureay is unquestionably isolated. Situated in a sparsely populated part of Caithness eight miles west of the

TABLE I—*Comparison of Thurso and Seascale with other areas of comparable category and population growth*

Index area	Type of area	Total no in country	No of other areas with an increase as great as index area
	Scotland		
Thurso small burgh	Small burgh	194‡	0
	England		
Seascale Parish	Parish in rural district	11 211	394
Seascale Parish	Parish in sparsely populated rural district†	2804	25
Millom rural district*	Rural district	475	51
Millom rural district	Sparsely populated rural district	118	1

* Includes Seascale; † 0·15 person per acre or less in 1951 (Millom rural district = 0·15/acre);
‡ Thurso also increased more than any other local authority district in Scotland (total 397).

small town of Thurso, it was then 160 miles by road north of Inverness and over 300 miles from Edinburgh. The isolation in the late 1940s and 1950s of Sellafield, near Seascale, is perhaps less obvious. Although quite close to the lake district, the west Cumbrian coastal strip was by comparison little visited by tourists. Always recognised as distinctive and somewhat separate by the people of Carlisle and lakeland, the small industrial towns of Whitehaven, Workington, and Maryport on the coast were nevertheless of sufficient size to make the west Cumbrian population fairly self sufficient. Sandwiched between the sea to the west and the lakeland mountains to the east, access to Seascale was mainly from the north along the coast, which in turn was reached from the main regional centre of Carlisle to the north east, 53 miles from Seascale. But in addition to their relative isolation, the populations of Thurso and Seascale were unusual in increasing greatly between the 1951 and 1961 censuses. Thurso increased more than any other burgh or indeed any other Scottish local authority district. Seascale increased more than 96% of the 11 211 parishes in rural districts of England and Wales (see table I). If account were taken of increase and isolation simultaneously, then their national positions would be even more extreme.

(3) The possibility that childhood leukaemia is of viral origin has often been raised. Indeed for two rare types of adult leukaemia, T cell leukaemia-lymphoma and the T cell variant of hairy cell leukaemia, there is mounting evidence for their causation by specific viruses—namely, HTLV-1 and HTLV-2, respectively. Furthermore, specific viruses are known to cause leukaemia in cats and other animals. Epidemiologists have made many

attempts to assess whether childhood leukaemia behaves as an infectious disease, particularly by looking for space-time clustering. The absence of consistent evidence of this does not, however, weigh strongly against a viral origin.[15] Spread of the agent may not depend mainly on persons with leukaemia but, as in infectious mononucleosis and Epstein-Barr virus infection, on a common infection in apparently healthy people to which leukaemia is a rare response.

The obvious test of the above hypothesis is to investigate whether there is an excess of leukaemia in other isolated areas that have seen a considerable influx of population but which lack any potential source of radiation made by humans. The population of Seascale parish increased by 50% from 1328 to 1990 between 1951 and 1961, while that of Thurso more than doubled, increasing by 147% from 3249 to 8037. Local authority districts, of which Thurso small burgh is an example, are the smallest category of area for which population details by age are available before 1971.

Table II shows details of all the 11 local authority districts of Scotland that experienced even a 25% increase in population between the 1951 and 1961 censuses.[16] No district increased proportionately as much as Thurso small burgh, the nearest being in the Clydeside central conurbation, the fifth district of Lanarkshire (110%) in which most of the new town of East Kilbride was created. But apart from showing smaller increases than Thurso, none of these areas approaches it in respect of its isolated situation. Most are in, or close to, major urban centres (see table II): Dollar, though moderately rural, is too small whereas Annan district of county must be excluded as it includes a nuclear power station. Only Kirkcaldy district of county is a possibly comparable area in that its population doubled, and in being at this time rural and moderately separated from a conurbation (table II).

COMPARISON AREA OF KIRKCALDY DISTRICT OF COUNTY AND GLENROTHES

Kirkcaldy district is the rural district of Fife in which the new town of Glenrothes was designated in 1948. In consequence of the growth of Glenrothes from 1100 in 1948 to 12 750 in 1961, the population of Kirkcaldy district doubled between the 1951 and 1956 censuses. Glenrothes is undoubtedly an example of a large influx of people into a rural area causing a greater population increase (20-fold by 1971) than in Thurso. It is far less isolated than Thurso and indeed no one would now regard them as similar. However, in the 1950s and early 1960s, before the opening of the Forth road bridge, Glenrothes was appreciably more isolated than at present. Away from the main roads to Dundee and other centres of population, in an area of gently wooded hills with Loch Leven to the west and the Lomond hills to the north, that part of Fife was much less exposed to outside contact than most places. With the opening of the Forth road bridge in 1964, the ensuing great increase in Lothian–Fife traffic,[18] the

TABLE II—*Local authority districts (LAD) of Scotland with a 25% or greater population increase from 1951 to 1961*

LAD and county	1951 Population	Increase (%) 1961–51	1971 Population	Rough distance to large centre* (road miles, 1955)	Geographical comment
Thurso SB, Caithness	3 249	147	9 085	240	In CCC; incl E Kilbride NT
No 5 DC, Lanark	24 255	110	Boundary change	8	Includes Glenrothes NT
Kirkcaldy DC, Fife	10 069	96	Boundary change	58	Edinburgh outskirts
Currie DC, Midlothian	5 743	66	14 390	7	Edinburgh outskirts
Newbattle DC, Midlothian	8 404	41	15 135	12	Rural: near Alloa DC
Dollar SB, Clackmannan	1 389	40	2 280	28	In CCC; became Bearsden SB
New Kilpatrick DC, Dumbarton	12 264	38	25 015	6	In CIB; incl Cumbernauld NT
Cumbernauld DC, Dumbarton	5 283	38	Boundary change	18	Includes nuclear power station
Annan DC, Dumfries	4 644	30	5 870	87	Near CIB†
Alloa DC, Clackmannan	11 377	27	17 590	28	Edinburgh outskirts
Musselburgh DC, Midlothian	6 477	26	8 465	7	

SB = small burgh; DC = district of county; CCC = central Clydeside conurbation; NT = new town; CIB = central industrial belt; * 100 000 population; † on route north from only road bridge over Forth east of Stirling.

increasing prevalence of car ownership, and the newly forged outside links associated with a thriving new town all combined to end its previous seclusion. The Glenrothes area, therefore, can only be regarded as having been moderately secluded in, say, the first half of the period covered by this study (1951–67). This, then, is the area predicted by the hypothesis as the most likely of all districts of Scotland apart from Thurso to show an increase of childhood leukaemia.

Methods

Leukaemia and lymphoma mortality at ages 0–24 has been investigated in Thurso and in the Glenrothes areas and also in the areas of high growth that were rejected from the outset as comparable to Thurso. Computerised details of deaths were obtained from the registrar general for Scotland for the maximum period—namely, 1953–83—to which were later added 1984–85. In addition, deaths from leukaemia in 1951 and 1952 were found by searching the death registers at register house and consulting a series of leukaemia death certificates provided many years previously for another study. Before 1964, deaths in landward areas (the collective term for the rural districts of county), were not routinely coded beyond the county of residence level. This meant that the certificates for *all* deaths outside the burghs of the relevant counties had to be traced in register house to decide whether they related to districts in the study.

The observed numbers of deaths from leukaemia and lymphoma in each five year age group and quinquennial period were compared with expected numbers, obtained by applying Scottish national mortality rates to the corresponding estimated person-years at risk. The last were derived by multiplying the fractions of the census population of a given area in each sex group and age group to the total population estimates in adjacent years as follows: 1951 fractions to the years 1952–55, 1961 to 1956–65, and so on. Population estimates were not available for individual districts before 1957, and were estimated by extrapolation from the 1951 census to the estimates for 1957. After the 1961 census, major boundary changes affected Lanark no 5 districts of county and Kirkcaldy districts of county, and, in addition, deaths in new towns of Scotland began to be coded to these areas by the registrar general. From 1962, therefore, Kirkcaldy district was replaced in the study by Glenrothes new town, and Lanark no 5 district by East Kilbride new town. As new town areas were not affected by the 1974 reorganisation, this change in definition also allowed the use of 1981 census data for the new towns. Local authority districts were abolished in 1974 but, by use of age-specific census small-area statistics for localities, parishes, and postcode areas, the 1981 populations of the former areas were obtained. After 1973 intercensal population estimates were derived by

TABLE III—*Observed (and expected) numbers of deaths from leukaemia, non-Hodgkin's lymphoma, and all lymphomas in Thurso and Glenrothes new town, previously Kirkcaldy district of county*

	1951–67			1968–85			Total: 1951–85		
	0–4	0–14	0–24	0–4	0–14	0–24	0–4	0–14	0–24
Leukaemia									
Thurso	0 (0·47)	2 (0·94)	2 (1·21)	0 (0·32)	1 (0·89)	2 (1·30)	0 (0·78)	3 (1·83)	4 (2·52)
Glenrothes	7 (1·49)*	8 (2·87)†	10 (3·60)‡	0 (1·30)	1 (3·50)	1 (5·18)	7 (2·79)§	9 (6·37)	11 (8·78)
Non-Hodgkin's lymphoma									
Thurso	0 (0·11)	0 (0·20)	0 (0·29)	1 (0·04)	1 (0·17)	1 (0·30)	1 (0·15)	1 (0·37)	1 (0·59)
Glenrothes	1 (0·32)	1 (0·58)	0 (0·78)	0 (0·17)	1 (0·64)	1 (1·16)	1 (0·48)†	2 (1·22)	2 (1·95)
All lymphomas‡									
Thurso	0 (0·11)	0 (0·25)	0 (0·51)	1 (0·04)	1 (0·19)	1 (0·51)	1 (0·15)	1 (0·44)	1 (1·01)
Glenrothes	1 (0·32)	1 (0·71)	3 (1·32)	0 (0·17)	1 (0·74)	1 (1·95)	1 (0·49)	2 (1·45)	4 (3·27)

*p < 0.002 (two sided); †p < 0.02 (two sided); ‡p < 0.01 (two sided); §p < 0.05 (two sided). Lymphoma data relate to the period 1953–85.

extrapolation, on the assumption that changes were proportional to those in the relevant local government district as a whole (though in fact there were no striking changes).

Results

The observed and expected numbers of deaths from leukaemia and lymphoma for the two periods 1951–67 and 1968–85 in Thurso and the Kirkcaldy district–Glenrothes area are shown in table III. In the first half (1951–67) of the study period and the part most relevant to the hypothesis, there is a significant excess of leukaemia deaths below age 25 in the Glenrothes area—10 observed and 3·60 expected (O/E ratio 2·78, p < 0·01). This is mainly due to an excess (seven observed, 1·49 expected; p < 0·001) at ages below 5, six being in the period 1954–59. In the second half (1968–85) there is no excess—indeed, a non-significant deficit, with one death observed and 5·18 expected. Corresponding details for leukaemia in the areas that were rejected from the outset as being comparable with Thurso are shown in table IV. With the exception of leukaemia at ages below 5 in Dollar in the second period (and based on one case) there was no significant increase in any area or in all areas combined.

Discussion

Ideally the above hypothesis should be tested in an area similar to Thurso. However, because the town increased more in population and is

TABLE IV—Observed (and expected) numbers of deaths from leukaemia in areas not considered comparable with Thurso

	1951–67			1968–85			Total: 1951–85		
	0–4	0–14	0–24	0–4	0–14	0–24	0–4	0–14	0–24
Lanark No 5 DC	1 (3·47)	1 (6·93)	3 (8·66)	0 (2·26)	2 (6·74)	5 (10·27)	1 (5·73)	3 (13·67)	8 (18·93)
Currie DC	1 (0·61)	1 (1·19)	3 (1·56)	0 (0·52)	0 (1·54)	0 (2·27)	1 (1·13)	1 (2·73)	3 (3·83)
Newbattle DC	1 (0·97)	2 (2·01)	3 (2·67)	0 (0·54)	0 (1·55)	2 (2·48)	1 (1·51)	2 (3·56)	5 (5·16)
Musselburgh DC*	0 (0·52)	1 (1·13)	1 (1·53)	0 (0·10)	0 (0·31)	0 (0·46)	0 (0·62)	1 (1·44)	1 (1·99)
Dollar SB	0 (0·08)	0 (0·24)	0 (0·32)	1 (0·05)†	1 (0·23)	1 (0·35)	1 (0·13)	1 (0·47)	1 (0·68)
Alloa DC	1 (1·00)	1 (2·14)	1 (2·84)	2 (0·63)	3 (1·83)	6 (2·90)	3 (1·63)	4 (3·97)	7 (5·74)
Bearsden SB	3 (0·90)	4 (1·92)	4 (2·50)	1 (0·77)	3 (2·22)	4 (3·27)	4 (1·67)	7 (4·14)	8 (5·77)
Cumbernauld DC	0 (0·72)	0 (1·45)	2 (1·89)	1 (1·61)	4 (4·38)	6 (6·34)	1 (2·33)	4 (5·83)	8 (8·23)
Annan DC	0 (0·40)	0 (0·84)	0 (1·10)	0 (0·16)	0 (0·49)	0 (0·75)	0 (0·56)	0 (1·33)	0 (1·85)
Total excluding Annan DC	7 (8·26)	10 (17·01)	17 (21·98)	5 (6·48)	13 (18·81)	24 (28·36)	12 (14·74)	23 (35·81)	41 (50·34)

DC = district of county; SB = small burgh.
* 1951–73. This area could not be separated from Musselburgh small burgh after 1973 on the basis of postcodes. †p < 0·05, two sided.

109

also further away from a sizeable centre than any other burgh, the comparison area had to be the *only* other rural area of Scotland to experience a large influx of people and which was even moderately separated from a conurbation—namely, the Glenrothes area of central Fife in the years 1951–67. Most of this period preceded the opening of the Forth road bridge in 1964, an event that had important economic and demographic effects on Fife.[18] The finding of a significant excess of childhood leukaemia in this area therefore supports the hypothesis. Chance is an unlikely explanation, as an excess was postulated before the data were collected; nor can it be attributed to underestimation of the population in the relevant age groups. Even if the official total population estimates of Kirkcaldy district of county in the years 1956–60 had been underestimated, and, most improbably, the 1961 census population had been reached five years sooner with no further increase until 1961, an excess would still have been evident at ages below 5 (five observed, 1·28 expected; $p < 0·005$, two sided). An excess of non-Hodgkin's lymphoma has been reported near Dounreay based on two cases below age 5, both of which were misdiagnosed cases of lymphatic leukaemia:[10] there was one death from non-Hodgkin's lymphoma below age 5 in Glenrothes in the first period (expected 0·3) (see table III).

The influx to Glenrothes (designated 1948) occurred before that in Thurso (Dounreay, operational 1958) but certain other differences are also relevant. The former (1951) residents of Thurso, on the present hypothesis, include most of the "susceptibles" whereas the incomers, most from urban areas (many from outside Scotland), include the carriers and infected people. By contrast, in Glenrothes the largest group of incomers came from other parts of Fife, many being as likely to be susceptible as the original inhabitants whose number represented a much smaller fraction (8·6%) of the 1961 population than in the case of Thurso (40·4%). Glenrothes was also notable in receiving, by 1961, a much smaller population of incomers from Glasgow and other urban centres than the other new towns of East Kilbride and Cumbernauld.

There are also differences between Thurso and Glenrothes in the age groups and time period that show the increases of leukaemia. The former may reflect differences in the ages of exposure of susceptibles. The recent persistence (or recurrence) of an excess near Dounreay (more striking in the incidence data)[5-7] is intriguing and may be due to both the continuing isolation of Thurso and the appreciable turnover in the workforce and their families, many of whom come from the south.

Classic epidemiological reasoning about infectious disease is applied here to childhood leukaemia, a disease often suspected of being viral in origin. The relevance of geographical isolation to the pattern of infectious diseases has been stressed previously. The Highland Region, in which Thurso lies, is a large and sparsely populated area, most of which is far removed from centres of population. This isolation can certainly influence the clinical course of one viral infection—namely, measles. Whereas in most of Britain the ubiquity of the virus and the many opportunities for transmission ensure that the vast majority of children have had measles before the age of 15, this is not so in the highlands and islands. Even since the second world war, deaths from measles above this age have been 19 times commoner there than in the rest of Scotland.[17]

This particular excess of leukaemia deaths within central Fife in the 1950s first came to light during the analyses for the present study, conducted to test the hypothesis as stated above. The absence of an excess of leukaemia in Glenrothes in the more recent period of the study weighs little against the hypothesis. The fact that there was actually a deficit of deaths from leukaemia in this latter period is itself of interest. This deficit might have been related to the earlier excess, as the later dearth of cases may represent the exhaustion of susceptible people that is typical of epidemic infections: on the other hand, it is barely significant ($p < 0.06$, one sided) and is more likely to be due to chance.

The previously reported excess of leukaemia under age 25 near Dounreay came from an elegant analysis of incidence by Heasman and colleagues.[4-7] Observed and expected numbers of leukaemia cases were compared within geographical zones delineated by circles with radii of 12·5 and 25 km centred on the Dounreay site, an exercise made possible by the use of postcodes in recent censuses. As stressed recently,[10] the choice of those boundaries was inevitably arbitrary. No such choice was possible in the present study for, whereas the 1981 populations can be calculated for areas similar to the former local authority areas, it is impossible to estimate the pre-1971 populations of postcode units. With improvements in survival, mortality has become an inefficient measure of childhood leukaemia incidence, but this was not so in the 1950s when the disease was uniformly fatal. The previous study of leukaemia incidence near Dounreay was based on four cases in, and two near, Thurso in the period 1968–84.[10] Of the four patients in Thurso, two have died and are included in the present study. The 1·78-fold increase in mortality from leukaemia over the whole period (1958–85) since the Dounreay reactor was completed is not appreciably different from the estimate based on incidence over the more restricted period 1968–84 (2·03-fold).[10]

The Glenrothes cluster of childhood leukaemia seems to be the first instance of a particular cluster being found as predicted by a hypothesis specified before the data were collected. It is difficult to escape the conclusion that at least some of the excesses near Dounreay and Sellafield have a similar (infective) explanation as they represent more extreme degrees of isolation combined with population influx. It is the locally born children near Sellafield[19] and also near Dounreay, as found in this study, who show the increase of leukaemia, and not those born outside but attending school there.[20] This is consistent with there being fewer outside contacts among the former, which produces more susceptible children among those born locally than among the children of incoming workers. It may also reflect an interaction between age at exposure and dose of virus, as seems to occur in feline leukaemia.[21] But the pattern of transmission even in cases of known infection can be extremely elusive.[22]

The absence of space-time clustering commonly reported in leukaemia is consistent with the notion that leukaemia is a rare response to a common, possibly subclinical, infection, the studies having been conducted mainly in fairly stable populations in which the virus-host equilibrium had not been disturbed. A viral cause for childhood leukaemia deserves renewed attention, including further investigations in situations of large scale population mixing. These might focus particularly on populations that include groups whose exposure to common viruses may plausibly be considered lower than average, such as those in (or from) rural areas. Examples will be easiest to find in the past, for improvements in communication must have severely reduced the differences in herd immunity between urban and rural areas.

I am grateful to the registrar general for Scotland and to Dr W H Price for their help; to Vicky Stephenson, Karen Sharp, Kathy Anderson, Kathy Chalmers, and Lyn Tatler for their work facilitated by Dr J Shaw in register house; to Marjorie MacLeod for abstracting population details; to Tony Willows and Kathy Chalmers for calculating expected numbers of deaths; to Susan Hill and Davina Patrizio for secretarial help; and to Dr Paula Cook-Mozaffari, Professor David Harnden, and Dr D A J Tyrrell for their valuable comments on an earlier draft of the paper.

1 Craft AW, Birch JM. Childhood cancer in Cumbria. *Lancet* 1983;**ii**:1299.
2 Urquhart J, Palmer M, Cutler J. Cancer in Cumbria: the Windscale connection. *Lancet* 1984;**i**:217–18.
3 Gardner MJ, Winder PD. Cancer in Cumberland during 1959–68 with reference to cancer in young people around Windscale. *Lancet* 1984;**i**:216–7.
4 Heasman MA, Urquhart JD, Black R, Kemp IW. *Leukaemia in young persons in Scotland: a study of its geographical distribution and relationship to nuclear installations.* (Recognitions submitted to Dounreay Inquiry.) Edinburgh: Scottish Health Service Common Services Agency, Information Services Division, 1986.
5 Heasman MA, Kemp IW, Urquhart JD, Black R. Childhood leukaemia in northern Scotland. *Lancet* 1986;**i**:266.
6 Heasman MA, Kemp IW, Urquhart JD, Black R. *Lancet* 1986;**i**:355.
7 Heasman MA, Urquhart JD, Black RJ, Glass S, Gray M. Leukaemia in young persons in Scotland: a study of its geographical distribution and relationship to nuclear installations. *Health Bull (Edinb)* 1987;**45**:147.
8 Black D for the Independent Advisory Group. *Investigation of the possible increased incidence of cancer in west Cumbria.* London: HMSO, 1984. (Black report.)
9 Committee on Medical Aspects of Radiation in the Environment (COMARE). *First report: the implications of the new data on the releases from Sellafield in the 1950s for the conclusions of the report on the investigation of the possible increased incidence of cancer in west Cumbria.* Chairman: Professor M Bobrow. London: HMSO, 1986.
10 Committee on Medical Aspects of Radiation in the Environment (COMARE). *Second report: investigation of the possible increased incidence of leukaemia in young people near the Dounreay nuclear establishment, Caithness, Scotland.* Chairman: Professor M Bobrow. London: HMSO, 1988.

11 Darby SC, Doll R. Fallout, radiation doses near Dounreay and childhood leukaemia. *BMJ* 1987;**294**:603.

12 Burnet M, White DO. *Natural history of infectious disease*. Cambridge: Cambridge University Press, 1972.

13 Yorke JA, Nathanson N, Pianigiani G, Martin J. Seasonality and the requirements for perpetuation and eradication of viruses in populations. *Am J Epidemiol* 1979;**109**:103.

14 Bartlett MS. Measles periodicity and community size. *Journal of the Royal Statistical Society [Series A]* 1957;**120**:48.

15 Smith PG. Spatial and temporal clustering. In: Schottenfeld D, Fraumani JR, eds. *Cancer epidemiology and prevention*. Philadelphia: WB Saunders, 1982.

16 General Register Office, General Register for Scotland, Office of Population Censuses and Surveys. *Census reports 1951, 1961, 1966, 1971, 1981*. London: HMSO.

17 Register General for Scotland. *Annual reports 1946–85*. London: HMSO.

18 MacGregor DR. A survey of the social and economic effects of the Forth road bridge with particular reference to the county of Fife. *Scottish Geographic Magazine* 1966;**82**:78.

19 Gardner MJ, Hall AJ, Downes S, Terrell JD. Follow up study of children born to mothers resident in Seascale, west Cumbria (birth cohort). *BMJ* 1987;**295**:822.

20 Gardner MJ, Hall AJ, Downes S, Terrell JD. Follow-up study of children born elsewhere but attending schools in Seascale, west Cumbria (schools cohort). *BMJ* 1987;**295**:819.

21 Francis DP, Essex M, Jakowski RM, Cotter SM, Lerer TJ, Hardy WD. Increased risk for lymphoma and glomerulonephritis in a closed population of cats exposed to feline leukaemia virus. *Am J Epidemiol* 1980;**111**:337.

22 Tyrrell DAJ. *Common colds and related diseases*. London: Arnold, 1965.

14: Infective cause of childhood leukaemia

Letter to the *Lancet*

ROBIN RUSSELL JONES

Dr Kinlen's hypothesis (*Lancet* 10 December 1988, p 1323, and preceding chapter) that the increased incidence of childhood leukaemia around reprocessing facilities in the United Kingdom can be explained by the large population influx into a susceptible community deserves serious consideration. However, it also begs questions, not least whether childhood leukaemia has a viral aetiology. Also the excess cases of leukaemia observed by Kinlen in a Scottish community remote from any nuclear facility occurred early in the period of population growth, whereas the only significant excess at Dounreay was confined to 1979–84, more than 20 years after the nuclear facility started operations.[1] Kinlen's mortality data also show a significant excess of deaths from non-Hodgkin's lymphoma around Dounreay (ratio of observed to expected deaths of 6 in the population aged under 25) but again this is confined to 1968–85. At Sellafield, excess cases of childhood leukaemia or lymphoma have been observed throughout the period of operation and show no signs of diminishing.[2] Thus eight cases of Hodgkin's or non-Hodgkin's lymphoma have occurred in Seascale since 1980, and in the under 25 population, three cases of non-Hodgkin's lymphoma have occurred since 1982, the last year analysed by the Black committee of inquiry. In a population of 2000 one might expect one young case of lymphoma or leukaemia every 30 years, so three in six years is significant (p < 0·001).

There is, however, a more fundamental objection to Kinlen's hypothesis. For the hypothesis to apply to Sellafield or Dounreay it would be necessary to show that the leukaemias occurred in the indigenous population and not in the migrants, unless of course the migrants happened to come from a remote area. For Sellafield we know that most of the affected children were born in the locality[3 4] but we are told nothing about their parents. In fact all of the Seascale children with leukaemia had at least one parent working at Sellafield, in all but two cases the parents had moved into the area, and the three recent cases of non-Hodgkin's lymphoma also occurred in migrant families. These observations virtually exclude Kinlen's hypothesis in relation to Sellafield.

My other concern with Kinlen's study is that it may detract attention from other more plausible explanations. Conventional radiobiology does not allow for the possibility that the doses received by the populations around Dounreay or Sellafield are sufficient to account for the excess leukaemias observed,[5 6] but such risk assessment models are fraught with uncertainty, particularly in relation to α-emitting radionuclides such as plutonium and americium.[7] Until recently the observation by Darby and Doll that national rates of childhood leukaemia did not change after the above ground weapons testing programme gave some confidence that the models were not completely useless,[8] but this observation has now been challenged. At a meeting at the Institute of British Geographers in Coventry (6 January 1989) G Bentham and R Haynes reported a peak in deaths from leukaemia in the 0–4 age group in the mid-1960s in regions of the United Kingdom with high rainfall.

These new data remove the remaining scientific obstacle to accepting that radioactive discharges from the two reprocessing facilities in the United Kingdom are responsible for the excess cases of leukaemia and lymphoma in the surrounding population. The only problem now is political: the recognition that British children are among the first victims of our independent nuclear deterrent.

1 Heasman MA, Kemp IW, Urquhart JD, Black R. Childhood leukaemia in northern Scotland. *Lancet* 1986;i:226.
2 Black D for the Independent Advisory Group. *Investigations of the possible increased incidence of cancer in west Cumbria.* London: HMSO, 1984. (Black report.)
3 Gardner MJ, Hall AJ, Downes S, Terrell JD. Follow up study of childhood born elsewhere but attending schools in Seascale, west Cumbria (schools cohort). *BMJ* 1987;**295**:819–21.
4 Gardner MJ, Hall AJ, Downes S, Terrell JD. Follow up study of children born to mothers resident in Seascale, west Cumbria (birth cohort). *BMJ* 1987;**295**:822–7.
5 Stather J, Wrixon A, Simmonds J. *The risks of leukaemia and other cancers in Seascale from radiation exposure.* London: HMSO, 1984. (Chilton NRPB-R 171).
6 Hill MD, Cooper JR. Radiation doses to members of the populations of Thurso. London: HMSO, 1986. (Chilton NRPB-R 195).
7 Crouch D. The rate of predictive modelling: social and scientific problems of radiation risk assessment. In: Russell Jones R, Southwood R, eds. *Radiation and health: the biological effects of low level exposure to ionising radiation.* Chichester: Wiley, 1987: 47–64.
8 Darby S, Doll R. Fallout, radiation doses near Dounreay, and childhood leukaemia. *BMJ* 1987;**294**:603–7.

15: Germ cell injury and childhood leukaemia clusters

Letter to the *Lancet*

T E WHELDON, R MAIRS, A BARRETT

The increased incidence of childhood leukaemia found near some United Kingdom nuclear establishments is not explicable by conventional models relating radiation dose to leukaemogenic risk.[1] One alternative hypothesis is parental germ cell injury by radiation or chemicals.[1] Germ cell injury by radiation and chemicals has been reported to predispose to malignancy in mice,[2] but human evidence is very sparse. Professor Greaves (*Lancet*, 14 January 1981, p 95) cites retinoblastoma as an instance where a causative molecular event (deletion or inactivation of the retinoblastoma gene) can occur either in germ or somatic cells, and he suggests a similar mechanism in some cases of childhood leukaemia.

The germ cell injury hypothesis in its most general form is as follows. Suppose that k molecular events (for example, mutations) are necessary to cause leukaemic transformation of a single cell and that, ordinarily, m of the resultant aberrations are transmitted via the germ line, leaving k-m to be acquired somatically. The hypothesis states that additional aberrations (for example, m + 1) are transmitted in the germ line because of presumed environmental injury to germ cells, so that fewer (k − [m + 1]) are required somatically for leukaemic transformation. Consequently, less time will be required until transformation of the first leukaemic cell, and the age distribution of the disease should be shifted to the left, to younger ages. This is a testable prediction. It is not necessary to assume, as in retinoblastoma, that exactly two molecular events are required, or that a familial subgroup will be prominent. It cannot be reliably concluded that an increased germ line component that predisposes to leukaemia must necessarily predispose to other malignancies; this will depend on the overlap of causative molecular events between different malignancies, but the possibility deserves consideration. Observation of age-incidence distributions and follow up studies of leukaemia cluster patients may provide indirect evidence on the germ cell injury hypothesis.

More direct evidence could also be sought. The likelihood of a germ line component in causing childhood cancer may be strengthened by the finding of chromosomal aberrations in non-malignant somatic cells of various tissues.[34] Similar evidence in the present context would be of great significance. Dr Nag and colleagues (*Lancet*, 4 February 1981, p 274) report a mutant H-ras gene in both malignant and non-malignant cells in a patient with bladder cancer and in the leucocytes of a healthy individual, implying that this oncogene may be transmitted via the germ line. This claim has been disputed (*Lancet*, 25 March 1981, p 668) but it is plausible that other oncogenes and genetic aberrations predisposing to malignancy are similarly transmitted. The finding of such aberrations in malignant and non-malignant somatic cells of unlike tissue type would suggest germ line transmission. These aberrations could be sought in patients in areas where clusters of leukaemia (or other childhood cancer) have occurred and compared with those found in non-cluster areas, or looked for whenever a raised incidence of leukaemia with unusually young ages of presentation has occurred over a wide area but within a limited time.[5]

The polymerase chain reaction method of amplifying specific DNA sequences has greatly simplified the investigation of allelic variation without the need for a genomic library, for screening, or for gene sequence mapping. Molecular studies will therefore become increasingly practicable in the investigation of cancer clusters in young children, and the results may provide evidence pertinent to the hypothesis of an increased component of germ cell injury in causing some cases of childhood malignancy.

1 Committee on Medical Aspects of Radiation in the Environment (COMARE) (chairman Professor M Bobrow). *Investigation of the possible increased incidence of leukaemia in young people near the Dounreay nuclear establishment, Caithness, Scotland*. London: HMSO, 1988.
2 Nomura T. Parental exposure to X-rays and chemicals induces heritable tumours and anomalies in mice. *Nature* 1982;**296**:575–7.
3 Moriyama M, Shuin T, Kubota Y, Satomi Y, *et al*. A case of rhabdomyosarcoma of the bladder with a (2;5) chromosomal translocation in peripheral lymphocytes. *Cancer Genet Cytogenet* 1986;**22**:177–81.
4 Brodeur GM, Caces J, Williams DL, Look AT, Pratt CB. Osteosarcoma, fibrous dysplasia and a chromosome abnormality in a 3 year old child. *Cancer* 1980;**46**: 1197–201.
5 Gibson B, Eden OB, Barrett A, Stiller CA, Draper GJ. Leukaemia in young children in Scotland. *Lancet* 1988;**ii**:630.

16: Geographical variation in mortality from leukaemia and other cancers in England and Wales in relation to proximity to nuclear installations, 1969–78

P J COOK-MOZAFFARI, S C DARBY, R DOLL, D FORMAN, C HERMON, M C PIKE, T VINCENT

The distribution of mortality from 11 causes of death (lymphoid leukaemia, other leukaemia, leukaemia of all types, Hodgkin's disease, other lymphomas, all lymphomas, multiple myeloma, lung cancer, other malignancies, all malignancies, and all other causes) has been examined in three age groups throughout England and Wales over the period 1969–78. The reorganisation of local authority administration in 1974 meant that the smallest areas that could be examined were 400 county districts or (in some cases) approximate county districts formed by aggregating pre-1974 local authority areas. The variation in the numbers of deaths observed about the numbers expected was assessed using log-linear models to estimate the effect on the relative risk in each district associated with social class, rural status, population size, health authority region, and proximity to one of 15 nuclear installations. Trends in risk with increasing proximity to an installation (as judged by the proportion of the population resident within 10 miles) were examined after adjustment for the other four variables. The results showed that in districts near to an installation there were significant excess mortalities from leukaemia in persons under 25 years of age (relative risk = 1·15, p = 0·01) and especially from lymphoid leukaemia (relative risk 1·21, p = 0·01) and from Hodgkin's disease (relative risk 1·24, p = 0·05) and a significant deficiency of mortality from lymphoid leukaemia in persons aged 25–64 years. No significant trends were observed with an increasing proportion of the population near to the installations and the greatest excess mortality from lymphoid leukaemia in young persons was observed in the districts with the intermediate proportion of the population (10·0–65·9%) near an installation.

Reports of an increased incidence of leukaemia in young people near certain nuclear installations have caused concern about the possible effect on communities that live near other such installations. The extent and localisation of the increase near Sellafield leaves no doubt about its reality,[1] but it is not clear how far many of the other reports represent selection of high rates that are bound to occur by chance, while low rates are neglected. To check this possibility the evidence relating to all the installations in the country needs to be examined. This, however, is not easy to do as the reorganisation of local government in 1974 altered the boundaries of most administrative units and made it difficult to obtain relevant figures for each area of interest over a long enough period.

In England and Wales the Office of Population Censuses and Surveys (OPCS) overcame this difficulty by using the pre-1974 local authority areas and allocating the cancer registrations and deaths that had been reported since 1974 to the old areas.[2] In that study, local authority areas with more than a third of their population within 10 miles of an installation were compared with control areas that were chosen to be more distant from the installations but of similar population size, urban/rural status, and, as far as possible, within the same standard region. The results supported the idea that in recent years the mortality from leukaemia, and especially lymphoid leukaemia, in young people tended to be relatively high in areas close to installations that began operations before 1955, but showed that in adults mortality from all cancers, considered as a group, tended to be relatively low.[3] Some of the relatively high rates around nuclear installations were, however, difficult to assess, as the main reason for them was unusually low rates in the control local authority areas.

We have therefore tackled the problem in another way. Like the OPCS we have limited ourselves to England and Wales but, instead of trying to select matched control areas, we have considered data for the whole country and have taken into account the effect of four factors that may influence the mortality from cancer (namely rural status, population size, socioeconomic distribution of the population, and health authority region). We have compared the mortality rates in areas close to nuclear installations with the rates in all other parts of the country, after making allowance for any effect that the above four factors might have. For this purpose, we have classed as nuclear installations all the 15 installations studied in the OPCS report; that is, the three installations of British Nuclear Fuels Ltd (BNFL) at Sellafield, Springfields, and Capenhurst, the two United Kingdom Atomic Energy Authority (UKAEA) installations at Harwell and Winfrith, the Ministry of Defence (MoD) installation at Aldermaston, Amersham International plc's installation at Amersham, and the eight Central Electricity Generating Board (CEGB) installations at Bradwell, Berkeley, Dungeness, Hinkley, Oldbury, Sizewell, Trawsfynydd, and Wylfa (see figure). All the installations operated by BNFL, UKAEA, MoD, and Amersham International began to discharge radioactive waste before 1955, with the exception of Winfrith which began to do so in 1964. Seven of the eight CEGB installations began operations between 1961 and 1965 and the eighth, Wylfa, began in 1971. Berkeley and Oldbury have been classed together as they are very near to each other. Other installations, the discharges from which have been at least an order of magnitude less than those from the CEGB installations, for example, Burghfield,[4] and installations with start up after the period for which cancer data have been analysed, have been omitted.

Analyses have used only mortality data. Since the mid-1960s these have become progressively less satisfactory as indicators of the incidence of some types of cancer, and particularly of leukaemia in young people, because treatment has improved and fatality has been reduced. We believe, nevertheless, that local variation in mortality was the best available indicator of local variation in the incidence of leukaemia and of most other cancers during the period of our study (1969–78) as registration of cancer was incomplete and consequently likely to be biased by local interest in local incidence.[5 6]

Materials and methods

Eleven causes of death (or groups of causes) have been examined separately within the three age bands, 0–24 years, 25–64 years, and 65 years and over. These age bands were chosen at the outset of the study, before the data were compiled, to include the band initially examined in the Black inquiry.[7] The 11 causes are listed in table I, together with the total number of deaths attributed to them in each age group in the period 1969–78. This

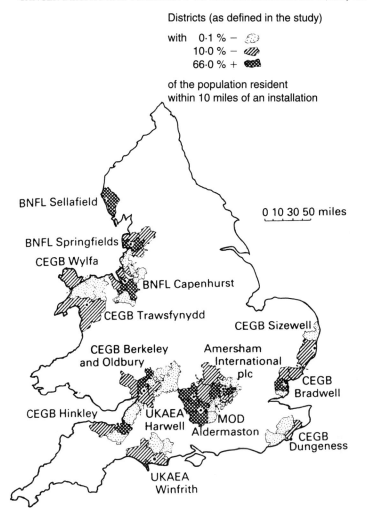

Districts (as defined in the study)

with 0·1 % –
 10·0 % –
 66·0 % +

of the population resident
within 10 miles of an installation

BNFL Sellafield

0 10 30 50 miles

BNFL Springfields
CEGB Wylfa

BNFL Capenhurst

CEGB Trawsfynydd

CEGB Sizewell

CEGB Berkeley
and Oldbury

Amersham
International
plc

CEGB
Bradwell

CEGB Hinkley   UKAEA
Harwell

MOD
Aldermaston

CEGB
Dungeness

UKAEA
Winfrith

Location of nuclear installations and installation districts included in the study.

limited period was chosen for study for three reasons: firstly, to concentrate on the period after the start up of almost all the installations, when any hazard with a latent period measured in years would be capable of detection; secondly, to be able to examine separately figures for lymphoid leukaemia which, until 1968, had not been possible as deaths from acute lymphoid and acute myeloid leukaemia had been classed together; and thirdly, because the OPCS was able to make available death rates for complete quinquennia only.

121

TABLE I—*Total number of deaths from selected causes: England and Wales 1969–78 by age*

Cause of death	ICD code*	Age		
		0–24	25–64	65+
Leukaemia—all types	204–207	4 230	10 412	16 466
Lymphoid leukaemia	204	2 401	2 329	6 315
Other leukaemia	205–207	1 829	8 083	10 151
All lymphomas	200–202	1 628	11 882	11 818
Hodgkin's disease	201	683	4 410	2 494
Other lymphomas	200, 202	945	7 472	9 324
Multiple myeloma	203	3†	4 290	8 128
Cancer of lung	162	112†	126 836	194 834
Other malignancies	other 140–207	6 214	278 766	523 690
All maligancies	140–207	12 187	432 186	754 936
All other causes	other	185 985	901 971	3 525 583
All causes	001–999	198 172	1 334 157	4 280 519

* International Classification of Diseases, 8th Revision[8]; † These have been grouped with "other malignancies" in the analyses.

To calculate mortality in the pre-1974 local authority areas during the period 1959–80, Cook-Mozaffari *et al* first had to estimate the mean population in each area using data obtained in the 1961, 1971, and 1981 censuses.[2] Figures were already available for each area after the earlier two censuses, but new calculations had to be made to build up from data for census wards and enumeration districts comparable population figures for 1981. This was possible for the limited number of pre-1974 areas studied in the OPCS report, but it was not practicable for us to obtain similar figures for all the 1316 local authority areas throughout the whole country. We have therefore been constrained by the need to use the 402 new post-1974 county districts as the smallest practicable units for which both 1971 and 1981 census data were available.

Information about cancer deaths is not available by county districts before 1974, but deaths can be summed into pre-1974 local authority areas up to 1980. To obtain areal units for which mortality rates could be compared for a period that straddles the 1974 boundary changes we have combined pre-1974 local authority areas so as to make them as nearly as possible coterminous with post-1974 county districts. For 249 districts the correspondence is exact. For the remaining 153 an approximation has been made and in two instances a pair of county districts has had to be combined. The resulting 400 areas—county districts, approximate county districts, and combined county districts—are the basic units of this study and are referred to in the remainder of the chapter simply as "districts".

For each district the population for 1971 by sex and age has been obtained by summation from the 1971 census. A similar population for 1976 has been derived by linear interpolation between the 1971 and 1981 censuses, with the assumption that in 1981 the relative size of the population in the approximate districts compared with the actual districts on which each was based was, for each age-sex group, the same as in 1971. This assumption was made possible by the fact that the 1971 census had been published for both the pre-1974 local authority areas and the post-1974 districts. The two sets of figures for 1971 and 1976 were then used to calculate average population figures for the period 1969–78.

The number of deaths that occurred in 1969–78 in each district was obtained in the same way: that is by building up from the allocations to the pre-1974 local authority areas. The numbers of deaths expected in each district were then calculated by multiplying the estimated populations by the corresponding 10 year England and Wales death rates for each sex and 5 year age group.

STATISTICAL ANALYSIS

The variation in the observed numbers of deaths in the 400 districts about the numbers expected has been assessed by log-linear regression analyses carried out using the GLIM computer program.[9] Preliminary analysis showed that for many diseases, including childhood leukaemia and most notably the lymphoid type, the residual variation was in excess of that expected from Poisson sampling theory, and allowance was therefore made for extra-Poisson variation using the method of Breslow.[10] In these analyses log-linear models were used to estimate the relative risk associated with the five variables described below. No account has been taken in this chapter of possible variation in mortality associated with external terrestrial γ radiation. Preliminary analyses, however, show no evidence of an association. Significance tests were carried out by comparing χ^2 goodness-to-fit statistics as recommended by Breslow,[10] or by comparing estimates of changes in log-relative risks with their standard errors. One sided tests in the direction of the observed difference were used throughout, apart from tests of heterogeneity which are necessarily many sided (see also note added in proof at end of this chapter). The five variables considered were social class, rural status, population size, health authority region, and proximity to a nuclear installation.

Social class

Data giving the number of persons in each of 15 socioeconomic groupings used in the 1971 census (excluding men and women in the armed forces and in unspecified occupations) have been summed to give for each

123

district the approximate proportion of the population in each of the six principal social class grades (I, professional; II, intermediate; IIIN, skilled non-manual; IIIM, skilled manual; IV, partly skilled; and V, unskilled).[11]

Rural status

Districts have been classified simply as rural and other, using Webber and Craig's categorisation,[12] and the characteristics of the county districts defined by Webber and Craig have been assumed to apply to the corresponding approximate county districts.

Population size

Districts have been grouped into those with a population of less than 50 000, 50 000–99 999, 100 000–149 999, 150 000–299 999, and 300 000 and over in 1971.

Health authority region

Districts have been grouped into the 15 health authority regions to allow for the effects of broad geographical differences and for possible effects of differing diagnostic practice or treatment regimens between health authority regions.

Proximity to a nuclear installation

The position of each nuclear installation has been located from its grid reference on large scale maps. Circles with a radius that represented 10 miles were drawn around each installation. The proportion falling within this radius was estimated using the method described for the OPCS study,[2] except that, where no parish had more than half its area within the 10 mile radius, the actual area of the parishes that had any part within the circle was assessed as a percentage of the area of the districts in which they lay, and it was assumed that this percentage of each district's population lay within the 10 mile radius.

NUCLEAR INSTALLATION DISTRICTS

In the course of the log-linear regression analyses, relative risks have been estimated for all districts that have at least 0·1% of the population within a 10 mile radius, relative to all other districts. Trends in risk with increasing proximity to an installation have been carried out by examining three categories of district: those with 66·0% or more of the population living within 10 miles of an installation (high proportion zone, 20 districts); those with 10·0–65·9% (middle proportion zone, 24 districts) and those with 0·1–9·9% within the 10 mile zone (low proportion zone, 26 districts) (see figure).

In this chapter the areas considered close to installations are broader than those considered in the OPCS report,[2] a condition dictated by the use of county districts as the basis of investigation. The precise relation between the two sets of areas is set out in table II. It can be seen that whereas 98% of the population resident in the high proportion zone of the present study was included in one of the four zones defined as close to an installation in the OPCS study, this was true of only about 30% of the middle proportion zone and of less than 1% of the low proportion zone.

All comparisons in which districts close to grouped installations are examined have been made separately including and excluding Copeland district, which is the only district with more than 0·1% of its population near Sellafield. The results can, therefore, be used to test hypotheses based on the original observations near Sellafield.[7]

Results

SOCIOECONOMIC AND GEOGRAPHICAL VARIATION

Districts that are near to nuclear installations were found to have, on average, a higher proportion of their population in social classes I, II, and IIIN and a lower proportion in social classes IIIM, IV, and V than other districts. These nearby districts also had somewhat smaller populations, very few having more than 150 000 inhabitants. There was little difference in the proportion classed as rural, but a substantial difference in the distribution by regional health authority, 86% (60 out of 70 districts) being located in seven of the 15 regions (North West, Mersey, Oxford, North West Thames, Wessex, South West, and Wales).

The variation in relative risk by these four variables is given in table III for all leukaemia and the leukaemia subtypes at ages 0–24. For all leukaemia there is an upward trend in risk with an increasing proportion of the population being of higher social class after adjustment for the other three variables ($p = 0.001$) but the effect is confined to lymphoid leukaemia ($p = 0.001$) and is not present for other types ($p = 0.24$). For lymphoid leukaemia also there is evidence of regional variation ($p = 0.02$). It should be noted that the estimated relative risks associated with social class in table III describe the relation between mortality and the social class structure of the districts. They do not describe the risk to an individual associated with belonging to a particular social class, but the ratio of the relative risks for any two social classes shows instead the overall effect on mortality in a district associated with a shift of 5% of the total population from the social class of the denominator to that of the numerator, when the proportions in the other classes remain the same. For example, the results for leukaemia of all types would indicate that a 3% shift from social class IV to social class I would tend to increase the number of deaths observed in the district by a factor of $(1·06/1·02)^{3/5}$.

TABLE II—*Relation between populations defined as living close to installations in the OPCS study[2] and in the present study (populations in thousands)*

Zones of the present study (characterised by the percentage of the population resident within 10 miles)	Discrete distance zones in the OPCS study				Control LAAs in the OPCS study	Other LAAs not in the OPCS study	Total population included in the present study
	1*	2†	3‡	4§			
	population in end category						
High proportion (66·0+)	493	326	865	165	12	23	1 884
Middle proportion (10·0–65·9)	71	96	213	438	211	1 713	2 742
Low proportion (0·1–9·9)	0	0	0	3	318	2 741	3 062
Other districts (<0·1)	0	0	0	0	2 117	39 348	41 465
Total population in 1971	564	422	1 078	606	2 658	43 825	49 153

OPCS = Office of Population Censuses and Surveys. LAAs = local authority areas. *Two thirds of the population resident within six miles of an installation; † Two thirds of the population resident within eight miles but excluding those resident in zone 1; ‡ Two thirds of the population resident within 10 miles but excluding those resident in zones 1 or 2; § One third of the population resident within 10 miles but excluding those resident in zones 1, 2, and 3.

TABLE III—*Variation in relative risk of death from selected causes at ages 0–24 by social class, rural status, population size, and health authority region. Relative risks for each variable are calculated after adjustment for the other three*

		Leukaemia all types	Lymphoid leukaemia	Other leukaemia
Social class	I	1·06	1·03	1·09
(relative risks associated	II	1·09	1·07	1·12
with a 5% shift)	IIIN	1·03	1·05	1·00
	IIIM	1·03	0·99	1·08
	IV	1·02	1·01	1·04
	V	1·00	1·00	1·00
p value for heterogeneity		0·07	0·07	0·35
p value for trend*		0·001	0·001	0·24
Rural/other (1·00)		1·09	1·07	1·11
p value for difference*		0·22	0·50	0·28
Population size	<50	1·00	1·00	1·00
(thousands)	50–100	1·14	1·23	1·04
	100–150	1·18	1·23	1·13
	150–300	1·22	1·22	1·22
	>300	1·18	1·14	1·24
p value for heterogeneity		1·00†	1·00‡	1·00§
p value for trend*		0·50‖	0·24	0·50¶
Health authority region	Northern	1·06	1·16	0·94
(England and	Yorkshire	0·93	0·89	0·98
Wales = 1·00)	North West	1·01	1·16	0·84
	Mersey	1·07	1·09	1·05
	Trent	1·04	1·09	0·98
	West Midlands	1·13	1·18	1·06
	East Anglia	0·97	1·02	0·92
	Oxford	1·16	1·17	1·15
	North West Thames	0·96	0·81	1·18
	North East Thames	0·97	0·96	0·99
	South East Thames	1·01	1·00	1·04
	South West Thames	1·00	1·02	0·96
	Wessex	0·90	0·83	1·02
	South West	0·90	0·87	0·95
	Wales	0·94	0·88	1·01
p value for heterogeneity		0·50	0·02	0·93

* One sided tests; † deviance based p value 0·40; ‡ deviance based p value 0·45; § deviance based p value 0·23; ‖ deviance based p value 0·10; ¶ deviance based p value 0·01 (see note added in proof at end of chapter).

VARIATION IN RISK NEAR NUCLEAR INSTALLATIONS

Table IV gives the relative risks at ages 0–24 and 25–64 for districts that have 0·1% or more of their population living within 10 miles of an installation. Values are given both with and without adjustment for the socioeconomic and geographical variables and both including and excluding Copeland district. At ages 0–24 there is a tendency for the relative risks to be slightly higher and for the significance levels to be slightly more extreme with the inclusion of Copeland, but the effect is small. At other

TABLE IV—*Relative risk of death from selected causes in districts with 0·1% or more of their population resident within 10 miles of a nuclear installation compared with other districts, by age at death. Unadjusted values are given, and also values adjusted for social class, rural status, population size, and regional health authority, both including and excluding Copeland district in which Sellafield is situated*

		Ages 0–24				Ages 25–64			
		All districts (including Copeland)		Excluding Copeland		All districts (including Copeland)		Excluding Copeland	
		Relative risk	p Value*	Relative risk	p Value*	Relative risk	p Value*	Relative risk	p Value*
Leukaemia—all types	unadjusted	1·12	0·005	1·11	0·008	0·98	0·33	0·99	0·34
	adjusted	1·15	0·01†	1·14	0·03‡	0·97	0·15	0·97	0·16
Lymphoid leukaemia	unadjusted	1·16	0·007	1·16	0·01	0·89	0·13	0·89	0·14
	adjusted	1·21	0·01§	1·20	0·02‖	0·86	0·05	0·87	0·06
Other leukaemia	unadjusted	1·06	0·34	1·06	0·36	1·01	0·35	1·01	0·34
	adjusted	1·07	0·50	1·06	0·50	1·00	0·49	1·00	0·46
All lymphomas	unadjusted	1·04	0·25	1·04	0·28	0·99	0·50	0·99	0·50
	adjusted	1·10	0·09	1·09	0·10	0·99	0·39	0·99	0·42
Hodgkin's disease	unadjusted	1·09	0·09	1·08	0·11	0·98	0·30	0·98	0·32
	adjusted	1·24	0·05	1·23	0·04	0·99	0·44	1·00	0·49
Other lymphomas	unadjusted	1·01	0·50	1·00	0·50	0·99	0·50	0·99	0·50
	adjusted	1·00	0·50	0·99	0·50	1·00	0·49	1·00	0·50
Multiple myeloma	unadjusted	—	—	—	—	1·05	0·13	1·04	0·15
	adjusted	—	—	—	—	1·04	0·21	1·04	0·24
Cancer of the lung	unadjusted	—	—	—	—	0·95	0·02	0·95	0·02
	adjusted	—	—	—	—	0·99	0·28	0·99	0·35
Other malignancies	unadjusted	1·00	0·50	0·99	0·44	0·99	0·19	0·99	0·16
	adjusted	1·03	0·27	1·02	0·31	0·99	0·26	0·99	0·24
All malignancies	unadjusted	1·04	0·06	1·04	0·09	0·98	0·06	0·98	0·05
	adjusted	1·07	0·03	1·06	0·05	0·99	0·21	0·99	0·23
Other causes	unadjusted	0·95	0·003	0·95	0·003	0·96	0·04	0·95	0·03
	adjusted	0·97	0·02	0·97	0·02	0·98	0·08	0·98	0·08

*One sided tests calculated by the method of Breslow to allow for extra-Poisson variation[10]; † deviance based p value 0·005; ‡ deviance based p value

ages the exclusion of Copeland makes practically no difference. In the following description of results, therefore, reference is made only to data including Copeland district.

Elevated relative risks occur at ages 0–24 for all leukaemia and for lymphoid leukaemia. The relative risks are highest for lymphoid leukaemia and slightly higher after adjustment than before (values after adjustment: all leukaemia relative risk = 1·15, p = 0·01; lymphoid leukaemia relative risk = 1·21, p = 0·01). Raised relative risks also occur for all malignancies and Hodgkin's disease that are significant after adjustment (relative risk = 1·07, p = 0·03 and relative risk = 1·24, p = 0·05 respectively). For non-malignant diseases there is a slight reduction of relative risk which is less pronounced after adjustment, but which still remains significantly low (relative risk = 0·97; p = 0·02).

At ages 25–64, no relative risks are significantly raised. For lymphoid leukaemia the relative risk is low after adjustment for the background variables (relative risk = 0·86; p = 0·05). For all other groups of disease the relative risks are close to, and not significantly different from, unity after adjustment (range of relative risks 0·97–1·04).

Calculations as in table IV have also been made for persons aged 65 and over. When all districts including Copeland were considered, no relative risks were significantly above unity either before or after adjustment.

In table V relative risks are given for those individual types of cancer that in table IV showed a significant deviation from unity after adjustment. Details are given for all installations, all installations excluding Sellafield (that is, excluding Copeland district), the four categories of installations that were used in the analyses of the OPCS study, and each of the 15 individual installations. Overall figures are given for all districts with at least 0·1% of their population resident within 10 miles of an installation (pooled installation districts) and separate figures are given for the high, middle, and low proportion zones, so that the trend in relative risk with increasing proportion of the population living within 10 miles of an installation can be examined.

For all leukaemia at ages 0–24, when the pooled installation districts are considered for the four categories of installations used in the OPCS study, there is a significant increase near Sellafield (relative risk = 1·85, p = 0·03). The relative risks for other pre-1955 installations (1·14) and for all CEGB installations combined (1·15) are also raised, although only that for the pre-1955 installations is significantly high (p = 0·03). For none of the three categories with districts in more than one zone is there evidence of a significant trend in relative risk with increasing proportion of the population living within 10 miles of an installation. When individual installations other than Sellafield are considered, the relative risk for the pooled installation districts is raised significantly above unity only for Springfields (relative risk = 1·25; p = 0·04).

For lymphoid leukaemia at ages 0–24, the results are similar except that the relative risks for the pooled installation districts in all four OPCS groupings are higher than they are for all leukaemia, although the relative risk is significantly greater than unity only for the pre-1955 installations other than Sellafield. For the individual installations, the relative risks are significantly raised for the pooled installation districts around Springfields ($p = 0.009$) and Sizewell ($p = 0.02$). Neither for the four categories nor for the individual installations is there any indication of trend apart from a decrease in risk with increasing proportion of the population near to Bradwell.

For Hodgkin's disease at ages 0–24, when the pooled installation districts are considered for the four categories, there is a raised relative risk for the CEGB installations (relative risk = 1.48, $p = 0.03$) but no clear indication of a trend. When the individual installations are considered, there is a raised relative risk for the CEGB installation at Wylfa (relative risk = 4.72, $p = 0.01$) and an increase in risk between the only two zones (low and middle proportion) that are near to Dungeness ($p = 0.02$).

For lymphoid leukaemia at ages 25–64, the relative risks for the pooled installation districts are below unity for each of the summary groupings used in the OPCS study and for all but one of the individual installations, although only for Dungeness is the pooled relative risk significantly low (relative risk = 0.53, $p = 0.04$). At Dungeness there is a trend of decreasing risk between the two zones that are near to this installation ($p = 0.05$), and at Winfrith and Trawsfynydd there are trends of increasing risk ($p = 0.02$ and $p = 0.01$ respectively).

Further analyses of the type presented in table V were made for non-malignant diseases at ages 0–24 but showed no significant deviation from unity and no significant trends either for the four categories of installations or for individual installations.

Discussion

COMPARISON WITH OPCS STUDY

For leukaemia of all types and for lymphoid leukaemia, the results of the present study echo and extend those derived from the OPCS study,[23] despite substantial differences in methodology. For example, when installation local authority areas with more than two thirds of their population resident within six miles of an installation were compared with their controls during the period for which information was available on leukaemia subtypes, there wws a 1.46-fold increase for leukaemia and a twofold increase in deaths from lymphoid leukaemia at ages 0–24,[3] whereas in the present study, after adjustment for four socioeconomic and demographic variables, there is a 15% increase in leukaemia and a 21% increase

TABLE V—*Relative risks of death from selected types of cancer at different ages in districts with 0·1% or more of their population resident within 10 miles of a nuclear installation compared with other districts, by installation and percentage of the population within 10 miles adjusted for social class, rural status, population size, and regional health authority*

	Leukaemia—all types ages 0–24					Lymphoid leukaemia ages 0–24				
	All districts with at least 0·1	Relative risks for districts with specified percentage of the population resident within 10 miles of an installation (number of deaths in parentheses)				All districts with at least 0·1	Relative risks for districts with specified percentage of the population resident within 10 miles of an installation (number of deaths in parentheses)			
		0·1–9·9	10·0–65·9	66·0§	p Value for trend§		0·1–9·9	10·0–65·9	66·0§	p Value for trend§
All installations	1·15†	1·16* (295)	1·19† (269)	1·09 (181)	0·36	1·21†	1·18* (165)	1·29† (160)	1·16 (112)	0·40
All excluding Sellafield	1·14*	1·15* (295)	1·18* (269)	1·05 (170)	0·26	1·20*	1·17 (165)	1·29† (160)	1·12 (105)	0·45
OPCS categories:										
BNFL Sellafield	1·85*	—	—	1·84* (11)	—	1·94	—	—	1·94 (7)	—
Other pre-1955 installations	1·14*	1·23* (185)	1·22* (183)	1·02 (151)	0·09	1·21*	1·21 (102)	1·32* (108)	1·13 (97)	0·37
UKAEA Winfrith	0·96	0·93 (6)	0·97 (12)	—	0·42	1·06	1·28 (4)	0·94 (6)	—	0·27
CEGB installations	1·15	1·09 (104)	1·18 (74)	1·42 (19)	0·09	1·20	1·12 (59)	1·32* (46)	1·11 (8)	0·20
Individual installations:										
BNFL Sellafield	1·81*	—	—	1·79* (11)	—	1·87	—	—	1·81 (7)	—
Springfields	1·25*	1·47 (39)	1·32 (22)	1·14 (39)	0·26	1·47†	1·69 (27)	1·45 (12)	1·47* (31)	0·44
Capenhurst	1·09	1·01 (54)	1·31 (102)	0·99 (22)	0·30	0·92	0·70 (23)	1·28 (60)	0·78 (11)	0·19
Amersham International	1·18	1·27 (67)	1·19 (47)	1·06 (51)	0·15	1·26	1·36 (37)	1·25 (26)	1·15 (29)	0·26
MoD Aldermaston	1·11	1·39 (25)	—	0·95 (32)	0·13	1·29	1·37 (15)	—	1·24 (23)	0·38
UKAEA Harwell	0·77	—	0·82 (12)	0·67 (7)	0·32	0·90	—	1·19 (10)	0·48 (3)	0·08
Winfrith	0·96	0·96 (6)	1·00 (12)	—	0·50	1·09	1·30 (4)	1·01 (6)	—	0·32
CEGB Bradwell	1·17	1·62 (9)	1·05 (19)	0·98 (3)	0·14	1·02	1·72 (6)	0·96 (10)	—	0·04
Berkeley and Oldbury	1·12	1·03 (43)	1·13 (23)	1·62 (8)	0·17	1·06	0·92 (22)	1·24 (15)	0·00 (0)	0·37
Hinckley	1·23	1·04 (19)	2·28 (4)	1·48 (8)	0·19	1·12	0·82 (9)	2·20 (2)	1·13 (3)	0·13
Trawsfynydd	1·21	1·08 (11)	1·65 (6)	—	0·17	1·46	1·36 (7)	1·81 (7)	1·65 (5)	0·39
Dungeness	0·93	0·96 (12)	0·91 (6)	—	0·39	0·97	1·11 (8)	0·75 (3)	—	0·28
Sizewell	1·44	1·29 (10)	1·65 (12)	—	0·30	1·88*	1·64 (7)	2·19* (9)	—	0·29
Wylfa	0·72	—	0·74 (4)	—	—	1·48	—	1·52 (4)	—	—

131

TABLE V—continued

	Hodgkin's disease ages 0–24					Lymphoid leukaemia ages 25–64				
All installations	1·24*	0·91 (33)	1·82‡ (58)	0·99 (24)	0·18	0·86*	0·88 (136)	0·92 (122)	0·76* (72)	0·25
All excluding Sellafield	1·23*	0·90 (33)	1·81‡ (58)	0·94 (22)	0·18	0·87	0·88 (136)	0·92 (122)	0·77* (70)	0·28
OPCS categories:										
BNFL Sellafield	1·86	—	—	1·81 (2)	—	0·53	—	—	0·52 (2)	—
Other pre-1955 installations	1·06	0·73 (17)	1·62* (36)	0·94 (21)	0·50	0·90	0·94 (79)	0·99 (80)	0·81 (65)	0·22
UKAEA Winfrith	1·39	0·94 (1)	1·57 (3)	—	0·20	0·52	0·19* (1)	0·74 (6)	—	0·01∥
CEGB installations	1·48*	1·13 (15)	2·10† (19)	0·56 (1)	0·07	0·86	0·89 (56)	0·87 (36)	0·58 (5)	0·50
Individual installations:										
BNFL Sellafield	1·87	—	—	1·74 (2)	—	0·52	—	—	0·50 (2)	—
Springfields	0·89	0·81 (3)	0·30 (1)	1·39 (7)	0·13	0·88	1·03 (16)	0·70 (9)	0·90 (20)	0·36
Capenhurst	1·27	1·11 (9)	1·64 (18)	0·88 (3)	0·36	0·83	0·91 (25)	0·99 (42)	0·51* (7)	0·13
Amersham International	1·25	0·51 (4)	2·74† (15)	0·91 (7)	0·32	0·98	0·94 (32)	1·17 (24)	0·84 (23)	0·37
MoD Aldermaston	0·67	0·42 (1)	—	0·84 (4)	0·50	0·96	0·83 (6)	—	1·02 (13)	0·41
UKAEA Harwell	0·65	—	1·33 (2)	0·00 (0)	0·07	0·78	—	1·03 (5)	0·48 (2)	0·18
Winfrith	1·36	0·82 (1)	1·52 (3)	—	0·21	0·53	0·19 (1)	0·74 (6)	—	0·02¶
CEGB Bradwell	1·41	2·35 (1)	1·42 (4)	0·00 (0)	0·14	0·67	0·57 (1)	0·75 (8)	0·41 (1)	0·39
Berkeley and Oldbury	1·22	1·19 (7)	0·55 (4)	0·00 (0)	0·50	0·98	1·09 (26)	0·95 (12)	0·34 (1)	0·21
Hinckley	0·92	0·82 (2)	0·00 (0)	1·73 (1)	0·43	0·90	0·82 (10)	1·21 (2)	0·98 (3)	0·50
Trawsfynydd	0·99	0·63 (1)	1·96 (1)	—	0·20	1·37	0·87 (8)	2·68† (9)	—	0·01
Dungeness	2·14	0·57 (5)	4·50† (5)	—	0·02	0·53*	0·72 (5)	0·18* (1)	—	0·05
Sizewell	1·57	1·61 (2)	1·50 (2)	—	0·47	0·71	0·99 (5)	0·43 (2)	—	0·17
Wylfa	4·72*	—	4·49† (3)	—	—	0·64	—	0·65 (2)	—	0·50

OPCS = Office of Population Censuses and Surveys; BNFL = British Nuclear Fuels Ltd; UKAEA = United Kingdom Atomic Energy Authority; CEGB = Central Electricity Generating Board; MoD = Ministry of Defence. * 0·05 > p > 0·01; † 0·01 ≥ p > 0·001; ‡ p ≤ 0·001; § One sided tests: Both Sellafield and Winfrith appear twice in this table for each disease, once under "OPCS categories" and once under "individual installations." In some cases the values under these two entries are different, especially at ages 0–24. This is because the estimates are derived from slightly different multiple regression models. In both models the background variables are included but in one case individual terms for the remaining installations are included, while in the other the remaining installations are grouped into "other pre-1955" and "CEGB" installations. In no case are the results obtained under the two models substantially different, although in some instances the significance levels are slightly affected; ∥ deviance based p value 0·07; ¶ deviance based p value 0·08 (see note added in proof at end of chapter).

in lymphoid leukaemia at ages 0–24 in districts that had any part within 10 miles of nuclear installations ($p = 0.01$ in both instances). The differences in the size of the observed effects between the two studies are the combined consequence of three major differences in methodology. Firstly, in the present study, all districts in England and Wales with less than 0.1% of their population within 10 miles of an installation have been included as controls, giving a total control population of over 40 million. In the OPCS study, control areas of roughly the same population size as the installation areas were selected, which gave a control group of some two and a half million overall and of only half a million for comparison with the six mile distance zone cited above. Secondly, differences in mortality because of region of the country, urban or rural status, population size, and social class structure have been taken into account by regression analysis, instead of by selective matching. Thirdly, to obtain data covering the whole of England and Wales, it has been necessary to base the study on larger geographical units, namely the 402 post-1974 county districts of England and Wales, rather than the 1316 pre-1974 local authority areas. The consequence of this is that we have had to consider larger areas surrounding the installations, so that a total population of nearly seven and a half million has been classified as living near a nuclear installation, while in the OPCS study the total "exposed" population was under three million (see table II).

A further finding of the OPCS study was that at ages 25–74 there was a deficit of 6% of deaths from lung cancer and a 4% deficit of deaths from all malignancies in local authority areas with at least two thirds of their population resident within eight miles of installations.[3] It does not seem likely that living near a nuclear installation can protect against the development of cancer, and it was concluded that the deficits of lung cancer and all malignancies in the installation local authority areas among adults were likely to have resulted from socioeconomic or other environmental differences between the installation and the control areas. In the present study, after adjustment for the four socioeconomic and geographical variables, the relative risks of death from lung cancer and all malignancies at ages 25–64 in the pooled installation districts compared with other districts are both very close to unity (lung cancer relative risk = 0.99, $p = 0.28$; all malignancies relative risk = 0.99, $p = 0.21$ (one sided tests)) and we conclude that the regression adjustments, together with the use of the more restricted age group, 25–64, have been highly successful in eliminating social, economic, and environmental differences, other than proximity to a nuclear installation, that may affect cancer mortality. For diseases other than cancer in the present study, the relative risks are also low before adjustment and move close to unity with adjustment, although the deficit for non-malignant diseases at ages 0–24 remains significant (relative risk = 0.97, $p = 0.02$).

The fact that the OPCS study, which was able to identify populations

133

living within six miles of an installation, gave a higher estimate of relative risk than the present study, which has considered broader geographical areas, might at first sight be thought to imply that the increases are concentrated very close to the installations. Three observations indicate that this may not be so: firstly, there is no suggestion of increasing trend in relative risk with an increasing proportion of the population near to an installation in the present study (see table V); secondly, the difference in the number of excess deaths estimated from the two studies implies that the increase may not be confined to the close geographical areas considered in the OPCS study and that the lower rate observed in the present study is not, therefore, merely a dilution effect (the estimated annual number of excess deaths associated with the relative risk of 1·21 for lymphoid leukaemia in the present study is about eight a year based on a total of 437 deaths or, if Copeland is excluded, seven a year based on a total of 430 deaths compared with one to two a year based on 44 deaths associated with the twofold relative risk in the OPCS study); and thirdly, the control local authority areas in the OPCS study had very low rates compared with the rates in the whole of the standard regions in which they were situated, which may have been at least in part a chance finding.

In the OPCS study, the increase in lymphoid leukaemia in young people appeared to be confined to installations other than Sellafield with start up date before 1955. In the present study the increase in the same category of installations is confirmed (relative risk = 1·21, p = 0·02, see table V) and there is also an increase around Sellafield (relative risk = 1·94) that is significant for all leukaemia (relative risk = 1·85, p = 0·03) but not specifically for lymphoid leukaemia (relative risk = 1·94, p = 0·06). The relative risk for the districts near the combined CEGB installations is of similar size to that around the pre-1955 installations other than Sellafield, but the number of deaths involved is small and the increase does not reach statistical significance either for all leukaemia or for lymphoid leukaemia.

The most significant results relating to leukaemia in table V are the increases at ages 0–24 in the middle proportion zone when all installations are combined. In carrying out a more detailed analysis of the districts which contribute to the increase in risk in the middle proportion zone, it emerged that the large urban conurbation of Liverpool county district makes up a major proportion of the excess risk in the middle proportion zone round Capenhurst. Seventy one of the leukaemias at ages 0–24 were from Liverpool district alone, and the adjusted relative risk for leukaemia in this district is 1·68 (p = 0·001) and 2·25 (p < 0·001) for lymphoid leukaemia. If Liverpool county district is subtracted from the all installations grouping in table V, then the relative risk for all leukaemia at 0–24 years falls from 1·19 (p = 0·01) to 1·12 (p = 0·08) in the middle proportion zone and from 1·15 (p = 0·01) to 1·14 (p = 0·03) over all zones. For lymphoid leukaemia the corresponding relative risks are 1·19 (p = 0·06) for the middle proportion zone and 1.20 ($p = 0.02$) over all zones. Liverpool county district is unique among the installation districts considered in this analysis in terms of its population size and social class composition, and the likelihood of some particular hazard in the district remains a possibility. However, this does not materially change the significance of the overall results.

Further differences from the OPCS study are the findings of an increase in Hodgkin's disease in the age group 0–24 (relative risk $= 1.24$, $p = 0.05$) and a deficit in lymphoid leukaemia in the age group 25–64 (relative risk $= 0.86$, $p = 0.05$) in the vicinity of nuclear installations. Neither has been reported previously. In installation districts the deficit of lymphoid leukaemia at ages 25–64 is not correlated inversely with the excess at ages 0–24, nor is there a general inverse correlation between mortality from lymphoid leukaemia in these two age groups when data for all districts are examined. Similarly, when mortality from lymphoid leukaemia and Hodgkin's disease at ages 0–24 are compared, there is no evidence of any correlation between the two, either when all districts are considered or when districts near a nuclear installation are excluded. Both the deficit of lymphoid leukaemia at ages 25–64 and the excess of Hodgkin's disease at younger ages may be the sort of chance finding that must be expected when many age-specific disease groups are examined.

REASONS FOR THE EXCESS OF LEUKAEMIA

Several explanations of the increase in leukaemia near the nuclear installations are possible. Firstly, it may be due to local environmental pollution by radiation. Against this explanation are the current assessments of annual radiation doses which, with estimates of the risks of leukaemia per unit dose, together imply that the doses received by populations living near nuclear installations are far below those that would cause any detectable increase in incidence.[13–16] The present data, moreover, fail to provide support for this explanation in two ways: no trend in relative risk is observed with increasing proximity to an installation as measured by the trend from low to middle to high proportion zones (see table V) and the difference in excess risk between the district round Sellafield and those around the other installations is less than a factor of six (relative risks 1.85 and 1.14), whereas the estimated annual doses received by children living in the vicinity of Sellafield are many orders of magnitude greater that those estimated for the other nuclear installations.[15] Similarly, no unusually high exposure to radioactive discharges has been noted in the discharges from Springfields and Capenhurst that could account for the concentration of high rates in the districts near Springfields or in Liverpool county district.

A second possibility is that the increase in leukaemia in young people associated with proximity to the nuclear installations is attributable to some other factor characteristic of the nuclear industry that might cause a hazard to children via the occupation of parents employed in the installations. This cannot be investigated by geographical studies alone but requires the detailed study of affected individuals and this is now being undertaken by several groups of research workers.

A third possibility is that the districts close to nuclear installations differ from those elsewhere in some other characteristic that is relevant to the aetiology of childhood leukaemia. That this should be so seems unlikely, as the adjustments that have been made for geographical variation in socio-economic and demographic factors that are known to influence mortality from cancer make the relative risks of death from leukaemia, lymphoma, multiple myeloma, lung cancer, all malignancies, and all non-malignant diseases in adults close to unity (relative risks all between 0·97 and 1·04) and, despite the large numbers in some instances, not significant. Nevertheless, the causes of different types of cancer differ greatly, and it is possible that there is some other factor that influences the incidence of childhood leukaemia that is not allowed for by these adjustments. In this respect the tendency for a higher mortality from leukaemia in young people in districts with relatively high proportions of their populations in social classes I and II (see table III) deserves further investigation partly because in Seascale, near Sellafield, where an increased mortality from childhood leukaemia was first established, the proportion of the population in social class I was most unusual, namely 47% of the economically active male population in 1971 compared with 5% nationally,[17] and partly because it is at odds with mortality data for children based on the social class of their parents, which showed no increased risk with social classes I and II.[11] It may be noted that any effect associated with social class appears to operate in the opposite way in Seascale than in Liverpool county district, which had a very low proportion of the population in social classes I and II.

Fourthly, the observed excess from leukaemia may be due to chance. This seems unlikely, however, as the excess observed in all districts other than Sellafield that were examined to test a hypothesis derived from independent observations in the district near Sellafield was such that an excess as large or larger would have been expected by chance only 3 times in 100. Nevertheless, a 3 in 100 chance may have turned up.

At present there are few data available from other countries with which to compare the increase in leukaemia at ages 0–24 seen in Britain around nuclear installations. Two studies are available from the United States.[18 19] In the first of these, cancer incidence was related to the Rocky Flats plant in Colorado. No association with the plant was found, but data were not shown separately for children. In the second, an increase of leukaemia was observed in a five town area of Massachusetts near a nuclear plant in Plymouth. Data were not presented separately by age, but it was reported that the excess was in adults and the elderly.

The results of the present study do not exclude the possibility that some substantial excesses of leukaemia in young people might be found in villages sited very close to the installations, as was observed in Seascale. Detailed investigation of such a possibility is currently being undertaken in the ICRF cancer epidemiology unit, Radcliffe Infirmary, Oxford, and elsewhere.

In the interpretation of these results, it has to be borne in mind that numbers of deaths from leukaemia in young persons were reducing throughout the period of the study, the mortality falling from 27·4 per 10 million persons aged under 25 years (standardised for age and sex) through 25·1 and 23·3 to 20·3 per 10 million a year in the quinquennia 1961–65 to 1876–80. The period of this reduction was a time when new and more effective treatment was being introduced, and the possibility has to be considered that the treatment of patients in the nuclear installation areas was worse than average. Leukaemia in young persons has mostly been treated in regional centres, and standardisation for health service region and rural status should have accounted for any major geographical difference in the efficacy of available treatment. Definitive studies need to be based on cancer incidence, but for this purpose standard registration data are inadequate and special efforts need to be made to ensure that coverage is complete.

In future studies of this sort, whether dealing with mortality or incidence data, analyses will need to take account of the fact that national rates may not provide appropriate expected numbers for local studies. This is due not only to the association between disease and the factors such as the four socioeconomic and demographic variables included in the present study, but also those due to further, at present unknown, factors that led to the extra-Poisson variation that we have observed for most of the 11 diseases, including childhood leukaemia and most notably childhood lymphoid leukaemia.

Conclusion

The results of this study confirm that there has been a small excess mortality from leukaemia and in particular from lymphoid leukaemia in persons aged 0–24 years in districts with some of their population resident within 10 miles of one or other of 15 nuclear installations in England and Wales during the period 1969–78 and suggest that the excess for lymphoid leukaemia in these districts is about eight deaths a year out of an average annual total of about 240 for England and Wales as a whole. They provide no evidence of any other excess mortality in the installation districts at ages 0–24 years or 25–64 years, except possibly for an increase in Hodgkin's disease in the younger age group. Analysis of the results does not provide any positive evidence that the increase in leukaemia is due to local environmental pollution from the installations.

The small excess mortality from Hodgkin's disease in persons aged 0–24 and the deficiency of lymphoid leukaemia at ages 25–64 years may both be due to random variation.

Note added in proof

Since we completed this paper Professor Breslow has informed us in a personal communication that a recent simulation study has shown significance tests based on a comparison of χ^2 goodness-of-fit statistics, as suggested in Breslow (1984), to perform poorly. We have therefore recalculated all the p values referred to in the chapter using a comparison of deviances and also, where the test involves only one extra parameter, by comparison of the parameter estimate with its estimated standard error. In all cases the p values calculated by a comparison of deviances were virtually identical to those calculated by comparison of the parameter estimate with its standard error. In the vast majority of cases these were not substantially different from those based on the χ^2 criterion. Three exceptions were: (i) in table III the test for trend with population size approached significance for leukaemia of all types and became highly significant for leukaemia other than lymphoid leukaemia; (ii) in table IV the p values for the relative risk of mortality from leukaemia and lymphoid leukaemia at ages 0–24 after adjustment for the four socioeconomic variables became smaller (that is, more highly significant), and (iii) in table V two of the tests for trend for lymphoid leukaemia at ages 25–64 were no longer significant (see footnotes to tables).

We are grateful to the National Radiological Protection Board for financial assistance towards this study, to Dr Paul Travers for extensive computing spadework that rendered the Office of Population Censuses and Surveys mortality data accessible, and to Mrs Sonia Busfield, Mrs Cathy Harwood, and Ms Sandra Connell-Hinkes for typing the text and the tables. Detailed data relative to: the identity and characteristics of the installation districts; relative risks for each disease category and age-group by the four socioeconomic and geographical variables; relative risks similar to those shown in table IV for each disease category at ages 65 and over; relative risks similar to those shown in table V for other disease categories at ages 0–24 and 25–64 and for all disease categories at ages 65 and over; and relative risks for all leukaemia and for lymphoid leukaemia at ages 0–24 for Liverpool county district and for pooled installation districts excluding Liverpool district are available on request from Ms Paula Cook-Mozaffari.

1 Gardner MJ, Winter PD. Mortality in Cumberland during 1959–78 with reference to cancer in young people around Windscale. *Lancet* 1984;i:216.
2 Cook-Mozaffari PJ, Ashwood FL, Vincent T, Forman D, Alderson M. *Cancer incidence and mortality in the vicinity of nuclear installations. England and Wales, 1959–1980.* London: HMSO, 1987. (OPCS studies on medical and population subjects, No 51).
3 Forman D, Cook-Mozaffari PJ, Darby S, *et al.* Cancer near nuclear installations. *Nature* 1987;**239**:499.
4 Roman E, Beral V, Carpenter L, *et al.* Childhood leukaemia in the West Berkshire and

Basingstoke and North Hampshire District Health Authorities in relation to nuclear establishments in the vicinity. *BMJ* 1987;**294**:597.

5 Swerdlow AJ. Cancer registration in England and Wales: some aspects relevant to interpretation of the data. *Journal of the Royal Statistical Society [Series A]* 1986;**149**:146.

6 Cook-Mozaffari PJ. Cancer near nuclear installations. *Lancet* 1987;**1**:855.

7 Black D for the Independent Advisory Group. *Investigation of the possible increased incidence of cancer in west Cumbria.* HMSO: London, 1984. (Black report.)

8 World Health Organisation. *International Classification of Diseases. Manual of the International Statistical Classification of Diseases, Injuries, and Causes of Death.* WHO: Geneva, 1967.

9 Payne CD, ed. *The GLIM System.* Royal Statistical Society: London, 1986. (Release 3.77.)

10 Breslow NE. Extra-Poisson variation in log-linear models. *Applied Statistics* 1984;**33**:38.

11 Office of Population Censuses and Surveys (1978). *Occupational Mortlity 1970–72 Decennial Supplement for England and Wales.* HMSO: London, 1978. (Series DS No 1.)

12 Webber R, Craig J. *Which local authorities are alike?.* HMSO: London, 1976. (OPCS Population Trends No 5:13.)

13 Hughes JS, Roberts GC. *The radiation exposure of the UK population—1984 review.* HMSO: London, 1984. (NRPB-R173.)

14 Dionian J, Wan SL, Wrixon AD. *Radiation doses to members of the public around Atomic Weapons Research Establishment, Aldermaston, Royal Ordnance Factory, Burghfield and Atomic Energy Research Establishment, Harwell.* HMSO: London, 1987. (NRPB-R202.)

15 Stather JW, Clarke RH, Duncan KP. *The risk of childhood leukaemia near nuclear establishments.* HMSO: London, 1988. (NRPB-R215.)

16 Darby SC, Doll R. Fallout, radiation doses near Dounreay, and childhood leukaemia. *BMJ* 1987;**294**:603.

17 Gardner MJ, Hall AJ, Downes S, Terrell JD. Follow up study of children born to mothers resident in Seascale, west Cumbria (birth cohort). *BMJ* 1987;**295**:822.

18 Crump KS, Ng T-H, Cuddihy RG. Cancer incidence patterns in the Denver metropolitan area in relation to the Rocky Flats plant. *Am J Epidemiol* 1987;**126**:127.

19 Clapp RW, Cobb S, Chan CK, Walker B. Leukaemia near Massachusetts nuclear power plant. *Lancet* 1987;**ii**:1324.

17: Cancer near potential sites of nuclear installations

PAULA COOK-MOZAFFARI, SARAH DARBY,
RICHARD DOLL

Mortality and census data for 400 districts of England and
Wales were analysed with respect to existing sites of nuclear
power stations and sites where the construction of such
installations had been considered or had occurred at a later
date (potential sites). Excess mortality due to leukaemia and
Hodgkin's disease in young people who lived near potential
sites was similar to that in young people who lived near
existing sites. Areas near existing and potential sites might
share unrecognised risk factors other than environmental
radiation pollution.

Introduction

In 1969–78 mortality from leukaemia, and especially from lymphoid
leukaemia, at ages 0–24 was higher in districts near nuclear installations
than in matched control districts[1 2] and in all other districts of England and
Wales.[3] In the latter study, we compared 70 districts that had any part of
their area within 16 km of an existing nuclear installation with 330 other
districts: relative risks near the installations were increased by 15% for
leukaemia of all types and by 21% for lymphoid leukaemia, after adjustment for social class, rural status, population size, and local regional health
authority of the districts. These increases corresponded to about eight
excess deaths from leukaemia annually. Mortality from Hodgkin's disease
at ages 0–24 was also increased near nuclear installations (relative
risk = 1·24), whereas mortality from lymphoid leukaemia at ages 25–64 was
reduced (relative risk = 0·86).

As annual radiation doses received by children living near nuclear
installations are much lower than those expected to cause any detectable

TABLE I—*No of deaths in districts with* $\geqslant 0.1\%$ *of their population within 16 km of an existing or potential nuclear installation in England and Wales, 1969–78*

	Ages 0–24 years			Ages 25–64 years		
	Existing*	Potential†	Both‡	Existing*	Potential†	Both‡
Leukaemia (all types)	635	189	110	1 367	419	267
Lymphoid leukaemia	372	104	68	284	88	48
Other leukaemia	263	85	42	1 083	331	219
All lymphomas	222	73	46	1 519	532	341
Hodgkin's disease	99	34	16	579	223	107
Other lymphomas	123	39	30	940	309	234
Multiple myeloma	—	—	—	587	209	115
Cancer of the lung	—	—	—	16 165	6 047	3 122
Other malignancies	845	304	160	36 128	12 327	7 410
All malignancies	1 702	566	316	55 766	19 534	11 255
All other causes	23 708	8 149	4 550	112 920	43 968	24 197

* Excluding districts near potential sites.
† Excluding districts near existing sites.
‡ Districts near both existing and potential sites.

increase in leukaemia, and many orders of magnitude so for installations other than Sellafield,[4–8] we must ask whether the observed increases are due not to the presence of the nuclear installations but to another feature of the areas in which installations have been built that was not adequately taken into account. To investigate this hypothesis we have considered the two Central Electricity Generating Board (CEGB) nuclear power stations that were established in England and Wales after the end of the period to which our mortality data referred (at Hartlepool, Cleveland in 1981 and at Heysham, Lancashire in 1983) and six other sites that, according to CEGB, were seriously considered for the construction of nuclear power stations (at Luxulyan, Nancekuke, and Gwythian, Cornwall; at Herbury, Dorset; at Portskewett, Monmouthshire; and at Druridge Bay, Northumberland). These eight sites will be referred to as potential sites of nuclear installations.

Methods

Mortality from 11 causes (or groups of causes) in 400 districts of England and Wales that approximate to the 402 county districts established in 1974 was analysed with census and mortality data from before and after the 1974 boundary changes as described in the preceding chapter.[3]

Thirty one districts, which had some part within a 16 km radius of the potential sites, had a total population of 3·37 million at the time of the 1971 national census compared with 7·67 million in the 70 districts near to existing nuclear installations. Eleven districts with a population of 1·29 million were in the vicinity of sites in both categories. The numbers of deaths from each of the causes in these three categories are shown in table I.

TABLE II—*Relative risk of death unadjusted/adjusted for social class, rural status, population size, and regional health authority*

Cause of death	At age 0–24 years		At age 25–64 years	
	Existing sites	Potential sites	Existing sites	Potential sites
Leukaemia	1·13**/1·16**	1·06/1·14	0·99/0·96	0·93/0·96
Lymphoid leukaemia	1·16**/1·20**	1·03/1·09	0·91/0·88*	0·86/0·80*
Other leukaemia	1·09/1·10	1·09/1·23	1·01/0·98	0·95/1·02
All lymphomas	1·03/1·06	1·04/1·31*	0·98/1·00	1·07/1·09
Hodgkin's disease	1·13/1·28*	1·18/1·50*	1·01/1·02	1·21**/1·23*
Other lymphomas	0·96/0·92	0·95/1·17	0·97/0·98	0·99/1·01
Multiple myeloma	—	—	1·07/1·07	1·15**/1·09
Cancer of lung	—	—	0·96/1·00	1·06/1·03
Other malignancies	1·00/1·04	1·11*/1·04	0·99/1·00	1·02/1·01
All malignancies	1·05*/1·08**	1·08/1·10	0·98/1·00	1·03/1·02
All other causes	0·94*/0·96*	1·03/1·02	0·96/0·98	1·13**/1·02

Existing sites: excluding districts near potential sites. As a result these figures differ slightly from those reported previously.[3]
Potential sites: excluding districts near existing sites.
* $p \leqslant 0.05$. ** $p \leqslant 0.01$.

Estimates of relative risk[3] were derived from log-linear regression by means of the "GLIM" computer program;[9] allowance for extra-Poisson variation was made with the method of Breslow,[10] except that significance tests were done with a comparison of deviances because the original χ^2 method performed poorly (Breslow, personal communication). One sided tests in the direction of the observed difference were used to evaluate the risk in districts near the sites of interest.

For simplicity of presentation, the districts in proximity both to existing and to potential sites have been excluded from the analyses. Alternative analyses, however, in which all districts were included and adjustment was made simultaneously for the two types of site gave results very similar to those presented. Relative risks for existing sites have been calculated with the inclusion of Copeland district, in which Sellafield is situated, because exclusion of this district made little difference to the overall results.[3]

Relative risks have been calculated both with and without adjustment for the four socioeconomic and demographic characteristics of districts that we have considered—namely, social class structure, rural status, population size, and health authority region. As in our previous study we have based our conclusions on the adjusted values.

Results

Relative risks for existing sites are strikingly similar to those of potential sites (table II), particularly for leukaemia of all types and for all malignancies at ages 0–24 years. However, the population near the potential sites is smaller and the increases in relative risks, though proportionally similar, are significant only in districts near the existing sites ($p = 0.008$ v $p = 0.10$ for leukaemia; $p = 0.01$ v $p = 0.06$ for all malignancies). For Hodgkin's disease at ages 0–24, both relative risks are significantly raised ($p = 0.05$), with a notably higher value for the potential sites than for the existing sites. The high relative risk for Hodgkin's disease near the potential sites contributes to a significant increases in risk also for all lymphomas ($p = 0.04$).

The increase in risk for leukaemia mortality in young people in districts near the existing sites is more pronounced for lymphoid leukaemia than for other types of leukaemia; this pattern is not repeated near the potential sites, although for both types of leukaemia the risks are again above unity.

At ages 25–64 years, the deficit in mortality from lymphoid leukaemia that was observed near the existing sites ($p = 0.04$) is repeated and is more striking in districts near the potential sites ($p = 0.03$). There was no material increase in risk for any of the causes of death analysed near the existing sites, but there was a significantly raised mortality from Hodgkin's disease near the potential sites at ages 25–64 years ($p = 0.01$), which echoes the finding at younger ages.

Discussion

Our hypothesis that, with the possible exception of Sellafield, an increased risk for leukaemia is not associated with local environmental radiation pollution is strengthened by our new findings—namely, that the death rate from leukaemia in areas where there were no nuclear installations, but where the construction of such installations was considered or actually occurred at a later date, was similar to that in areas near existing nuclear installations.

In our previous study,[3] the increased death rate at young ages near nuclear installations was particularly pronounced for lymphoid leukaemia, whereas in the present study the relative risk is greater for other types of leukaemia. This difference may reflect sampling variation or the inaccuracy of the classification of leukaemia types on death certificates at the time of the study. However, it is noteworthy that by no means all of the leukaemias diagnosed among young people in the vicinity of Sellafield and Dounreay were recorded as the lymphoid type: in Millom rural district, near Sellafield, leukaemias were certified as acute lymphoid (5), chronic lymphoid (1), acute myeloid (5), chronic myeloid (1), erythroleukaemia (1), and unspecified (1),[11] whereas in Dounreay the cases were registered as acute lymphoid (9) and acute myeloid (3).

New treatments that reduced the mortality from leukaemia in young people should be considered in the interpretation of our new findings.

During 1961–65 (just before our study) and 1976–80 (at the end of the period covered) mortality fell from 27·4 to 20·3 per 10 million people aged under 25 years (standardised for age and sex). That the treatment of patients near the sites of existing and, perhaps also, potential installations was possibly less effective than average has to be considered. However, we have standardised for health authority region and for rural status, and this should have accounted for any major difference in the efficacy of available treatment. Definitive studies need to be based on cancer incidence but, during the period studied, standard registration data were unfortunately inadequate.

Recent data from new towns in Scotland[13] and from England and Wales[14] are compatible with an earlier suggestion[8] that the increased incidence of leukaemia around Sellafield and Dounreay might be attributable to a cluster of cases caused by an infective agent associated with a large influx of people to these areas. However, census data for 1961 and 1971 in the districts near potential installations show that, by comparison with England and Wales as a whole, the population of young people increased less whereas the population of adults of working age decreased more. This does not obviously support a hypothesis that rests on the intermingling of populations brought about by the sudden influx of a new labour force and their families.

Exposure to radon may also be a significant cause of leukaemia,[15] particularly in Cornwall, where three of the potential sites are situated and where the average exposure indoors is more than five times higher than that in the UK as a whole.[16] For adults, an effect of radon seems to be unlikely as there was no increase in the incidence of leukaemia in underground miners who were occupationally exposed to high levels of radon.[17] In Sweden, radon levels in the homes of children with cancer were slightly lower than in the homes of control children.[18] To investigate the issue further in our data we have subdivided the potential sites into those situated in Cornwall and those elsewhere. For districts near the three potential installations in Cornwall, the relative risk for leukaemia mortality at ages 0–24 was 1·18 (based on 32 deaths), whereas for districts near the remaining potential installations it was slightly lower (1·13, based on 157 deaths). Thus, although our data for Cornwall are consistent with the hypothesis that indoor radon exposure may slightly increase the risk of leukaemia among young people, clearly this factor could not, on its own, explain our findings.

We had previously believed it to be unlikely that districts close to existing nuclear installations might differ from those elsewhere in another characteristic relevant to the development of childhood leukaemia. This was because the adjustment for geographical variation in the socioeconomic and demographic factors that influence mortality from cancer had brought close to unity the relative risks of death at ages 25–64 from most malignancies studied, including lung cancer, and also from all non-malignant diseases. By contrast, our new findings point to systematic differences between districts near existing or potential installations and other districts with respect to some important, unrecognised risk factors.[19]

We thank the CEGB for making available to us the grid references of sites at which they have seriously considered building nuclear power stations and Paul Dolin for help with data analysis.

1 Forman D, Cook-Mozaffari PJ, Darby SC, *et al.* Cancer near nuclear installations. *Nature* 1987;**329**:499–505.
2 Cook-Mozaffari PJ, Ashwood FL, Vincent T, Forman D, Alderson M. *Cancer incidence and mortality in the vicinity of nuclear installations. England and Wales, 1959–1980.* London: HMSO, 1987. (OPCS Studies on Medical and Population Subjects 51).
3 Cook-Mozaffari PJ, Darby SC, Doll R, *et al.* Geographical variation in mortality from leukaemia and other cancers in England and Wales in relation to proximity to nuclear installations, 1969–78. *Br J Cancer* 1989;**59**:476–85.
4 Hughes JS, Shaw KB, O'Riordan MC. *The radiation exposure of the UK population 1988.* Chilton: National Radiological Protection Board, 1988. (Review NRPB-R227).
5 Dionian J, Wan SL, Wrixon AD. *Radiation doses to members of the public around Atomic Weapons Research Establishment, Aldermaston, Royal Ordnance Factory, Burghfield and Atomic Energy Research Establishment, Harwell.* London: HMSO, 1987. (NRPB-R202).
6 Stather JW, Clarke RH, Duncan KP. *The risk of childhood leukaemia near nuclear establishments.* London: HMSO, 1988. (NRPB-R215).
7 UN Scientific Committee on the Effects of Ionizing Radiation. *Sources, effects and risks of ionizing radiation.* New York: United Nations, 1988.
8 Darby SC, Doll R. Fallout, radiation doses near Dounreay, and childhood leukaemia. *BMJ* 1987;**294**:603–07.
9 Payne CD, ed. *The GLIM system.* London: Royal Statistical Society, 1986. (Release 3.77).
10 Breslow NE. Extra-Poisson variation in log-linear models. *Applied Statistics* 1984;**33**:38–44.
11 Black D for the Independent Advisory Group. *Investigation of the possible increased incidence of cancer in west Cumbria.* London: HMSO, 1984. (Black report.)
12 Committee on Medical Aspects of Radiation. *Investigation of the possible increased incidence of leukaemia in young people near the Dounreay Nuclear Establishment, Caithness, Scotland.* London: HMSO, 1988. (COMARE 2nd report).
13 Kinlen L. Evidence for an infective cause of childhood leukaemia: comparison of a Scottish new town with nuclear reprocessing sites in Britain. *Lancet* 1988;**ii**:1323–26.
14 Kinlen L. The relevance of population mixing to the aetiology of childhood leukaemia. In: Crosbie WA, Gittus JH, eds. *Proceedings of a conference on medical response to the effects of ionising radiation.* London: Elsevier, 1989.
15 Lucie NP. Radon exposure and leukaemia. *Lancet* 1989;**ii**:99–100.
16 Clarke RH, Southwood TRE. Risks from ionizing radiation. *Nature* 1989;**338**:197–8.
17 Committee on the Biological Effects of Ionizing Radiations (BEIR IV). *Health risks of radon and other internally deposited alpha-emitters.* Washington DC: National Academy Press, 1988.
18 Stjernfeldt M, Samuelsson L, Ludvigsson J. Radiation in dwellings and cancer in children. *Pediatric Hematology and Oncology* 1987;**4**:55–61.
19 Greaves MF. Aetiology of childhood acute lymphoblastic leukaemia: a soluble problem? In: Gale RP, Moelzer D, eds. *Acute lymphoblastic leukaemia. UCLA symposium on molecular and cellular biology.* New York: Alan R Liss (in press). (New series 108).

18: Review of reported increases of childhood cancer rates in the vicinity of nuclear installations in the United Kingdom

MARTIN J GARDNER

During the past few years several studies of childhood cancer near nuclear installations in the United Kingdom have been undertaken. These studies have looked in particular at leukaemia rates around specific nuclear sites but also around groups of installations. The original suggestion of a raised level of cancer in young people based on cases around Sellafield has been supported by the findings, but the overall magnitude of the relative excess is much less than first found. Attempts to control for potential confounding variables in some of the analyses have not explained the excess, and its cause—whether related to radiation or to other factors—is still not clear.

Introduction

For many years before 1983 there had been concern that radioactive emissions from nuclear installations could be a health hazard to local communities, and some scientific studies assessing this possibility had been initiated.[1] However, substantial public interest was raised only with the showing on national network of the Yorkshire Television documentary *Windscale: the Nuclear Laundry* on 1 November 1983.

The background to the potential for concern was the awareness that

146

ionising radiation is a known cause of cancer in humans, and therefore any unnecessary exposure might lead to an increase in risk. Exposures to radiation from many sources, such as medical, occupational, and military related, have been found to lead to an increase in cancer in adults and children.[2] Thus (a) medical examples include the associations of radiotherapy for ankylosing spondylitis with an increase in leukaemia and cancers of irradiated organs, and of prenatal diagnostic irradiation of mothers with increased leukaemia in their children; (b) occupational examples include earlier members of the radiological profession having experienced raised levels of leukaemia, uranium miners exposed to radon gas decay products having high rates of lung cancer, and nuclear workers having raised levels of multiple myeloma; and (c) military related examples are Japanese atomic bomb survivors who have suffered excesses of leukaemia and other cancers, and servicemen involved in atomic bomb testing who have shown possible increases of leukaemia.

The concern about health effects to populations living near nuclear installations had been somewhat minimised by the belief, particularly among those involved in assessing the biological effects of radiation, that the likely risk from known emissions was negligible. Even though it had been firmly established that radiation exposure at high levels carried a risk of cancer developing some time afterwards, it was believed that the relatively low levels associated with the environment around nuclear power plants were unlikely to prove a hazard. Thus, little scientific or medical effort had been directed towards examining the health of populations near nuclear installations. However, the television documentary generated a large amount of such activity—including an independent inquiry headed by Sir Douglas Black.[3]

This chapter reviews various aspects of the findings. A description is given of the initial observations and the difficulty in their interpretation, followed by a summary of the main results of ensuing investigations—including studies of areas around particular as well as groups of nuclear sites in the country. Problems of geographical studies, as well as comments on their improved methodology, are discussed. Finally, studies of individuals aimed at further clarification of the situation are mentioned.

Background to the concern: television programme

It is instructive and important to consider the origin of the television programme to help with interpretation of the available evidence. The producer of the documentary had previously made a programme on the effects of asbestos on health. It was called *Alice: a Fight for Life* and was instrumental in implementing proposed legislation to reduce allowable levels of exposure to asbestos in the workplace. The success of this programme encouraged him to make another on occupational health and safety.

The producer approached British Nuclear Fuels Ltd (BNFL) at Windscale (now called Sellafield) with a request to make a documentary on the health effects of occupational exposure to radiation in the nuclear power industry. At the time there were no indications of any health risks on the basis of an internally conducted epidemiological study of the BNFL workers.[45] (A later independent study of the workforce, which showed no excess mortality from cancer compared with the general population and similar cancer rates in both radiation and non-radiation workers, has since been reported by Smith and Douglas.[6] However, some associations between accumulated radiation dose and specific cancers were found—for example, for multiple myeloma—which is consistent with other findings.) While in the area of Sellafield making his enquiry, the producer heard from local people about cases of leukaemia and other cancers in children which had occurred at what they thought was an unusually high rate for a rare disease. This information, together with an awareness of the scale of the Windscale discharges, resulted in the focus for the new programme being changed from the Windscale workforce to the local children—particularly those living in the village of Seascale on the coast of west Cumbria about 2 km south of the Sellafield site.[3] The "cluster" of cancer cases was moreover possibly linked with Windscale by the programme, both indirectly through its title and directly through its content.

Difficulties of interpretation

CONFIRMATION OF CASES

The identification of cases of cancer by the television programme was based partly on anecdotal evidence. However, a check was satisfactorily made that the reported cases were known to registered medical sources.[3]

CONFIRMATION OF EXCESS

The suggestion that the number of cancers, and particularly leukaemia, was in excess among children in the neighbourhood of Sellafield was examined by two subsequent analyses. First, it was shown that in Millom rural district (the local authority area containing Seascale) there had been raised leukaemia mortality among persons aged 0–24 years during 1968–78—six deaths compared with 1·4 expected at national rates—but not during 1959–67, and not in adjacent Ennerdale rural district (the local authority area containing Sellafield) during either period of time.[7] These particular calendar years were used to correspond to series of the International Classification of Diseases. Rates for other cancers at these ages were not raised, nor were either leukaemia or total cancer rates in the adult populations. The total cancer rates might have been expected to be raised also if radiation was the cause—unless some special argument relating to increased child susceptibility, possibly involving a particular route of exposure, is invoked. Secondly, Craft et al reported four cases of lymphoid malignancy among children 0–14 years old in Seascale during 1968–82 compared with 0·25 expected at registration rates for the overall northern region of England.[8] Cancer registration started in this region in 1968.

STATISTICAL ASPECTS OF UNEXPECTED FINDING

One difficult question is how to interpret this excess. If we start out on an investigation and find, not what we are expecting (in this case a health risk to the workforce), but something different—unintentionally—how should we react? Is it a chance event that we have stumbled across or is it an exposure-related observation waiting to be discovered? Standard statistical hypothesis testing applied to this situation is unhelpful, because it is primarily designed for a priori hypotheses rather than a posteriori hypotheses where the interpretation of the p value becomes complex. The particular excess discussed in the television programme and the linking of it to Windscale was certainly a post hoc argument.

An a priori hypothesis could have been set up given the knowledge that Windscale had discharged vastly more radioactive waste materials into the environment than any other nuclear site in the United Kingdom,[3] and given its known record of accidental releases, of which the Windscale fire in 1957 was the worst. However, although there was known to have been some previous local concern, for example, by the district medical officer, no detailed study had been launched.

BOUNDARY DEFINITIONS

The difficulty of interpretation is increased by the possible selection of geographical boundaries, calendar years, age groups, and diagnostic categories for analysis that maximise the numerical size of the excess—rather than specification of these defining characteristics in advance of data examination. The potential difficulties raised by this possibly data-guided selection of boundaries are indicated, for example, by the choice of the age group 0–9 years for a hypothesis test by the television programme collaborators (Urquhart et al), when traditionally the age group 0–14 years has been used and indeed was also considered by Urquhart et al themselves.[9] The exclusion of the ages 10–14 years was clearly not for lack of information but was possibly influenced by the knowledge that only one case was known at these older ages.

This particular problem was expanded in the Black report.[3] By variations of definition of boundaries it is possible to manipulate, if desired, the numerical size of any reported "excess" and also the associated p value from a test of statistical significance. If this procedure is followed, bias is introduced and the p value will not be a valid measure of its purpose—that is, to measure the role of chance in producing the observations. The problem is succinctly described as "moving the goalposts" or as the "Texas sharp-shooter effect".[10]

PUTTING FIGURES INTO CONTEXT

Another difficulty associated with the interpretation of such an excess is that alone it cannot be seen in the context of other similar geographical areas. With a rare disease like leukaemia in children it can be anticipated that during a limited time period some individually unpredictable areas with small populations will have high observed rates, and others low rates, by the play of chance alone. An examination of areas other than those around Sellafield can help to take the argument further, and some such data were provided.[38]

These studies have shown that the immediate areas around Sellafield do have high rates compared with those elsewhere, but not uniquely so. This is an appropriate and helpful approach—because rates in other localities, regionally and nationally, can be contrasted without any further redefinition of the area basis, calendar years, age, and diagnostic groups. Thus, was the rate in Millom extreme or, even though $p < 0.05$, was it in the main part of the distribution? In fact, Millom rural district had the second highest rate of leukaemia mortality at ages 0–24 years during 1968–78 among 152 similar sized rural districts around England and Wales (table I). The area with the highest rate was in Norfolk, not geographically close to Millom or near a nuclear installation. Seascale had the third highest registration rate of lymphoid malignancy at ages 0–14 years during 1968–82 among the 675 electoral wards in the northern children's malignant disease registry region (see fig 1 and the Black report[3]). If the associated Poisson probabilities are used in the latter case, rather than rates, that for Seascale is the lowest of the 675 wards (that is, Seascale had the lowest one sided p value).

RATES VERSUS p VALUES

The differential, and which of these is the preferred approach, was the subject of debate on whether the requirements for an excess should be a high risk estimate or a low p value.[11 12] If the numbers of cases involved are large, such that sampling error becomes a small component of the overall variance, rates would clearly be the choice. Argument arises if the numbers of cases are small and population sizes variable. One of the critiisms of the use of rates for a rare condition in small populztions has been that the rate is merely an inverse reflection of the population size, and hence any ranking that is based on rates is too closely connected to population size to be sensible or useful.[11] This criticism, however, applies equally to the associated Poisson probability, which is similarly related to population size.

The objections to rates may have arisen because Seascale was found to be

TABLE I—*Leukaemia mortality in people under 25 years of age during 1968–78 in 152 similar sized rural districts of England and Wales**

Standardised mortality ratio[†]	Number of districts	
	Observed	Predicted[‡]
0 –	35	36
50 –	43	50
100 –	26	26
150 –	26	23
200 –	14	9
250 –	5	5
300 –	1	2
350 –	0	1
400 +	2[§]	0·4
Total	152	152

* Based on the Black report.[3]
† Ratio (times 100) of the number of deaths in each rural district to the expected number at national rates.
‡ On the basis of Poisson distributions with parameters equal to the expected numbers of deaths within each district.
§ Millom rural district is included in this group with a standardised mortality ratio of 435.

the most extreme in terms of Poisson probability but not in terms of rate. However, because Seascale had a larger population than some electoral wards in the northern region, the statistical power to detect an excess rate of any given value is greater than for smaller wards. However, the probability of obtaining a high rate by chance is greater for wards with smaller populations than for those with larger populations.

Maybe empirical Bayes estimators should be incorporated (see, for example, Clayton and Kaldor[13]). An alternative, as discussed later (see section on Dounreay), is to remove the difficulty associated with the variable sizes of populations at risk in small areas and to develop areas of equal size population (or, perhaps preferably, "expected" numbers of cases). Ranking of disease levels by area can then be carried out on the numbers of observed cases alone—and the same ranking would also be given by the p values.

IS OVERALL DISTRIBUTION RANDOM?

Table I shows, alongside the observed distribution, the predicted distribution of leukaemia mortality in the 152 rural districts if cases occurred at random among the combined populations—that is, assuming uniform risk. It can be seen that, by and large, the observed and predicted distributions are similar. This comparison, however, is only of limited value as a test of spatial randomness as rates in contiguous areas were not

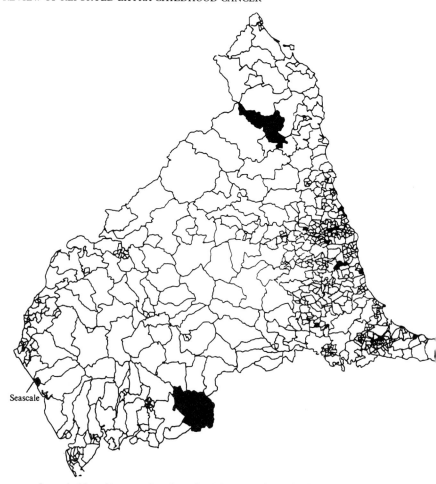

FIG 1—*Lymphoid malignancy levels under 15 years of age during 1968–82 among the 675 electoral wards in the northern children's malignant disease registry region: shaded wards (n=19) are those with statistically significant (p < 0·05, one-sided) raised rates (source: Craft et al[14]; reproduced by permission of the editor, J Epidemiol Community Health)*

examined. It is also of limited value as a test of whether the Sellafield area has a raised risk from some local factor whereas a uniformly lower rate operates in the other rural districts.

NUMBER OF SIGNIFICANT FINDINGS

The map shown in fig 1 from Craft *et al*[14] used a one sided Poisson probability level of 0·05 to define an electoral ward as having a high rate. Craft *et al* found 19 such wards, whereas we might have expected about 675 × 0·05—that is, 33 or 34—by chance alone. So what can be made of the

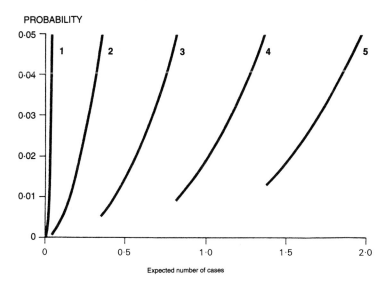

PROBABILITY

Expected number of cases

FIG 2—*Probability of obtaining a statistically significant, at the one-sided $p = 0.05$ level, excess of observed cases (that is equal to or greater than the critical number shown on each curve) over the expected number assuming uniformly distributed risk*

fact that fewer high areas were found than could naively be expected? Are all the high areas simply due to chance variation—including Seascale?

Figure 2 shows that, for the Poisson distribution, the answer is not straightforward because of its discrete nature. The actual probability associated with $p < 0.05$ can be very much lower and depends on the size of the population in a somewhat irregular manner. It can be seen that for any critical number (the minimum needed to achieve $p < 0.05$) of observed cases the associated probability increases to 0.05 as the number of expected cases increases—the range shown in fig 2 for the expected number of cases, from zero to 2, covers those found in the northern region electoral wards. After each change point, where the critical number increases by unity, there is a marked fall in the associated Poisson probability to values much lower than 0.05. Some of these are even lower than 0.01 and so, depending on the distribution of population size (or expected numbers) among the 675 electoral wards, the number of areas satisfying $p < 0.05$ by chance could be expected to be less than 675×0.05, and 19 may be a reasonable number.

Among the areas shown in table I, four of the 152 rural districts had standardised mortality ratios that were significantly raised using a one sided p value of 0.05. Again, for the same reasons, the expected number of areas statistically significant at this level arising by chance assuming a uniform distribution of risk will be less than $152 \times 0.05 = 7.6$. When the appropriate calculation is carried out it gives an expected number of 4.6 out of the 152 rural districts—that is, only 3% rather than 5% of areas. It is not possible from these figures to say whether one or more of the four significantly raised areas are due to the presence of a non-uniform risk, or whether these are simply four of the 4·6 expected by chance under a null hypothesis distribution of uniform risk.

Developing the evidence

A natural extension, to test a hypothesis generated from one set of data, is to examine other opportunities for addressing the same question.[15] This has been carried out in two ways. One was to look at cancer rates around other nuclear sites in the UK in general (fig 3), taking account of their nature and duration of operation, and the second was to look around individual nuclear sites. The other nuclear sites have discharged much lower levels of radiation to the environment than the Sellafield plant,[3] but none the less add further information for assessment. However, they do not form ideal situations for attempting to test the hypothesis in an experimental sense.

OTHER NUCLEAR SITES

A study that looked at nuclear sites generally within England and Wales resulted in an extensive report,[16] which has been summarised to identify the main findings.[17] This study essentially involved a more detailed continuation of that initiated by Baron[1] and examined cancer rates during 1959–80 in local authority areas near 14 established nuclear sites compared with rates in selected control areas. Some more recently initiated nuclear installations shown in fig 3 were left out as having minimal relevant experience. Areas included as being close to nuclear sites were defined in four increasingly broad distance zones, from a requirement of having at least two thirds of their population at the 1971 census within six miles of a nuclear installation to having at least one third of their population within 10 miles of an installation. Control areas were taken as being further removed from the same nuclear installations but matched to the installation areas in terms of population size, urban or rural status, and being located wherever possible within the same standard region as that containing the nuclear site.

Leukaemia registration and mortality figures for people under 25 years of age for the 10 mile distance measure are shown in table II for groupings of the installations. Overall there is a suggestion of raised registration rates in installation areas compared with control areas, but greater around Sellafield than the other sites. This pattern is not found for death rates, which are not affected by the known varying completeness of cancer registration data, particularly during the early years of this period.[18] Although some significant high and low rates were found for other areas, it is difficult to interpret these given the large numbers of comparisons that were made.

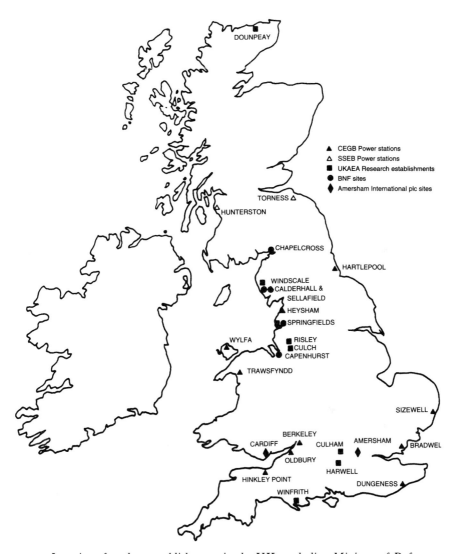

FIG 3—*Location of nuclear establishments in the UK, excluding Ministry of Defence sites (source: Black[3]).*

Additionally, some concerns were expressed by the researchers themselves about the appropriateness of some of the control areas based both on the difficulties in their selection and the tendency for cancer rates overall to be lower in the installation areas.[17]

Partly for these reasons at least, a subsequent regression analysis of

155

TABLE II—*Leukaemia registration (1961–80) and mortality (1959–80) in people under 25 years of age in local authority areas with at least one third of their population at the 1971 census within 10 miles of one of 14 nuclear installations and control areas by grouping of installation**

					Installation to control areas	
Nuclear installation	Installation area		Control area		Ratio of SR(M)Rs	95% confidence interval
Registration	Cases	SRR	Cases	SRR		
BNFL Sellafield	26	1·76	13	0·93	1·89	0·96 to 4·01
Pre-1955 sites†	442	1·10	406	0·98	1·12	0·98 to 1·29
CEGB sites‡	91	1·16	73	0·95	1·22	0·89 to 1·68
UKAEA, Winfrith	23	1·04	22	0·96	1·09	0·58 to 2·05
All minus Sellafield	556	1·11	501	0·97	1·14	1·01 to 1·28
All sites	582	1·12	514	0·97	1·16	1·03 to 1·30
Mortality	Deaths	SMR	Deaths	SMR		
BNFL Sellafield	20	1·26	21	1·43	0·88	0·46 to 1·71
Pre-1955 sites†	409	0·99	447	1·06	0·94	0·82 to 1·07
CEGB sites‡	87	1·11	77	0·99	1·13	0·82 to 1·55
UKAEA, Winfrith	22	1·13	25	1·25	0·90	0·49 to 1·67
All minus Sellafield	518	1·02	549	1·06	0·96	0·85 to 1·09
All sites	538	1·02	570	1·07	0·96	0·85 to 1·08

SR(M)R, standardised registration (mortality) ratio; BNFL = British Nuclear Fuels Ltd; CEGB = Central Electricity Generating Board; UKAEA = United Kingdom Atomic Energy Authority.
* Based on Cook-Mozaffari et al[16]; † Includes BNFL Springfields (start 1948), BNFL Capenhurst (1953), Amersham International plc (1946), Aldermaston (1952) and UK Atomic Energy Authority Harwell (1947); ‡ Includes Bradwell (start 1961), Berkeley and Oldbury (1961), Hinkley Point (1964), Trawsfynydd (1964), Dungeness (1965), Sizewell (1965) and Wylfa (1971).

cancer mortality during 1969–78 in all the county districts of England and Wales by the same research group has recently become available.[19] This has adjusted for social class, population size, urban or rural status, and health authority region in examining areas near the same nuclear plants, and some of the results are shown in table III. Registration rates were not examined in this study. The findings overall suggest excess leukaemia mortality among people aged under 25 years of about 15% (20% for lymphoid leukaemia) in districts with at least 0·1% of their population resident within 10 miles of a nuclear installation. A similar result was found for Hodgkin's disease, but not for other cancers or at other ages. In this analysis the rates for childhood leukaemia were particularly high around Sellafield but were also raised in other areas. Cook-Mozaffari et al also examined leukaemia mortality for any trends with increasing percentage of the population resident within either six or 10 miles of an installation, but found no overall relation.[19]

TABLE III—*Leukaemia mortality in people under 25 years of age during 1969–78 in county districts with at least 0·1% of their population at the 1971 census resident within 10 miles of one of 14 nuclear installations**

Installation area†	No of deaths	Relative risk of death‡		Relative risk of death‡	
		Unadjusted	95% confidence interval	Adjusted	95% confidence interval
BNFL Sellafield	11	1·72 (p<0·05)§	0·93 to 3·18	1·85 (p<0·05)§	0·98 to 3·49
Pre-1955 sites	519	1·14 (p<0·05)§	1·04 to 1·26	1·14 (p<0·05)§	1·00 to 1·31
CEGB sites	197	1·08	0·92 to 1·25	1·15	0·97 to 1·36
UKAEA, Winfrith	18	0·87	0·54 to 1·39	0·96	0·58 to 1·58
All areas–Sellafield	734	1·11 (p<0·01)§	1·02 to 1·21	1·14 (p<0·05)§	1·02 to 1·26
All areas	745	1·12 (p<0·01)§	1·03 to 1·22	1·15 (p<0·01)§	1·04 to 1·28

BNFL = British Nuclear Fuels Ltd; CEGB = Central Electricity Generating Board; UKAEA = United Kingdom Atomic Energy Authority.
* Based on Cook-Mozaffari *et al*[19] and Cook-Mozaffari (personal communication).
† See footnote to table II.
‡ From log-linear regression analysis of the observed number of deaths against the expected number in the 400 county districts—unadjusted and adjusted for social class, urban or rural status, population size, and health authority region.
§ In these analyses Cook-Mozaffari *et al*, have adopted the unusual practice of carrying out one sided tests of the null hypothesis in the direction of the observed difference.[19]

SPECIFIC NUCLEAR SITES

Other studies that have been reported have concentrated on examining cancer rates around specific nuclear installations. Some, but not all, of these were excluded from the analyses just described—for example, Dounreay as it is in Scotland and Burghfield as its reported emissions are an order of magnitude or more lower than those from other sites.[16]

Dounreay

The installation at Dounreay on the north coast of the Scottish mainland is the only site in the UK apart from Sellafield that has a nuclear waste reprocessing facility. The duration and level of discharges from the plant have been much lower than from Sellafield, however. When information was requested by the Black inquiry in 1984 for this site, the leukaemia figures were reported as three cases observed and 2·56 expected under the ages of 25 years during the period 1968–81 in postcode sectors falling totally or partly within a 10 mile radius of the plant—not suggestive of any increase. However, later data, somewhat prompted by the public inquiry into the possible development of the site, revised this view.[20]

In the updated study the analysis made use of the more detailed coding of area of residence in the Scottish information systems, compared with

TABLE IV—*Leukaemia registrations for people under 25 years of age during 1968–84 in the postcode area containing Dounreay by distance from site**

Area	Number of cases		Ratio	95% confidence interval
	Observed	Expected†		
< 12·5 km from Dounreay	5	1·53	3·26	1·06 to 7·61
12·5–25 km from Dounreay	1	1·42	0·70	0·02 to 3·92
Other mainland	4	3·49	1·15	0·31 to 2·93
Orkney	2	3·11	0·64	0·08 to 2·32

† Based on Committee on Medical Aspects of Radiation in the Environment.[21]
† Calculated using rates for Scotland.

England and Wales, both for cancer registration and census data. By using the postcodes of residential addresses it is possible to amalgamate the disease information in ways that are more appropriate to answering epidemiological questions than the administrative areas that have been the basis of other studies described so far. Thus, if suitable data were available—for example, from environmental monitoring programmes—it would be possible to analyse cancer registration rates within relevant exposure contours. For Dounreay, in the absence of exposure measurements, circular areas centred on the Dounreay plant have been examined. Table IV shows leukaemia registrations during 1968–84 for people under the age of 25 years who were resident within 12·5 km and 25 km of the site, as well as in other more remote districts of the same postcode area on the mainland and the Orkney islands. It can be seen that the only figures of concern are those for the inner circle.

Questions can be asked about the choice of the 12·5 km radius and how critical this is to the apparent excess, especially as the circle's circumference passes through the middle of Thurso which is the main town in the region. To address these points a "sensitivity analysis" was carried out in which varying radii and other geographical areas were examined. This established that the choice of 12·5 km was not crucial to showing the existence of an excess (Committee on Medical Aspects of Radiation in the Environment, second report[24]). When the original researchers subdivided the calendar period of observation into three they found that the five cases within the circle with a 12·5 km radius had all been diagnosed during the last six years of the 17 year period for which data were available.[20]

In addition to these analyses, the Scottish researchers have also produced a means of putting the findings in the circle with a 12·5 km radius into the context of other artificially defined areas of similar population size throughout Scotland as a whole.[21] This was carried out using an algorithm which, from an arbitrary starting point, combines adjacent census enumeration districts until their joint population is as near as possible to that within the

TABLE V—*Leukaemia registrations for people under 25 years of age during 1968–84 in 634 areas of Scotland**

Number of cases	Number of areas	
	Observed	Predicted†
0	135	137
1	224	210
2	150	161
3	78	82
4	29	31
5	13‡	10
6	3	2·5
7	2	0·5
8	0	0·1

* Based on Committee on Medical Aspects of Radiation in the Environment:[21] the areas are that within 12·5 km from Dounreay plus 633 areas, of roughly equal population size and with 1·53 expected cases, formed by aggregating adjacent enumeration districts.
† Derived from the Poisson distribution with mean 1·53, taking account of the slight inequality of populations in the areas used.
‡ The area within 12·5 km from Dounreay is included in this group.

circle with 12·5 km radius—giving roughly 1·53 expected leukaemia cases during 1968–84 in each area. The numbers of observed cases in the 634 "equal areas" so formed are shown in table V.

It can be seen that the position of the Dounreay area is in the upper tail of the distribution, with 18 (2·8%) of the 634 areas having the same or more leukaemia cases. The one sided Poisson probability of five or more cases being observed given an expected number of 1·53 is 0·020, the same as the value obtained using the results in the predicted values column of table V. These values were calculated from the Poisson distribution under the assumption of uniform risk in each of the 634 areas and are similar to the results in the observed values column—indicating little departure from randomness. These results were generated by only one run of the algorithm, and the spatial distribution of the areas was not considered. The same analysis as in table V carried out for the years 1979–84 only, when all five cases of leukaemia within the circle around Dounreay with a 12·5 km radius were registered, showed an extreme result.[21] No other of the 612, in this instance, equal areas with expected number 0·49 had more than three cases. This finding, however, was made without a prior expectation that these particular six years would be the period to show an excess of leukaemia.

A recent suggestion has been made that the raised childhood leukaemia rate around Dounreay, and other nuclear installations situated in remote areas, may be caused by an increased susceptibility to a virus introduced into the local community by the large influx of workers.[22] Although a viral hypothesis has long been considered for childhood leukaemia, the evidence is not strong and the data produced to support this possible explanation are not yet convincing.[22]

Aldermaston, Burghfield, and Harwell

Three nuclear installations that have been jointly the subject of specific investigations are Aldermaston, Burghfield, and Harwell. This particular study arose as the consequence of a clinical suspicion at the Royal Berkshire Hospital in Reading that childhood leukaemia rates were high in west Berkshire.[23] The topic was also addressed in another television programme, *Inside Britain's Bomb*, screened in December 1985. Aldermaston and Harwell were included in the study described earlier in the section on other nuclear sites.

A subsequent analysis investigated childhood leukaemia registration rates within the West Berkshire and the Basingstoke and North Hampshire District Health Authority areas in more detail, in particular in relation to distance from the Aldermaston, Burghfield, and Harwell sites.[23] Relevant findings are shown in table VI. Although results for other distances were presented, particular a priori focus was on electoral wards with half or more of their area within 10 km of at least one of the three sites compared with all other wards within the district health authority areas. The main analysis was for the age range 0–14 years. It can be seen that leukaemia registration ratios are somewhat higher within the 10 km radius circles than outside, and higher overall in the district health authority areas than in England and Wales nationally. The raised rate seems to be limited to the age group 0–4 years—a group, however, that was not of particular defined interest before data analysis.

Data have since become available for other childhood cancers in a similar manner and are also shown in table VI (Committee on Medical Aspects of Radiation in the Environment, third report[24]). The same general findings as for leukaemia are repeated. These similarities could reflect real differences in incidence rates, but it needs to be satisfactorily established that they are not at least partly related to varying registration practices in the various areas. Cancer registration is not a legal requirement and is known to have been more complete in some regions than in others.[18] Thus, although registration (incidence) rates are more relevant to the questions raised, particularly for childhood leukaemia where survival has been much improved, mortality rates are possibly more valid for comparisons. The quality of cancer registration information is currently the subject of review by the Office of Population Censuses and Surveys and its investigation has also been recommended in the third report of the Committee on Medical Aspects of Radiation in the Environment[24].

TABLE VI—*Leukaemia (1972–85) and other cancer (1971–82) registrations in children under 15 years of age in the West Berkshire and the Basingstoke and North Hampshire District Health Authority areas by distance of the electoral ward of residence from Aldermaston, Burghfield, and Harwell**

| | Wards < 10 km away | | | Wards ⩾ 10 km away | | | Comparison of two distances | |
| | No of registrations | | | No of registrations | | | | 95% CI for ratio of < 10/⩾ 10 km O/E ratios |
Age group (years)	Observed (O)	Expected (E)†	O/E ratio	Observed (O)	Expected (E)†	O/E ratio	Ratio of < 10/⩾ 10 km O/E ratios	
				Leukaemia				
0–4	29	14·4	2·01	24	19·6	1·23	1·64	0·92 to 2·94
5–14	12	14·2	0·85	24	21·2	1·13	0·75	0·34 to 1·56
0–14	41	28·6	1·43	48	40·8	1·18	1·22	0·78 to 1·89
				Other cancers				
0–4	30	19·4	1·55	33	26·3	1·25	1·24	0·73 to 2·09
5–14	31	28·1	1·10	49	42·0	1·17	0·94	0·58 to 1·51
0–14	61	47·5	1·28	82	68·3	1·20	1·07	0·75 to 1·51

* Based on Committee on Medical Aspects of Radiation in the Environment.[24]
† Expected numbers based on age-specific registration rates in England and Wales.

Winfrith and Hinkley Point

Separate reports of increased childhood cancers around other specific nuclear establishments in England and Wales have been made independently—although some of these establishments are included in the combined analysis described earlier. The report for around Winfrith (South Coast Radiation Elimination Action Movement[25]) should be considered scientifically inadequate, and relevant information should be taken from tables II and III in this chapter. Further details are given in the paper by Barclay.[26] The first study relating to Hinkley Point[27] has been updated and extended.[28] A raised incidence of leukaemia and non-Hodgkin's lymphoma is now reported within 12·5 km of the installation compared with the remainder of Somerset for ages under 25 years during the 10 years (1964–73) after operations began, but no subsequent excess up to 1986. Overall the figures for leukaemia within 12·5 km of Hinkley Point were 13 observed cases compared with 9·5 expected at Somerset rates (separately—11 observed, 3·7 expected; and 2 observed, 5·8 expected during the two periods). This nuclear plant is included among the Central Electricity Generating Board sites in tables II and III—in addition, results compatible with those of Ewings and Bowie[28] are reported in the installation and calendar period specific leukaemia registration rate tables of Cook-Mozaffari et al[16] and the adjusted relative risk estimate for Hinkley Point (see table III for details) is 1·23 from Cook-Mozaffari et al.[19]

OTHER NUCLEAR INSTALLATIONS IN SCOTLAND

As well as the data on childhood leukaemia for areas around Dounreay,

161

which were discussed earlier, reports have been made of the rates around other nuclear installations in Scotland.[29][30] In the initial findings there was a suggestion of a raised registration rate of leukaemia for ages under 25 years during 1968–81 for people living in postcode sectors that fell partly or totally within 10 miles of Hunterston compared with the rest of Scotland, but rates in similarly defined sectors around Dounreay and Chapelcross were reported as being close to those expected. This was before the inclusion of the years 1982–84, during which three of the five cases mentioned earlier near Dounreay were registered. The later publication included results in a similar manner to those given in table IV for Dounreay, and the figures for Hunterston (14 observed, 10·21 expected) and Chapelcross (5 observed, 3·65 expected) were slightly above expectation within a circle with 12·5 km radius.

NORTHERN IRELAND

Although there are no nuclear installations in Northern Ireland, because of local concern about radioactive emissions from Sellafield a special investigation was set up in 1985, and its report has appeared.[31] The results were negative—with, in particular, rates of leukaemia during 1968–85 among children under 15 years of age living in coastal areas being no higher than those living inland.

OTHER COUNTRIES

For the USA two papers are relevant. Firstly, a study around the nuclear weapons Rocky Flats site in Denver suggested that there was an excess cancer risk downwind of the installation,[32] but its findings are controversial.[33][34] Secondly, a study around the San Onofre nuclear power plant in California reported that rates of childhood leukaemia were no higher in neighbouring areas than elsewhere.[35] Thirdly, a study from Massachusetts reported higher leukaemia registration rates in adults but not children during 1982–84 in an area around a nuclear power plant in Plymouth.[36] Fourthly, Goldsmith has presented data for 1950–79 for counties around the Hanford and Oak Ridge nuclear installations showing an excess leukaemia mortality among children 0–9 years old in the earlier years but not more recently.[37] Similar investigations in France, where there is heavy investment in nuclear energy, are under way.

Further investigations

Some further epidemiological investigations recommended in the Black report[3] to supplement the information then available have now been reported.

MORE GEOGRAPHICAL ANALYSIS

A more refined study of the geographical pattern of childhood cancer in the northern region was proposed—in particular to use 1961, 1971, and 1981 census population figures rather than only 1981 counts as denominators for rates covering the period 1968–82. The first results following this recommendation were given in the paper of Openshaw,[38] although they did not address the denominator concern. By using postcoded addresses of children with leukaemia, grid referenced to a level of 100 m resolution and similarly grid referencing the centroids of census enumeration districts, Openshaw et al have, as in Scotland, been able to move away from the use of administrative areas. They have also devised a method of analysis based on circular areas, but incorporating multiple overlapping circles of varying size based on a large series of grid points systematically covering the region. The results support the earlier findings in relation to the Sellafield area, but Openshaw et al identified further clusters in other areas that they suggest must be due to non-radiation related factors.

COHORT STUDIES

There are many potential problems of interpretation with the geographical approach to looking at cancer rates. Among these are the inclusion of cases in people who may only have moved into an area immediately before diagnosis—which would make the attribution of their illness unlikely to be due to a local factor—and the use of population denominators based on decennial censuses, without always adequate consideration of migration, for the calculation of rates. Such aspects warn against the introduction of increasingly sophisticated statistical methods as a necessary improvement to the interpretation of current geographical data.

Because of these difficulties the Black report recommended cohort studies of the child population of Seascale—both of children born and of children attending schools in the village since 1950.[3] The results of these studies confirmed that Seascale children had experienced a raised rate of cancer both while living in the village and also after moving away (Gardner et al[39 40]). This was concentrated among those born in Seascale, with 12 cases of cancer being reported up to 1986 compared with 2·8 expected, in contrast with the corresponding figures of 4 and 4·0 for children born outside but attending schools in the village.

CASE-CONTROL STUDIES

As another epidemiological method of seeking further understanding of the current position,[41] case-control studies are currently under way around Sellafield, Dounreay, Aldermaston, and Burghfield. Their aim is to collect relevant information on individual cases and appropriate control children to assess whether or not there is a link between the raised cancer rates and the nuclear sites. In the study around Sellafield controls taken at random from the same birth register into which each case was entered will be used to examine geographical residence at birth in relation to the nuclear site, and maternal *x* ray data during pregnancy and parental occupational histories of cases and controls will be compared. These studies are simultaneously examining other possible reasons for the apparent excess rates.

Conclusions

The original claim in a television documentary that there was an excess of leukaemia and other cancer among children near Windscale (Sellafield) on the north west coast of England has been confirmed, particularly in the neighbouring village of Seascale. An excess of childhood leukaemia has similarly been shown in the area around Dounreay on the north coast of Scotland, the only other site in the UK that has reprocessed nuclear waste—although the scale of operations and level of emissions have been much smaller. Depending on which statistics are quoted up to tenfold or even greater excesses of leukaemia can be described, but these are based on small absolute numbers of cases. Both areas are isolated from main centres of population and are inhabited largely by employees of the nuclear installations and their families. In areas near other nuclear sites in England and Wales, again with much lower levels of radioactive emissions than Sellafield, there is also a suggestion of an excess rate of leukaemia in young persons. However, the size of the reported increase is much smaller— around 15% rather than tenfold.

The raised cancer rates that have been described appear to be limited to children and other young people under the age of 25 years. However, the particular age groups within this range that seem to have had the highest rates, and the time trends reported, have not been consistent across nuclear sites. Rates of cancer overall have not been higher in adults—and, in particular, not for known radiation-related cancers. Although some other specific cancers have been found at higher rates among adults living in areas near nuclear installations, their meaning is not certain especially as large numbers of comparisons have been made.

For various reasons, including the manner of the original observation, interpreting the findings in children, particularly in causal terms, is at present difficult. A role for radioactive discharges and emissions influencing the increased rates is thought unlikely, as shown by conventional radiobiological models,[42] although a link to the nuclear operations including radiation exposure through other routes, such as parental employment, cannot at present be excluded. This possibility as well as the role of established risk factors for childhood leukaemia—such as antenatal *x* rays (see Doll[43])—in the reported excesses are currently being investigated in case-control studies.

1 Baron J. Cancer mortality in small areas around nuclear facilities in England and Wales. *Br J Cancer* 1984;**50**:815–24.
2 Schottenfeld D, Fraumeni JF, eds. *Cancer epidemiology and prevention*. Philadelphia: Saunders, 1982.
3 Black D for the Independent Advisory Group. *Investigation of the possible increased incidence of cancer in west Cumbria*. London: HMSO, 1984. (Black report.)
4 Clough EA. The BNFL radiation-mortality study. *Journal of the Society for Radiological Protection* 1983;**3** No 1:24–7.
5 Clough EA. Further report of the BNFL radiation-mortality study. *Journal of the Society for Radiological Protection* 1983;**3** No 3:18–20.
6 Smith PG, Douglas AJ. Mortality of workers at the Sellafield plant of British Nuclear Fuels. *BMJ* 1986;**293**:845–54.
7 Gardner MJ, Winter PD. Mortality in Cumberland during 1959–78 with reference to cancer in young people around Windscale. *Lancet* 1984;**i**:216–7.
8 Craft AW, Openshaw S, Birch J. Apparent clusters of childhood lymphoid malignancy in northern England. *Lancet* 1984;**i**:96–7
9 Urquhart J, Palmer M, Cutler J. Cancer in Cumbria: the Windscale connection. *Lancet* 1984;**i**:217–8.
10 Rothman KJ. *Modern epidemiology*. Boston: Little Brown, 1986.
11 Pomiankowski A. Cancer incidence at Sellafield. *Nature* 1984;**311**:100.
12 Gardner MJ. Seascale hazard. *Nature* 1984;**312**:10.
13 Clayton D, Kaldor J. Empirical Bayes estimates of age-standardized relative risks for use in disease mapping. *Biometrics* 1987;**43**:671–81.
14 Craft AW, Openshaw S, Birch J. Childhood cancer in the Northern Region, 1968–82: incidence in small geographic areas. *J Epidemiol Community Health* 1985;**39**:53–7.
15 Wakeford R, Binks K, Wilkie D. Childhood leukaemia and nuclear installations. *Journal of the Royal Statistical Society [Series A]* 1989;**152**:61–86.
16 Cook-Mozaffari PJ, Ashwood FL, Vincent T, Forman D, Alderson M. *Cancer incidence and mortality in the vicinity of nuclear installations, England and Wales, 1959–80*. London: HMSO, 1987.
17 Forman D, Cook-Fozaffari PJ, Darby S, Davey G, Stratton I, Doll R, *et al*. Cancer near nuclear installations. *Nature* 1987;**329**:499–505.
18 Swerdlow AJ. Cancer registration in England and Wales: some aspects relevant to interpretation of the data. *Journal of the Royal Statistical Society [Series A]* 1986;**149**:146–60.
19 Cook-Mozaffari PJ, Darby SC, Doll R, Forman D, Hermon C, Pike M, *et al*. Geographical variation in mortality from leukaemia and other cancers in England and Wales in relation to proximity to nuclear installations, 1969–78. *Br J Cancer* 1989;**59**:476–85.
20 Heasman MA, Kemp IW, Urquhart JD, Black R. Childhood leukaemia in northern Scotland. *Lancet* 1986;**i**:266.
21 Committee on Medical Aspects of Radiation in the Environment. *Investigation of the possible increased incidence of leukaemia in young people near the Dounreay nuclear establishment, Caithness, Scotland*. London: HMSO, 1988. (2nd COMARE report.)
22 Kinlen LJ. Evidence for an infective cause for childhood leukaemia: a Scottish new town compared to nuclear reprocessing sites. *Lancet* 1988;**ii**:1323–6.
23 Roman E, Beral V, Carpenter L, Watson A, Barton C, Ryder H, *et al*. Childhood leukaemia in the West Berkshire and Basingstoke and North Hampshire District Health Authorities in relation to nuclear establishments in the vicinity. *BMJ* 1987;**294**:597–602.
24 Committee on Medical Aspects of Radiation in the Environment. *Investigation of the possible increased incidence of childhood cancer near Aldermaston and Burghfield*. London: HMSO, 1989. (3rd COMARE report.)
25 South Coast Radiation Elimination Action Movement. *Report proposing a causal link between radioactive discharges from the UK Atomic Energy's Establishment at*

Winfrith, Dorset and leukaemia excesses in the vicinity. Isle of Wight: South Coast Radiation Elimination Action Movement, 1984.

26 Barclay R. Childhood leukaemia in Wessex. *Community Med* 1987;9:279–85.

27 Bowie C, Ewings P. *Leukaemia in the west of Somerset—a second report.* Taunton: Somerset Health Authority, 1986.

28 Ewings PD, Bowie C. *Leukaemia incidence in Somerset with particular reference to Hinkley Point.* Taunton: Somerset Health Authority, 1988.

29 Heasman MA, Kemp IW, MacLaren AM, Trotter P, Gillis CR, Hole DJ. Incidence of leukaemia in young persons in west of Scotland. *Lancet* 1984;i:1188–9.

30 Heasman MA, Urquhart JD, Black RJ, Kemp IW. Leukaemia in young persons in Scotland: a study of its geographical distribution and relationship to nuclear installations. *Health Bull (Edinb)* 1987;45:147–51.

31 Lowry S. *Investigation into patterns of disease with possible association with radiation in Northern Ireland.* Belfast: HMSO, 1989.

32 Johnson CJ. Cancer incidence in an area contaminated with radionuclides near a nuclear installation. *Ambio* 1981;10:176–82.

33 Crump KS, Ng T-H, Cuddihy RG. Cancer incidence patterns in the Denver metropolitan area in relation to the Rocky Flats plant. *Am J Epidemiol* 1987;126:127–35.

34 Johnson CJ. Re: cancer incidence patterns in the Denver metropolitan area in relation to the Rocky Flats plant. *Am J Epidemiol* 1987;126:153–5.

35 Enstrom JE. Cancer near a California nuclear power plant. *Lancet* 1985;ii:1249.

36 Clapp RW, Cobb S, Chan CK, Walker B. Leukaemia near Massachusetts nuclear power plant. *Lancet* 1989;ii:1324–5.

37 Goldsmith J. Childhood leukaemia mortality before 1970 among populations near two US nuclear installations. *Lancet* 1989;i:793.

38 Openshaw S, Craft AW, Charlton M, Birch JM. Investigation of leukaemia clusters by use of a geographical analysis machine. *Lancet* 1988;i:272–3

39 Gardner MJ, Hall AJ, Downes S, Terrell JD. Follow up study of children born elsewhere but attending schools in Seascale, west Cumbria (schools cohort). *BMJ* 1987;295:819–22.

40 Gardner MJ, Hall AJ, Downes S, Terrell JD. Follow up of children born to mothers resident in Seascale, west Cumbria (birth cohort). *BMJ* 1987;295:822–7.

41 Gardner MJ. Epidemiological studies of environmental exposure and specific diseases. *Arch Environ Health* 1988;43:102–8.

42 Wheldon TE. The assessment of risk of radiation-induced childhood leukaemia in the vicinity of nuclear installations. *Journal of the Royal Statistical Society [Series A]* 1989;152:327–39.

43 Doll R. The epidemiology of childhood leukaemia. *Journal of the Royal Statistical Society [Series A]* 1989;152:341–51.

19: Results of case-control study of leukaemia and lymphoma among young people near Sellafield nuclear plant in west Cumbria

MARTIN J GARDNER, MICHAEL P SNEE,
ANDREW J HALL, CAROLINE A POWELL,
SUSAN DOWNES, JOHN D TERRELL

An excess of childhood leukaemia and lymphoma near the Sellafield nuclear plant has been observed. To examine whether the excess is associated with established risk factors or with factors related to the plant, a case-control study was undertaken of 97 people aged under 25 born in west Cumbria health district and diagnosed during 1950–85 as having leukaemia (52), non-Hodgkin's lymphoma (22), or Hodgkin's disease (23) compared with 1001 controls matched for sex and age taken from the same birth registers as the cases. Factors studied included antenatal abdominal x ray examinations, viral infections, lifestyles, proximity to Sellafield, and employment risks of parents working at Sellafield.

Expected associations with prenatal exposure to x rays were found, but little information about viral illnesses was available. Relative risks for leukaemia and non-Hodgkin's lymphoma were higher in children born near Sellafield and in children of fathers employed at the plant, particularly those with high radiation dose recordings before their children's conception. For example, the relative risks compared with area controls were 0·17 (95% confidence interval 0·05 to 0·53) for being born further than 5 km from Sellafield, 2·44 (1·04 to 5·71) for children of fathers employed at Sellafield at their conception, and 6·42 (1·57 to 26·3) for children of fathers receiving a total preconceptual ionising radiation dose of 100 millisieverts (mSv) or more. Other factors, including exposure to x rays, maternal age, employment elsewhere, eating seafood, and playing on the beach did not explain these relations.

Focusing on Seascale, where the excess incidence has predominantly been reported, showed (for the four out of five patients with leukaemia and one with non-Hodgkin's lymphoma whose fathers were employed at Sellafield and for whom dose information was obtained) that the fathers of patients had higher radiation doses before their children's conception than the fathers of matched controls; the father of the other Seascale patient (with non-Hodgkin's lymphoma) was not employed at the plant. These results seem to explain statistically the geographical association. For Hodgkin's disease neither geographical nor employment associations with Sellafield were found.

The raised incidence of leukaemia and (to a lesser extent) non-Hodgkin's lymphoma among children near Sellafield was associated with paternal recorded external dose of whole body penetrating radiation during work at the plant before conception. The association can explain statistically the observed geographical excess. This result suggests that ionising radiation of fathers may be leukaemogenic in their offspring, though other, less likely, explanations are possible. There are important potential implications for radiobiology and for protection of radiation workers and their children.

Introduction

There has been concern about levels of childhood cancer around nuclear installations in the United Kingdom since 1983, when a Yorkshire Television programme (*Windscale: the Nuclear Laundry*) suggested that there was an excess of leukaemia near Sellafield. Several studies have been carried out since,[1] and the one reported here was a direct consequence of a recommendation of the Black committee (of which MJG was a member).[2] This investigation was a case-control study of leukaemia and lymphoma among young people in west Cumbria, which specifically asked whether known causes or factors associated with the nuclear site might have been responsible for the observed excess.

Methods

The design of the study, methods of data collection, and basic information are described in detail in the next chapter.[3] Essentially all identified cases of leukaemia and lymphoma among people born in west Cumbria and diagnosed there at ages under 25 during 1950–85 were compared with controls matched by sex and date of birth selected—both unmatched (area controls) and matched (local controls) for civil parish of residence—from the same birth register in which the case child's birth was entered. For both types of control up to eight controls were included in the analysis for each case, some of whom were both area and local controls. Comparisons were carried out using data from birth and medical records, from questionnaires to parents of case and control children, and from employment and radiation records held by British Nuclear Fuels.

The analysis was carried out within the sets of cases and area or local controls, and findings are presented as relative risks with confidence intervals. The results were calculated using conditional logistic regression analysis,[4] which produces estimates of odds ratios that approximate closely to relative risks, with the computer program EGRET.[5] Unless otherwise stated the relative risks are for presence compared with absence of each factor; where specifically mentioned in tables relative risks are for the first compared with the second grouping, except in ionising radiation dose categories, where the risks are relative to the unexposed group.

Results and comment

Findings are shown for leukaemia alone and for leukaemia and non-Hodgkin's lymphoma combined (see next chapter) for area and local controls separately. Because some controls, who were entered closely adjacent to a case in the birth register, were both area and local controls these two analyses by control type were not completely independent statistically—for example, for the 52 leukaemia cases there were 217 area only controls, 207 local only controls, and 140 who were both (see table III of next chapter[3]). Results for non-Hodgkin's lymphoma are presented here only in combination with leukaemia for the reasons given in the next chapter and because the numbers were smaller. Numbers of individuals included in the analyses for different factors varied with the availability of

TABLE I—*Numbers of cases and controls with relative risks for leukaemia and non-Hodgkin's lymphoma in children by maternal exposure to abdominal x rays in pregnancy according to medical records and questionnaires*

Source of x ray information	Type of control	Cases		Controls		Relative risk	95% Confidence interval
		Total	No exposed to x rays	Total	No exposed to x rays		
Leukaemia							
Medical	Area	20	3	116	15	1·15	0·31 to 4·28
	Local	20	3	109	13	1·21	0·31 to 4·66
Questionnaire	Area	35	4	116	9	1·74	0·44 to 6·82
	Local	34	4	104	11	1·19	0·33 to 4·31
Leukaemia and non-Hodgkin's lymphoma							
Medical records	Area	28	5	167	25	1·19	0·43 to 3·32
	Local	28	5	153	20	1·34	0·46 to 3·88
Questionnaire	Area	47	5	152	14	1·32	0·43 to 4·08
	Local	45	5	143	15	1·14	0·37 to 3·53

data, and the number of case-control sets is given by the total number of cases. Results for Hodgkin's disease are not given in detail as they did not show any important associations with analysed factors in the same way as leukaemia and non-Hodgkin's lymphoma.

ANTENATAL X RAYS

Table I shows relative risks for leukaemia and non-Hodgkin's lymphoma associated with maternal abdominal radiographic examinations according to whether the information was obtained from obstetric records or questionnaire responses. The relative risks ranged from about 1·2 to 1·7, comparable to levels reported in earlier studies. This study was too small for meaningful analysis by number of films or trimester of exposure.

For cases of Hodgkin's disease a report of an abdominal x ray examination was made for none of the six mothers for whom we located obstetric records and by two of the 12 parents who responded on the questionnaire.

VIRAL INFECTIONS AND OTHER SUSPECTED RISK FACTORS

Only one episode of viral infectious illness during pregnancy was recorded in the hospital records examined, so analysis was restricted to data from the questionnaires. Results for any episode of chickenpox, shingles, influenza, measles, or rubella are given in table II, with no strong finding. Also shown are relative risks, again based on small numbers, for delivery by caesarean section based on information from obstetric records.

Findings are given for social class based on parental occupation at birth as recorded on each of birth certificates and questionnaires, and the similar results reflect the high level of agreement between the data sources. Table II shows relative risks around unity for a broad higher social class category

TABLE II—*Numbers of cases and controls with relative risks for leukaemia and non-Hodgkin's lymphoma in children by some suspected risk factors*

Suspected risk factor	Type of control	Cases Total	Cases Positive	Controls Total	Controls Positive	Relative risk	95% Confidence interval
Leukaemia							
Maternal viral infection in pregnancy	Area	35	2	119	7	1·12	0·22 to 5·67
	Local	35	2	103	6	1·23	0·22 to 7·04
Caesarean delivery	Area	20	2	116	8	1·38	0·27 to 6·99
	Local	20	2	109	9	1·17	0·24 to 5·81
Social class* (birth certificate)	Area	44	9	293	54	1·14	0·50 to 2·60
	Local	44	9	287	75	0·61	0·25 to 1·47
Social class* (questionnaire)	Area	20	5	51	16	0·90	0·24 to 3·34
	Local	19	5	54	21	0·60	0·17 to 2·10
Mother's age ($\geqslant 25$ v < 25 years)	Area	52	32	351	220	0·94	0·51 to 1·72
	Local	52	32	344	213	0·96	0·52 to 1·78
Mother's age ($\geqslant 40$ v < 25 years)	Area	52	4	351	6	4·94	1·11 to 21·85
	Local	52	4	344	8	3·38	0·88 to 13·03
Father's age ($\geqslant 25$ v < 25 years)	Area	46	38	287	220	1·42	0·63 to 3·18
	Local	46	38	276	213	1·43	0·61 to 3·33
Father's age ($\geqslant 40$ v < 25 years)	Area	46	6	287	26	1·87	0·59 to 5·91
	Local	46	6	276	24	2·27	0·66 to 7·76
Birth weight ($\geqslant 3·5$ v $< 3·5$ kg)	Area	18	7	99	42	0·88	0·32 to 2·42
	Local	18	7	94	41	0·84	0·29 to 2·42
Leukaemia and non-Hodgkin's lymphoma							
Maternal viral infection in pregnancy	Area	47	2	156	12	0·69	0·15 to 3·24
	Local	46	2	144	8	0·94	0·18 to 4·87
Caesarean delivery	Area	28	2	167	15	0·75	0·16 to 3·56
	Local	28	2	153	11	0·95	0·20 to 4·50
Social class* (birth certificate)	Area	64	14	418	75	1·33	0·68 to 2·59
	Local	64	14	408	100	0·70	0·33 to 1·49
Social class* (questionnaire)	Area	26	7	70	20	1·11	0·34 to 3·64
	Local	25	7	75	30	0·61	0·21 to 1·79
Mother's age ($\geqslant 25$ v < 25 years)	Area	74	47	492	311	0·99	0·60 to 1·65
	Local	74	47	484	305	0·99	0·59 to 1·66
Mother's age ($\geqslant 40$ v < 25 years)	Area	74	7	492	10	5·08	1·66 to 15·53
	Local	74	7	484	12	4·03	1·41 to 11·52
Father's age ($\geqslant 25$ v < 25 years)	Area	66	52	403	318	0·95	0·50 to 1·79
	Local	66	52	389	304	1·00	0·51 to 1·93
Father's age ($\geqslant 40$ v < 25 years)	Area	66	9	403	34	1·51	0·60 to 3·78
	Local	66	9	389	34	1·58	0·60 to 4·16
Birth weight ($\geqslant 3·5$ v $< 3·5$ kg)	Area	26	11	149	62	1·01	0·44 to 2·34
	Local	26	11	137	64	0·86	0·37 to 2·01

* Social class of father at child's birth: I, II, III non-manual v III manual, IV, V.

in relation to area controls but lower values for local controls. More detailed analysis did not identify any strong trends by social class.

Relative risks around unity were also found for maternal age of 25 or older compared with under 25 years at the child's birth. For mothers of 40 or older, however, when examined in a comparison of all age groups—that is, < 25, 25–29, 30–34, 35–39, and $\geqslant 40$ years—relative risks were about 4. The latter finding was much less strong for fathers. Birth weight, from obstetric records, showed no particular relation in either the broad categories listed or smaller groups.

TABLE III—*Numbers of cases and controls with relative risks for leukaemia and non-Hodgkin's lymphoma in children by family habit factors from parental questionnaire*

Habit factor	Type of control	Cases		Controls		Relative risk	95% Confidence interval
		Total	Positive	Total	Positive		
Leukaemia							
Play on beach	Area	28	13	94	47	0·89	0·37 to 2·17
(more *v* less often than monthly)	Local	28	13	92	57	0·62	0·24 to 1·59
Play on fells	Area	27	3	77	23	0·29	0·06 to 1·39
(more *v* less often than monthly)	Local	24	3	71	18	0·53	0·14 to 2·07
Eating fish	Area	29	16	97	49	1·26	0·50 to 3·21
(more *v* less often than weekly)	Local	28	16	93	49	1·16	0·45 to 3·00
Eating shellfish	Area	15	2	36	1	7·03	0·61 to 80·43
(more *v* less often than weekly)	Local	15	2	29	3	1·11	0·15 to 7·91
Grow own vegetables	Area	35	15	123	54	0·98	0·45 to 2·13
	Local	35	15	112	45	1·07	0·46 to 2·48
Seaweed as fertiliser	Area	11	1	25	1	1·73	0·10 to 30·76
	Local	13	1	25	1	2·00	0·13 to 31·98
Leukaemia and non-Hodgkin's lymphoma							
Play on beach	Area	40	18	131	61	0·95	0·45 to 2·00
((more *v* less often than monthly)	Local	39	18	131	78	0·66	0·31 to 1·40
Play on fells	Area	36	4	103	28	0·33	0·09 to 1·21
(more *or* less often than monthly)	Local	32	4	98	31	0·36	0·11 to 1·17
Eating fish	Area	39	20	126	62	1·03	0·45 to 2·37
(more *v* less often than weekly)	Local	36	19	127	67	0·86	0·38 to 1·98
Eating shellfish	Area	19	2	44	2	2·99	0·40 to 22·11
(more *v* less often than weekly)	Local	18	2	39	5	0·82	0·14 to 5·01
Grow own vegetables	Area	47	20	161	71	0·99	0·52 to 1·93
	Local	46	20	154	72	0·87	0·42 to 1·81
Seaweed as fertiliser	Area	15	1	30	1	1·73	0·10 to 30·76
	Local	17	1	36	1	2·00	0·13 to 31·98

For Hodgkin's disease there were no important relations with any of the above factors including parental ages.

QUESTIONNAIRE HABIT FACTORS

Table III shows findings based on the behavioural data obtained by questionnaire. The factors included, particularly those for which there were data on substantial numbers of cases, did not show any important relations with leukaemia and non-Hodgkin's lymphoma. Results for playing on the beach are shown in the table with all cases for whom information was available. Children aged under 5 years at diagnosis were less likely because of their illness to have played in the sand, and excluding these cases and their controls made little difference, with the relative risks against area controls for leukaemia alone and combined with non-Hodgkin's lymphoma becoming 0·83 and 1·04 respectively. The relative risks for play on the fells were particularly low.

Analysis by fish eating habits did not indicate any associated risk. For shellfish eating the relative risks were raised compared with area controls but not compared with local controls; the raised relative risks were,

TABLE IV—*Numbers of cases and controls with relative risks for leukaemia and non-Hodgkin's lymphoma in children by distance from Sellafield of residence at birth for area controls*

	Leukaemia				Leukaemia and non-Hodgkin's lymphoma			
Distance (km)	Cases (n=51)	Area controls (n=350)	Relative risk	95% Confidence interval	Cases (n=73)	Area controls (n=491)	Relative risk	95% Confidence interval
≤4	5	14	1		8	16	1	
5–9	5	31	0·35	0·08 to 1·62	6	43	0·21	0·06 to 0·78
10–14	14	117	0·21	0·05 to 0·92	22	160	0·17	0·05 to 0·56
15–19	5	35	0·22	0·04 to 1·22	8	50	0·16	0·04 to 0·67
20–24	9	52	0·22	0·03 to 1·59	11	84	0·07	0·01 to 0·38
25–29	8	66	0·14	0·02 to 0·91	12	100	0·06	0·01 to 0·31
≥30	5	35	0·17	0·02 to 1·88	6	38	0·11	0·02 to 0·80

however, based on only two exposed cases (both diagnosed before 1980). Restriction of these analyses to cases born during periods when discharges from Sellafield were highest did not show any important differential relative risks. Finally, there was no evidence of any increased risk in conjunction with families growing their own vegetables or using seaweed as a fertiliser.

There were no important relations of Hodgkin's disease with these factors.

GEOGRAPHY OF CASES AND CONTROLS RELATIVE TO SELLAFIELD

Distances of addresses of cases and controls from Sellafield were calculated by taking the grid reference of the plant to be NY 027 039 as used by the National Radiological Protection Board in its analysis of atmospheric discharges (J Stather, personal communication). The results given here are for area controls using addresses at birth. Table IV shows findings in circles of increasing 5 km radiuses moving away from Sellafield, and risks are given relative to the inner circle (which completely contains Seascale and some other smaller villages). All five cases of leukaemia and two of the three cases of non-Hodgkin's lymphoma in the inner circle occurred in children born to parents resident in Seascale. There was a large fall in relative risk in moving to outside the inner circle to levels of about one third and smaller, with some suggestion also of a decreasing risk with further distance. For leukaemia and non-Hodgkin's lymphoma combined the relative risks away from the inner circle were lower than for leukaemia alone. The relative risk of luekaemia for all children born outside the inner circle was 0·26 (95% confidence interval 0·07 to 1·01) and for leukaemia and non-Hodgkin's lymphoma together it was 0·17 (95% confidence interval 0·05 to 0·53). These latter results also applied when analysis was limited to cases born in the birth registration district containing Sellafield rather than all west Cumbria. None of the 23 cases of Hodgkin's disease in

173

TABLE V—*Numbers of cases and controls with relative risks for leukaemia and non-Hodgkin's lymphoma in children by paternal occupation and industry recorded on birth certificates*

Father's occupation/industry	Type of control	Cases	Controls	Relative risk	95% Confidence interval
Leukaemia					
Total	Area	46	286		
	Local	46	277		
Sellafield	Area	9	29	2·82	1·07 to 7·40
	Local	9	41	2·03	0·69 to 5·93
Coal mining	Area	2	33	0·37	0·09 to 1·61
	Local	2	31	0·35	0·08 to 1·60
Iron and steel	Area	5	18	1·84	0·60 to 5·60
	Local	5	16	2·36	0·71 to 7·78
Farming	Area	5	19	1·98	0·66 to 5·96
	Local	5	11	2·63	0·77 to 8·95
Chemicals	Area	5	25	1·39	0·49 to 3·97
	Local	5	23	1·58	0·52 to 4·84
Leukaemia and non-Hodgkin's lymphoma					
Total	Area	64	393		
	Local	64	383		
Sellafield	Area	10	38	2·02	0·87 to 4·67
	Local	10	54	1·32	0·51 to 3·43
Coal mining	Area	5	53	0·51	0·19 to 1·39
	Local	5	53	0·46	0·16 to 1·30
Iron and steel	Area	9	31	2·06	0·88 to 4·82
	Local	9	25	3·20	1·23 to 8·28
Farming	Area	6	27	1·54	0·57 to 4·11
	Local	6	16	2·15	0·71 to 6·51
Chemicals	Area	7	27	1·90	0·75 to 4·78
	Local	7	25	2·15	0·80 to 5·77

the study had an address at birth within the 5 km radius inner circle. Of the 95 total cases with complete information 79 (83%) remained in the same 5 km sector from birth to diagnosis.

FATHER'S OCCUPATION AND EMPLOYMENT AT SELLAFIELD

Three separate sources of parental occupational information were used: birth certificates, questionnaires, and the computer file of past and present workers at Sellafield. Maternal occupation is generally recorded on a birth certificate only in the absence of paternal occupation, questionnaire data were available for only about half the study members, and relatively few women have worked at Sellafield, so results given here are restricted to father's employment.

Table V shows the relative risks for leukaemia and non-Hodgkin's lymphoma associated with various paternal employment categories. These data were taken from birth certificates rather than questionnaires because of the greater completeness of information—for example, data for the 74 fathers of children with leukaemia and non-Hodgkin's lymphoma were available from 64 (86%) birth certificates but only 32 (43%) questionnaires. Results are given for the main industrial groups in west Cumbria which employed more than 5% of control fathers. Raised relative risks were associated with fathers working at Sellafield and in iron and steel, farming, and chemicals, with children of coal miners having low relative risks but based on small numbers. Similar results were found using the questionnaire data and when examining employment on the questionnaire at conception rather than birth, although then relative risks were somewhat higher in relation to Sellafield and farming than those shown in table V.

For Hodgkin's disease the relative risks associated with fathers working at Sellafield according to data from birth certificates were low—for example, for local controls the relative risk was 0·71 (95% confidence interval 0·08 to 6·03). This result was based on only one positive case, as, although we had records that four fathers altogether were Sellafield workers, for three this employment occurred after the birth of their children.

RADIATION DOSIMETRY AT SELLAFIELD

Table VI shows relative risks for leukaemia and non-Hodgkin's lymphoma in children associated with their fathers' employment and exposure to ionising radiation obtained through linkage with the Sellafield workforce file. As well as analysing the total radiation dose recorded before conception (taken as nine months before birth) we looked at that during the immediately preceding six months, as it has been suggested that this is the most sensitive period for the induction of transmissible genetic damage.[6] The six monthly doses were estimated proportionally from the recorded annual doses of the father and the date of birth of his child.

For paternal employment at the plant relative risks were higher for leukaemia alone than for leukaemia and non-Hodgkin's lymphoma combined and were higher for employment at conception than at any other time. Relative risks for leukaemia and non-Hodgkin's lymphoma were higher for fathers with a radiation dose record at conception than for those with a radiation dose record at any time before conception or diagnosis. The highest relative risks—about sixfold—were for fathers with total radiation doses of 100 mSv or more before the date of their child's conception or doses of 10 mSv or more during the six months before conception. Figures for all the control fathers in this study indicated that about 9% of the workforce had accumulated preconceptual doses over 100 mSv and about 13% had had doses over 10 mSv during the six months before conception.

The results shown in table VI relate to all fathers in the study for whom we could make a definite positive or negative linkage to the Sellafield file.

The same analysis limited to fathers positively linked to the Sellafield file showed similar relations to ionising radiation dose but with larger relative risks in the highest categories. For example, there was a relative risk of 17·2 for leukaemia compared with area controls in children of fathers with total radiation doses before conception of 100 mSv or more with a 95% confidence interval of 1·1 to 278, the wide interval reflecting that the analysis was based on a total of 11 case-control sets rather than 46 as in the table.

TABLE VI—*Numbers of cases and controls with relative risks for leukaemia and non-Hodgkin's lymphoma in children by timing of paternal employment and external ionising radiation dosimetry at Sellafield*

Father's employment/ radiation group	Type of control	Cases	Controls	Relative risk	95% Confidence interval
		Leukaemia			
Total	Area	46	288		
	Local	46	276		
Employed:					
Before conception	Area	9	36	1·97	0·82 to 4·78
	Local	9	45	1·39	0·53 to 3·65
At conception	Area	8	25	2·79	1·04 to 7·52
	Local	8	32	2·07	0·69 to 6·14
At birth	Area	8	27	2·51	0·95 to 6·67
		8	33	1·92	0·66 to 5·56
Before diagnosis	Area	9	53	1·17	0·49 to 2·76
	Local	9	58	0·89	0·36 to 2·18
Ever	Area	12	65	1·35	0·61 to 2·96
	Local	12	65	1·22	0·54 to 2·74
Dose record:					
Before conception	Area	8	35	1·71	0·68 to 4·26
	Local	8	40	1·40	0·50 to 3·94
At conception	Area	8	24	3·07	1·09 to 8·65
	Local	8	30	2·43	0·80 to 7·41
Before diagnosis	Area	8	48	1·11	0·45 to 2·72
	Local	8	54	0·81	0·31 to 2·10
Total dose before conception:					
1–49 mSv	Area	3	19	1·12	0·31 to 4·05
	Local	3	26	0·77	0·20 to 3·00
50–99 mSv	Area	1	11	0·69	0·08 to 5·73
	Local	1	11	0·78	0·08 to 7·73
⩾100 mSv	Area	4	5	6·24	1·51 to 25·76
	Local	4	3	8·38	1·35 to 51·99
Dose during 6 months before conception:					
1–4 mSv	Area	3	18	1·30	0·32 to 5·34
	Local	3	24	1·10	0·25 to 4·91
5–9 mSv	Area	1	3	3·54	0·32 to 38·88
	Local	1	3	3·04	0·28 to 32·61
⩾10 mSv	Area	4	5	7·17	1·69 to 30·44
	Local	4	3	8·21	1·62 to 41·73

TABLE VI—*continued*

Father's employment/ radiation group	Type of control	Cases	Controls	Relative risk	95% Confidence interval
	Leukaemia and non-Hodgkin's lymphoma				
Total	Area	66	404		
	Local	66	389		
Employed:					
Before conception	Area	11	47	1·77	0·82 to 3·85
	Local	11	62	1·08	0·47 to 2·52
At conception	Area	10	34	2·44	1·04 to 5·71
	Local	10	46	1·48	0·59 to 3·75
At birth	Area	10	37	2·14	0·93 to 4·92
	Local	10	50	1·26	0·48 to 3·28
Before diagnosis	Area	11	72	0·97	0·46 to 2·03
	Local	11	83	0·64	0·28 to 1·45
Ever	Area	14	88	1·01	0·51 to 2·02
	Local	14	93	0·81	0·39 to 1·69
Dose record:					
Before conception	Area	10	45	1·63	0·73 to 3·64
	Local	10	58	1·00	0·40 to 2·51
At conception	Area	10	32	2·71	1·12 to 6·60
	Local	10	45	1·58	0·60 to 4·18
Before diagnosis	Area	10	66	0·95	0·44 to 2·05
	Local	10	78	0·60	0·25 to 1·41
Total dose before conception:					
1–49 mSv	Area	4	27	1·06	0·35 to 3·21
	Local	4	41	0·53	0·16 to 1·78
50–99 mSv	Area	2	13	1·16	0·24 to 5·46
	Local	2	14	0·95	0·17 to 5·28
⩾100 mSv	Area	4	5	6·42	1·57 to 26·32
	Local	4	3	8·30	1·36 to 50·56
Dose during 6 months before conception:					
1–4 mSv	Area	5	22	1·80	0·59 to 5·53
	Local	5	33	0·97	0·28 to 3·41
5–9 mSv	Area	1	4	2·41	0·25 to 23·43
	Local	1	7	1·12	0·13 to 9·93
⩾10 mSv	Area	4	8	4·33	1·16 to 16·12
	Local	4	5	5·01	1·13 to 22·24

For cases of Hodgkin's disease none of the four fathers employed at Sellafield had a record of occupational radiation exposure before their child's conception.

SEASCALE

Earlier studies have concentrated on the geographical excess of childhood leukaemia in the neighbourhood of the Sellafield plant. This excess was found in Seascale particularly and was based on around five cases compared with fewer than one expected, depending on which age group and calendar period were reported. A pertinent question is to what degree this excess may be explained statistically by the demonstrated relation with paternal radiation dose during employment.

Three of the five Seascale cases in this study were among the four cases of leukaemia with fathers in the highest total radiation dose group (table VI), with doses of 102 mSv (over about seven years' employment), 162 mSv (about six years), and 188 mSv (about seven years). The one case in the intermediate group was also from Seascale, with a paternal total dose of 97 mSv (over about 13 years). The fifth Seascale leukaemia case was not, however, linked with the Sellafield computer file owing to our being unable to trace a date of birth for his father, although we know from the child's birth certificate and the mother's questionnaire that the father worked at Sellafield. Thus, we know that three of the five Seascale cases had fathers whose accumulated preconceptual radiation dose was in the group with an estimated sixfold to eightfold relative risk of leukaemia and the father of the fourth was in the group just below the cut off value used. These five Seascale leukaemia cases were precisely those in the inner circle of table IV, where the risk was highest.

If the exposure of the father to ionising radiation was the cause of leukaemia in the children then the reported geographical excess could effectively be explained on this basis. If, alternatively, the fact of living in Seascale itself were responsible for the excess then it would not be expected that three of the four fathers linked to the Sellafield workforce file would have a total radiation dose before conception in the highest category, whereas 16 out of 20 fathers of the local controls for these four cases (also born to mothers resident in Seascale) had a radiation record with only one in the highest category (the other four had not been employed at Sellafield). Moreover, in no father of the 20 local controls was their total preconceptual dose as high as in the father of their related case. For fathers of the area controls the corresponding figures were 9 out of 27 with a radiation record but none in the highest category (17 of the other 18 had not been employed at Sellafield), and all the total preconceptual doses of the fathers of the 27 area controls were lower than those of the father of their related case. These comparisons are shown in table VII and graphically in the figure, where case 1 was in the intermediate dose category of table VI and cases 2, 3, and 4 in the highest category. Similar results were found for radiation dose during the six months before conception, except that two of the 18 fathers of the total of 43 controls with a radiation record during this period had higher doses than the father of their associated case. Two mothers of the five leukaemia cases had been employed at Sellafield; neither worked there at the time of conception of their child, but one had experienced previous exposure to radiation (of 26 mSv) at the plant.

None of the 23 cases of Hodgkin's disease had an address at birth in Seascale.

TABLE VII—*Numbers of Seascale leukaemia cases and their controls by paternal employment and total external ionising radiation dose at Sellafield before their child's conception**

Paternal employment/ preconceptual radiation dose at Sellafield	Cases	Controls	
		Local	Area
Not employed	0	4	17
No dose record	0	0	1
1–49 sMv	0	8	6
50–99 mSv	1	7	3
⩾100 mSv	3	1	0
Total	4	20	27

* One Seascale case (and associated controls) is omitted from this table owing to lack of information on the father (see text). The 20 local controls, as the four cases, were all born to mothers resident in Seascale but only four of the 27 area controls.

Discussion

The main finding of this study is that the recorded external dose of whole body ionising radiation to fathers during their employment at Sellafield is associated with the development of leukaemia among their children. As radiation badge recording will reflect gonadal dose we interpret this finding to suggest an effect of the radiation exposure on germ cells producing a mutation in sperm that may be leukaemogenic in subsequent offspring. Other explanations may be possible, such as exposure to internally incorporated radionuclides or other concomitant exposures in the workplace: it has not been possible to examine the first of these so far, and the second seems unlikely (see below). Additionally, contamination of the home with radioactive or other material through occupational exposure may be relevant, although there is no evidence to support this.

The results suggest highest risks in those with the highest accumulated ionising radiation doses before conception, either over their total duration of exposure or during the preceding six months. For both periods of exposure the same four cases of leukaemia were in the highest groups, three of them in children born in Seascale, and none were lymphomas. We have not yet examined any other duration of exposure period. Comparison of the relative size of various calculated risks associated with fathers' being employed or having a radiation record at Sellafield either at any time or before the diagnosis of their children's illness supports the relevance of preconceptual exposure.

Other factors that we examined indicated smaller relations with leukaemia. Some of those were expected, such as antenatal exposure to *x* rays,

179

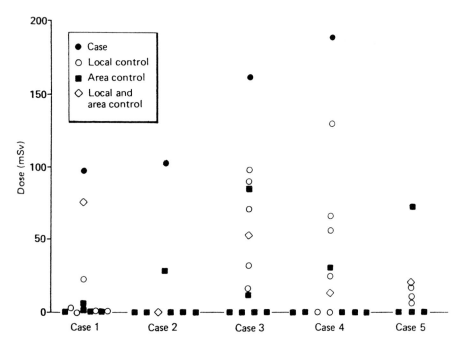

Total external ionising radiation dose during employment at Sellafield before the child's conception in fathers of Seascale leukaemia cases and in fathers of their controls (case 5 not linked to Sellafield workforce file). The different numbers of controls for each case are due to loss from the study of original controls who had moved from Seascale before their case's diagnosis and varying success in identifying fathers and obtaining information to attmpt their linkage to the Sellafield file (see next chapter[3]). The local and local and area controls were born to mothers resident in Seascale at the time (as were the five cases); the area controls were born outside Seascale but resident in the same birth registration district.

but the high relative risk in mothers aged over 40 was at least twice that previously reported.[7] This was not due to an excess of Down's syndrome as none of the cases in our study born to mothers in this age group had trisomy 21. The question arises whether any of these other factors explain the relation with paternal radiation dose. The one well established cause of childhood leukaemia, exposure in utero to x rays, is considered to have a relative risk of around 1·5 and be responsible alone for some 5% of cases. This level of increase is not sufficient to explain the observed relative risks for the highest occupational radiation doses. Moreover, each mother of the four cases in the highest exposure category reported on her questionnaire that she had not had an abdominal x ray examination during pregnancy, although we could trace the hospital record of only one mother to verify this information. The high risk found in mothers aged over 40 was also not an explanation as only one of the four cases in the highest radiation dose group was born to a mother of this age, as was one of three in the lowest group. Neither of these two cases born to mothers aged 40 or over with paternal radiation exposure at Sellafield was born in Seascale.

Of the four cases of leukaemia in the highest radiation dose group three were acute lymphatic leukaemia. The father of the non-Seascale case in this group had a total preconceptual dose of 370 mSv (over about 10 years). On their children's birth certificates two of the fathers were described as process workers, one as an analytical chemist, and the other as a fitter's mate. Although we have not yet examined jobs in detail, these various occupations do not suggest common non-radiation exposures that might be relevant to these findings. We are limited in the identification of individual cases that we can give both from our own ethical considerations and also from our undertakings to the British Medical Association ethical committee and British Nuclear Fuels.

The results for non-Hodgkin's lymphoma, for which the number of cases was much smaller, were less suggestive than for leukaemia. However, one of the two Seascale cases in this study had a father with a total preconceptual radiation dose of 97 mSv (during about 15 years' employment), higher than all 11 related control fathers, of whom six had a radiation record before their child's conception. The father of the other case was not employed at Sellafield. There were no cases of Hodgkin's disease with paternal ionising radiation dose records at Sellafield before their conception nor among Seascale children; this lack of association with radiation exposure is as could be expected (see next chapter) and strengthens the findings in this chapter.

One of the weaknesses of this study might be considered to be the relatively low quality information on potential confounding factors such as antenatal exposure to x rays and infectious illnesses in the mother during pregnancy. Nevertheless, the strength of the observed finding, together with the mothers of the relevant cases not reporting having had an abdominal x ray examination, would suggest that the imperfections in measuring confounders of lower and uncertain risk are not detrimental. Additionally the potential for low quality data on children playing on the beach and families' seafood eating habits, for example, is acknowledged, but this would be a more serious criticism if there had been a trend for positive answers by parents of cases. We recognise also the possibility of bias from the absence of information on some factors for a number of cases and controls, but this is due to the unavailability of old records and our failure to trace parents as well as to parents' failures to respond to the questionnaire. Also this absence of data did not greatly affect what seems to be the important risk variable.

These findings support the hypothesis, incorporated as part of this study, that exposure of fathers to ionising radiation before conception is related to the development of leukaemia in their offspring. The observed finding (the first of its kind with human data), however, is stronger than could have been expected from past knowledge, although relevant studies have largely not been undertaken. In a study of the offspring of 7387 men irradiated to an estimated mean dose of 493 mSv as a result of exposure to atomic bombs in Japan there was no excess of leukaemia (five cases observed, 5·2 expected).[8] Nevertheless, the radiation doses in Hiroshima and Nagasaki were instantaneous as opposed to accumulated over years in the Sellafield workers; the different dose rates may be important. Studies of high doses (360–5040 mSv) in mice have, none the less, indicated that paternal (as well as maternal) exposure to x rays induces heritable tumours in their first and second generation progeny, the tumours mainly being in the lung (papillary adenomas) but including lymphocytic leukaemia as well as leading to an increase in anomalies.[9] It was suggested that this effect might operate through germ line mutations, and the finding lends biological plausibility to the pathway suggested here.

Further data relevant to the results shown here are expected from two other British case-control studies currently in progress. These are in areas around other nuclear installations where excesses of childhood leukaemia in particular, but also of other childhood cancers in one instance, have been reported—Dounreay in Caithness and Aldermaston and Burghfield in Berkshire.[10 11] In the latter report the raised incidence in the neighbourhood was much less than around Sellafield or Dounreay (as it has also been much less around other nuclear plants[1]), but this would be expected if the results reported here are applicable as there is no dominant settlement of workers equivalent to Seascale or Thurso. The occupational radiation doses, however, have been somewhat less at these two establishments than at Sellafield. Consideration is currently being given to setting up cohort studies to examine the incidence of cancer among the offspring of nuclear plant workers, as well as other radiation workers, and these are also relevant to provide support or otherwise for the findings shown in this chapter.[10 11]

The results here are of interest in relation to those in the cohort studies of Seascale children.[12 13] These showed increased rates of leukaemia and total cancer among children born in Seascale (six observed cases of leukaemia compared with 0·6 expected and 12 cases of total cancer compared with 2·8) but not among children moving in after birth and attending the local schools (none compared with 0·6 and four compared with 4·0 respectively). If there is a causal role for radiation operating through paternal occupational exposure then these very different findings among children born in Seascale and those attending school there are as would be expected, apart possibly from the fact that some at least of the Seascale immigrants came from other nuclear establishments. It seems important now not only to extend the cohort studies in time forward from 1983 and backwards before 1950, which is currently being done, but also to carry out for all parents of children born in Seascale a similar linkage exercise as in this study with the Sellafield workforce file and radiation dose records. Additionally, we are planning to examine recent cases diagnosed in the Seascale area in the same manner as in this study. Furthermore, data on internally incorporated radionuclides will be analysed when these become available. Possibly men with high external doses also have high internal exposure. Certainly some degree of correlation between cumulative radiation dose and monitoring for possible internal contamination by specific radionuclides, including plutonium and tritium, was found among workers at United Kingdom Atomic Energy Authority establishments and the Atomic Weapons Establishment.[14 15]

One of the considerations made at the time of the Black inquiry was that the levels of radioactive discharges from Sellafield to atmosphere and sea were too low to account for the number of excess cases of leukaemia being observed in the Seascale area.[2] This was based on the relatively small additional contribution from Sellafield to total radiation exposure from natural background, medical, and other sources. This conclusion would be supported by the results in this study for playing on the beach and eating seafood. The findings here in relation to occupational radiation exposure of the father suggest a totally different pathway and do not conflict with that reasoning. These results also make other alternative hypotheses that have been proposed unlikely to be the explanations—for example, that epidemics of common infections produce a leukaemic response by mixing of populations[16] and that areas chosen as nuclear sites, existing or potential, share unrecognised risk factors.[17]

The range of total preconceptual external radiation doses of fathers in this study was from 0 to 383 mSv, the worker with the highest dose being employed over seven years. The range of estimated radiation doses during the six months before conception was 0 to 31 mSv. An annual dose limit of 50 mSv for radiation workers was recommended in 1965 by the International Commission on Radiological Protection,[18] and this figure still operates in the United Kingdom, although in 1987 the National Radiological Protection Board recommended a reduction to 15 mSv per year.[19] During 1987 in the United Kingdom some 1100 workers received annual doses above 15 mSv from artificial sources; most of these worked in nuclear fuel processing, with fewer than 10 being, for example, health professionals.[20]

If the associations reported in this paper are causal they need to be explored further to help assess which period of exposure may be most relevant. Although the two measures we have examined so far are highly correlated and show similar relations, there is a more convincing trend of increasing relative risks of leukaemia for paternal radiation dose during the six months preceding conception than for total exposure (table VI). The findings here contrast with those in the mortality follow up of Sellafield radiation workers themselves, among whom there were no excess deaths from leukaemia and only a limited suggestion of an association of death from leukaemia with dose of ionising radiation when considering a lag period of 15 years.[21] However, if these results have causal significance then they are of much importance to radiological protection of potential parents and their children.

We thank the registration division of the Office of Population Censuses and Surveys, the West Cumbria District Health Authority, the Cumbrian Family Practitioner Committee, and other sources mentioned in the text for their cooperation in identifying records on subjects included in the study; the National Health Service central register for providing follow up and tracing details and, with the generous collaboration of local general practitioners, for forwarding questionnaires to parents; the parents for completing them; the Ordnance Survey and British Nuclear Fuels for making relevant information available to us; and many staff of the Medical Research Council Environmental Epidemiology Unit for their help, particularly Mick Merwood, Carol Wickham, and Paul Winter for computer analyses and Gill Strange for preparing the manuscript. Professor Geoffrey Rose kindly commented on an earlier version of the chapter, and Professor Peter Smith and Allison Douglas helped with a sample check of the radiation dosimetry data. The study was approved by the British Medical Association ethical committee and the west Cumbria ethics of research committee and was supported partially by a grant from the Department of Health.

1 Gardner MJ. Review of reported increases of childhood cancer rates in the vicinity of nuclear installations in the UK. *Journal of the Royal Statistical Society [Series A]* 1989;**152**:307–25.

2 Black D for the Independent Advisory Group. *Investigation of the possible increased incidence of cancer in west Cumbria.* London: HMSO, 1984. (Black report.)

3 Gardner MJ, Hall AJ, Snee MP, Downes S, Powell CA, Terrell JD. Methods and basic data of case-control study of leukaemia and lymphoma among young people near Sellafield nuclear plant in west Cumbria. *BMJ* 1990;**300**:429–34.

4 Breslow NE, Day NE: *Statistical methods in cancer research. Vol 1. The analysis of case-control studies.* Lyon: International Agency for Research on Cancer, 1980:Chapters V and VII.

5 Anonymous. *EGRET.* Seattle: Statistics and Epidemiology Research Corporation, 1989.

6 Hall EJ. *Radiobiology for the radiologist.* Philadelphia: Harper and Row, 1978:Chapter 19.

7 Doll R. The epidemiology of childhood leukaemia. *Journal of the Royal Statistical Society [Series A]* 1989;**152**:341–51.

8 Ishimaru T, Ichimaru M, Mikami M. *Leukaemia incidence among individuals exposed in utero, children of atomic bomb survivors and their controls, Hiroshima and Nagasaki, 1945–79.* Hiroshima: Radiation Effects Research Foundation, 1981. (RERF Technical Report 11–81.)

9 Nomura T. Parental exposure to x rays and chemicals induces heritable tumours and anomalies in mice. *Nature* 1982;**296**:575–7.

10 Committee on Medical Aspects of Radiation in the Environment. *Investigation of the possible increased incidence of leukaemia in young people near Dounreay Nuclear Establishment, Caithness, Scotland.* London: HMSO, 1988. (COMARE 2nd report.)

11 Committee on Medical Aspects of Radiation in the Environment. *Report on the incidence of childhood cancer in the West Berkshire and North Hampshire area, in which are situated the Atomic Weapons Research Establishment, Aldermaston and the Royal Ordnance Factory, Burghfield.* London: HMSO, 1989. (COMARE 3rd report.)

12 Gardner MJ, Hall AJ, Downes S, Terrell JD. Follow up study of children born to mothers resident in Seascale, west Cumbria (birth cohort). *BMJ* 1987;**295**:822–7.
13 Gardner MJ, Hall AJ, Downes S, Terrell JD. Follow up study of children born elsewhere but attending schools in Seascale, west Cumbria (schools cohort). *BMJ* 1987;**295**:819–22.
14 Beral V, Inskip H, Fraser P, Booth M, Coleman D, Rose G. Mortality of employees of the United Kingdom Atomic Energy Authority, 1946–1979. *BMJ* 1985;**291**:440–7.
15 Beral V, Fraser P, Carpenter L, Booth M, Brown A, Rose G. Mortality of employees of the Atomic Weapons Establishment, 1951–82. *Br Med J* 1988;**297**:757–70.
16 Kinlen LJ. The relevance of population mixing to the aetiology of childhood leukaemia. In: Crosbie WA, Gittus JH, eds. *Medical response to effects of ionising radiation.* London: Elsevier, 1989:272–8.
17 Cook-Mozaffari P, Darby S, Doll R. Cancer near potential sites of nuclear installations. *Lancet* 1989;**ii**:1145–7.
18 International Commission on Radiological Protection. *Recommendations of the International Commission on Radiological Protection.* Oxford: Pergamon Press, 1966. (ICRP Publication Number 9.)
19 National Radiological Protection Board. *Interim guidance on the implications of recent revisions of risk estimates and the ICRP 1987 Como statement.* London: HMSO, 1987:4. (NRPB-G59.)
20 National Radiological Protection Board. *Radiation exposure of the UK population—1988 review.* London: HMSO, 1989:86 (NRPB-R227.)
21 Smith PG, Douglas AJ. Mortality of workers at the Sellafield plant of British Nuclear Fuels. *BMJ* 1986;**293**:845–54.

20: Methods and basic data of case-control study of leukaemia and lymphoma among young people near Sellafield nuclear plant in west Cumbria

MARTIN J GARDNER, ANDREW J HALL,
MICHAEL P SNEE, SUSAN DOWNES,
CAROLINE A POWELL, JOHN D TERRELL

An excess of childhood leukaemia and lymphoma near the Sellafield nuclear plant has been observed. To examine whether the excess is associated with established risk factors or with factors related to the plant, a case-control study was undertaken of 97 people aged under 25 born in west Cumbria health district and diagnosed during 1950–85 as having leukaemia (52), non-Hodgkin's lymphoma (22), or Hodgkin's disease (23) compared with 1001 controls matched for sex and age of birth taken from the same birth registers as the cases. Factors studied included antenatal abdominal x ray examinations, viral infections, lifestyles, proximity to Sellafield, and employment risks of parents working at Sellafield.

Ascertainment of cases through multiple sources was as complete as possible, and the diagnosis was established for nearly all cases from hospital records and by independent pathological review when suitable material (60% (58) of cases) was available. Identification and tracing of the parents of patients and controls enabled questionnaires to be forwarded to 730 (66%), and 467 (64%) of the questionnaires were returned completed. Obstetric records were located for 481 (44%) of the relevant births, more often in recent years. Linkage of study subjects to the Sellafield workforce file enabled dates of employment and records on external doses of whole body ionising radiation to be obtained. Concordance of information from duplicate sources (when available) was reasonably high, with no indications of bias.

It was concluded that overall the collected data were sufficiently reliable for detailed analysis and careful interpretation.

Introduction

In November 1983 a Yorkshire Television programme (*Windscale: a Nuclear Laundry*) suggested that there was an excess incidence of childhood leukaemia and other cancers in the village of Seascale and some neighbouring areas close to the Sellafield nuclear site on the coast of Cumbria. The Black committee (of which MJG was a member) was set up to investigate this suggestion and made recommendations for four epidemiological studies related to childhood cancer in west Cumbria.[1] Three of these, two reporting the occurrence of cancer among children born or attending schools in Seascale[2 3] and one examining the distribution of childhood cancer in the northern region,[4] have been published.

Part of the rationale behind the recommendations was that geographical studies of incidence or mortality include little or no direct information on individuals with or without the disease. Thus the Black report recommended that "a study should be carried out on the records of those cases of leukaemia and lymphoma which have been diagnosed among young people up to the age of 25, resident in west Cumbria. These cases should be compared with suitable controls in respect of factors that could be relevant to the development of leukaemia and lymphoma."

This study, carried out in response to that recommendation, addressed the following hypotheses: firstly, that the raised rates within the area are due to a high frequency of known causes of childhood leukaemia and lymphoma and, secondly, that the raised rates are associated with some aspect or aspects of the Sellafield plant. More specifically, the identified cases and controls served the following four predetermined study aims.

(1) To examine maternal exposure to medical x rays and the occurrence of infectious diseases during pregnancy, as x rays are an accepted cause of leukaemia in children[5-9] and infection is a suspected cause.[9-11]

(2) To examine the geographical distribution at birth, in particular to obtain information on proximity to Sellafield.

(3) To examine habits that might have enhanced exposure to radio-nuclides released from Sellafield—for example, consumption of fresh seafood and playing on the beach.

(4) To examine the occupations of the parent population, in particular to obtain information on employment at Sellafield and occupational radiation dose.

Using west Cumbria for the study included a larger area than that (mainly Seascale) in which the excess incidence (mainly of leukaemia) had been reported.[1] Nevertheless, it contains stretches of coastline, including estuaries, where concerns had been raised about potential risks from radiation contamination as well as inland regions away from the coast. In addition, west Cumbria was chosen partly to cover the places of residence of the Sellafield workforce. Non-Hodgkin's lymphomas were included because there is evidence of some relation with radiation and also because non-Hodgkin's lymphoma could have been confused with leukaemia during the early years of this study. Hodgkin's disease was included, although it is not thought to be related to radiation. Thus we decided in advance to examine leukaemia and non-Hodgkin's lymphoma separately from Hodgkin's disease in the main analysis and also to look at Seascale particularly. This paper reports the methods and some basic data of the case-control study.

Methods

IDENTIFICATION OF STUDY SUBJECTS

The cases

We started by compiling a definitive list of cases of leukaemia and lymphoma diagnosed from 1 January 1950 to 31 December 1985 among people aged under 25 years with a residential address in the area served by West Cumbria District Health Authority. This area runs down the coast from above Maryport to Millom, including Workington, Whitehaven, and Seascale, and inland for some 20 km. Various sources were used to identify the relevant cases, and other tumours, including—*notification* of cases to the Black inquiry; *case records* from a childhood cancer survey initiated in west Cumbria at the time of the Black inquiry; *pathology records*, using the histological diagnosis card index at the West Cumberland Hospital; *death entries* for 1950–8 for the registration divisions of Cumbria, Newcastle, and Manchester (the last two because patients are referred to these centres from west Cumbria); *death certificates* for 1959 onwards for Cumbria at the health authority office in Carlisle; *death entries* for districts that could have registered west Cumbrian deaths at the Office of Population Censuses and

TABLE I—*Numbers of cases by sex, independent pathological review, and diagnostic category*

Diagnosis	Classification number*	Sex		Independent pathological review		
		Male	Female	Yes	No	Total
Leukaemia		30	22	25	27	52
Lymphoid	1	17	13	15	15	30
Non-lymphoid	2 + 3	11	8	10	9	19
Unspecified	4	2	1	0	3	3
Lymphoma		20	25	33	12	45
Hodgkin's disease	5	9	14	18	5	23
Non-Hodgkin's	6	11	8	13	6	19
Histiocytosis X	29	0	3	2	1	3

* See annex 1 of Draper et al.[12]

Surveys; *death certificates* mentioning leukaemia from 1959 onwards (L J Kinlen, personal communication); *cancer registrations* in the northern region children's malignant disease registry; *cancer registrations* in the northern region cancer registry from 1969 onwards; *circular letters* to general practitioners in west Cumbria asking them to notify any known eligible cases; *preschool illness notifications* in the Flatt Walks Clinic records in Whitehaven; and *cancer registrations* held by the Oxford Childhood Cancer Survey (G J Draper, personal communication).

For this report we included only cases in people born and diagnosed in west Cumbria and omitted six cases of leukaemia and eight of lymphoma in people born outside. The residential addresses were determined from hospital records, questionnaires. death certificates, or the Cumbria Family Practitioner Committee records.

Table I shows the numbers of cases by sex and diagnostic category, where diagnosis was taken in order from the following sources as available: pathological review, hospital records, cancer registrations, and death certificates. Thus 52 cases of leukaemia, 22 of non-Hodgkin's lymphoma, and 23 of Hodgkin's disease make up the main study group; 95 other tumours were also identified and subjected to pathological review but are not reported on further in this chapter. Table II shows the numbers of cases by diagnostic category, calendar period, and age at diagnosis. The pattern of cases over time was fairly consistent, and the decreasing numbers of cases of leukaemia and increasing numbers of cases of Hodgkin's disease with age concur with known relations.

The controls

The selection of controls was from registers of live births at the Office of Population Censuses and Surveys. Two groups of eight controls of the same sex as the case were taken from the register into which the case's birth

TABLE II—*Numbers of cases by diagnostic category, calendar period, and age at diagnosis*

Group	Leukaemia	Non-Hodgkin's lymphoma	Hodgkin's disease
Period of diagnosis			
1950–4	4	3	1
1955–9	7	2	3
1960–4	8	4	2
1965–9	8	3	2
1970–4	7	4	2
1975–9	10	3	7
1980–5	8	3	6
Age (years) at diagnosis			
≤4	17	6	0
5–9	13	2	1
10–14	7	3	0
15–19	12	7	9
20–24	3	4	13
Total	52	22	23

was entered. The appropriate register was identified with the help of the National Health Service central register when necessary.

For one group (area controls) searches were made backwards and forwards from the case's entry in the birth register until the nearest four appropriate controls in each direction were found. Only births to mothers with a west Cumbria address were included. For the second group (local controls) the residence of their mothers was matched for residence (civil parish) of the mothers of the case at the date of birth, although otherwise the procedure was as for the first group. Date of birth matching was within six months for 99% of area controls and 92% of local controls. The area controls were particularly relevant to the geographical analysis mentioned in study aim 2, although their selection was stratified by birth registration district.

There was thus effectively matching of controls on sex and date of birth and each group of controls was registered in the same district or subdistrict (12 in number over the 35 years) as their case. This method of control selection was used for ease of procedure, to obtain close matching for date of birth, and because there is not thought to be an area of residence bias in the order of births within any register. The same individual could have been used as a control in both groups. Thus, if any one of the four adjacent births of the same sex to a case was also from the same civil parish then this control would have been in each group.

For each control a check was made at the National Health Service central register to see whether they were still alive and for any cancer registration

TABLE III—*Numbers of cases of leukaemia and lymphoma by numbers of controls of area or local type*

No of controls	Leukaemia		Non-Hodgkin's lymphoma		Hodgkin's disease	
	Area	Local	Area	Local	Area	Local
8	16	18	5	4	1	2
7	24	16	5	7	6	4
6	4	8	9	6	5	8
5	5	7	2	3	7	6
4	3	1	—	2	3	2
3	—	1	1	—	1	1
2	—	—	—	—	—	—
1	—	1	—	—	—	—
0	—	—	—	—	—	—
Cases	52	52	22	22	23	23
Controls	357	347	142	140	130	133
Both area and local controls	140		56		52	
Total controls	564		226		211	

particulars. Thirty four controls who were found to have died (25 infant deaths) before the date of diagnosis of their matched cases were excluded, but no controls were found to have been registered as having cancer by, or died from cancer within 10 years of, the date of diagnosis of their matched case.

Additionally, to have the potential to be a case in this study at the appropriate time, controls had to have been resident in west Cumbria at the date of diagnosis of their associated case. This information was obtained initially at the National Health Service central register by reference to the family practitioner committee area of registration at the appropriate date. In total 195 controls registered outside Cumbria were thus excluded. Residence particulars for controls with a Cumbrian registration or no registration were examined in questionnaires sent to parents (see later) and a further 13 controls were excluded. Those left out from the questionnaire part of the study, together with non-responders, were reviewed within the Cumbria Family Practitioner Committee records at the relevant date with no subsequent exclusions.

Table III shows the numbers of cases by their number of controls. Although not shown in the table, we were able originally to select from the birth registers eight area and eight local controls for all cases except one of leukaemia. When the other criteria for control definition were incorporated the numbers of included controls per case decreased as shown in the table.

TABLE IV—*Numbers of cases of leukaemia and lymphoma by parental vital status at date of study*

Parental vital status	Leukaemia	Non-Hodgkin's lymphoma	Hodgkin's disease
Mother			
Alive	45	18	18
Dead	7	4	5
Father (only when mother dead)			
Alive	3	1	2
Dead	4	3	3

In total 1001 of 1243 originally selected controls for the 97 cases remained. Of these 248 served as both area and local controls.

Parents of cases and controls

Identifying particulars for the parents of each case and control were found from the child's birth certificate and elsewhere, such as obstetric and general medical records. The aim was to identify uniquely the parents in the National Health Service central register and thus ascertain whether they were still alive. For parents found to be alive, and if they were eligible for the questionnaire part of the study (see below), their current family practitioner committee registration was traced to enable them to be contacted through their own general practitioner. Local family practitioner committees were able to identify the parent's general practitioner's name and address, as well as the parent's recorded residential particulars.

Table IV shows the numbers of mothers and fathers traced as being alive in the records of the National Health Service central register. Of the 97 cases the mothers of 81 were alive. Of the remaining 16 cases the fathers of six were alive. Both parents of 10 cases were recorded as having died.

DATA COLLECTED ON CASES AND CONTROLS

Hospital records

Hospital records were examined for two purposes: firstly, to obtain detailed information on the case's diagnosis and, secondly, to extract data from the relevant obstetric notes on the mother's pregnancy for both cases and controls.

Hospital records were available for all but two of the cases. As well as abstracting relevant clinical details, we ascertained whether or not a histological diagnosis had been made and whether histological material was available. When material was available the cases were the subject of an independent pathological review for the purposes of the northern region children's malignant disease registry (Drs M Reid and A Malcolm, personal communication) and we used their results in our classification.

Table I shows the numbers of cases whose diagnoses were established through the independent pathological review: 25 (48%) of the leukaemias and 33 (73%) of the lymphomas. In none of these was a major change in classification made as a result.

Antenatal data were available from obstetric records on the mothers of 35 (36%) of the cases and 446 (45%) of the controls. We extracted details on exposure to x rays during the pregnancy, including parts of the body examined and dates. For abdominal x ray examinations the number and type of examination were also noted. We also obtained any recorded information on viral infections that the mother suffered during pregnancy—for example, chickenpox, influenza, or rubella. Some further data, such as birth weight, were also collected. For those mothers who had had their babies at home we could not obtain any documents on the pregnancy.

Questionnaire

Procedure—The study included a questionnaire, with information being sought direct from parents of cases and controls. This was carried out through parents' general practitioners. The questionnaire was sent to the case's mother if she was still living and her current residence could be established. For such cases the questionnaire was sent to the associated controls' mothers if they were traced as being alive and registered with a general practitioner. For other cases and their controls the questionnaires were forwarded to their fathers if registered. In this way responses from within case-control sets were obtained from parents of the same sex. When both of a case's parents were dead or untraced questionnaires were not sent for either the cases or their controls.

The National Health Service central register posted the questionnaires together with covering letters to the family practitioner committee and the general practitioner explaining the study and asking for their cooperation. Also included were a letter and questionnaire to be addressed to the parent by the family practitioner committee or general practitioner. The general practitioner was asked to return an "action slip" to let us know what he or she had done. In particular, the general practitioners were asked to consider whether there were any reasons for not posting the questionnaire to the parent—for example, if the parent was known to be ill or the questionnaire might cause unacceptable stress—and if so to return the package to the central register with a note to this effect. Before the questionnaires were posted the district medical officer (JDT) wrote to all general practitioners in west Cumbria explaining the study and requesting their cooperation, and this was accompanied by a request in the local newspapers seeking parents' participation. If replies were not received from parents within three months a reminder package was sent, with a "reply slip" for the parents to return if they did not want to complete the questionnaire. No further attempts were made to obtain replies.

193

TABLE V—*Numbers of questionnaires forwarded to general practitioners and parents and whether or not completed and returned to Medical Research Council (MRC)*

	Cases			
Questionnaire	Leukaemia	Non-Hodgkin's lymphoma	Hodgkin's disease	Controls
Not forwarded to GP	4	3	4*	274
Forwarded to GP	48	19	19	727
Forwarded to parent	42	18	16	654
Returned to MRC (from mothers/fathers)				
Completed	35/2	12/1	13/1	392/11
Not completed	2/0	2/0	1/0	39/5
Not returned to MRC	3	3	1	207

* The mother of one case of Hodgkin's disease, although believed alive (table IV), could not be traced and the father had died.

Content—The purpose of the questionnaire was both to obtain information that had been partly collected through the methods described earlier, but now direct from parents, and to request data otherwise unavailable. Thus we asked the parent about antenatal care, including x ray examinations and infectious illnesses, during the relevant pregnancy. Also we asked for the residential and occupational histories of both parents from the time they left school, as well as the residential history of their child. Other data requested included the child's birth weight, childhood activities on the beach and in the lake district, and family habits in eating fresh seafood and home grown vegetables.

Response—Table V shows the numbers of questionnaires sent to general practitioners and to parents of cases and controls with their outcome. For the 97 cases 86 questionnaires were forwarded to general practitioners and 76 (78%) to parents. Of the latter, 64 (84%) were returned completed by the relevant parent and a further 5 (7%) were returned without being completed. For the 1001 controls 727 questionnaires were forwarded to general practitioners and 654 (65%) to parents. Of the latter 403 (62%) were returned completed by the relevant parent and a further 44 (7%) were returned without being completed. There was thus a higher response rate for cases than for controls, with the overall proportion of questionnaires forwarded being 66%, of which 64% were completed. A total of 29 parents replied saying that they did not want to complete the questionnaire. We were not informed of the general practitioner's action for only one of the 86 cases and 17 (2%) of the 727 controls.

Geographical data

One aspect of the study was to compare the geographical distributions of the cases and controls in relation to Sellafield. For this purpose residential addresses at birth for cases and controls were identified on Ordnance Survey maps, and national grid references accurate to 100 metre squares were obtained for most (87%) addresses. For the remainder the accuracy was less, and in some instances addresses were untraceable, mainly those from the earlier years covered by the study. This method permitted a modified approach to the geography of cases rather than simply examining routine mortality and cancer registration statistics.[13-15] The differences in approach are at least twofold: firstly, the use of controls rather than census figures to represent the population and, secondly, location at birth rather than diagnosis. In fact, the cases tended to be diagnosed at the same address or at one close to where they had been born.

Occupational data

Occupational data on the parents of cases and controls were obtained from three different sources. Firstly, we abstracted parental (mainly fathers') occupations from the birth certificates of their children. Secondly, we obtained occupational histories by questionnaire. These sets of data were coded to both occupation and industry using standard classifications[16 17] with local additions. Thirdly, we cross matched our computer file of study subjects with that of the past and present Sellafield workforce to indentify people who appeared on both files. This linkage was carried out using surname, initials, and date of birth, with incorporation of forenames and National Health Service numbers when available on both files. For those subjects identified as having worked at Sellafield, British Nuclear Fuels subsequently supplied us with dates of employment at the site and external whole body ionising radiation dosimetry on an annual basis. The radiation dose in each year had been estimated from monitoring with dose meters worn on the trunk, and our figures came from the data on which satisfactory quality checks have been reported.[18 19] No details of exposure to internally incorporated radionuclides are yet available, though they will become so. This information was used to examine the relative frequency of employment and radiation exposure at Sellafield among parents of cases and controls and also to examine relations with other occupations and industries.

Table VI shows the extent to which job data were available. Job descriptions were entered on birth certificates for most fathers (97%) but for only few mothers (about 2%, as expected from birth registration practice). Data from questionnaires, however, were obtained to a similar degree on both fathers and mothers (about 40% overall).

CONCORDANCE OF DATA

Antenatal x ray exposure—Table VII shows data on abdominal x ray examinations during pregnancy obtained from hospital obstetric records compared with data from the questionnaire for cases and controls separ-

TABLE VI—*Numbers of cases and controls by diagnostic category and availability of parental employment data by source*

Presence of employment data and source	Cases			Controls
	Leukaemia	Non-Hodgkin's lymphoma	Hodgkin's disease	
Birth certificate				
Father				
Yes	48	20	23	969
No	4	2	0	32
Mother				
Yes	2	1	0	17
No	50	21	23	984
Questionnaire				
Father				
Yes	36	12	13	386
No	16	10	10	615
Mother				
Yes	35	10	13	378
No	17	12	10	623

TABLE VII—*Data on maternal abdominal x ray examination during pregnancy from hospital records and postal questionnaires among cases and controls*

X ray examination according to hospital record	X ray examination according to questionnaire response			
	Yes	No	No response	Total
Cases				
Yes	1	2	1	5
No	1	20	9	30
No records	5	30	27	62
Total	8	52	37	97
Controls				
Yes	18	13	29	60
No	8	171	207	386
No records	9	155	391	555
Total	35	339	627	1001

TABLE VIII—*Data on paternal employment at Sellafield at child's birth from birth certificate, questionnaire, and from British Nuclear Fuels file of past and present workers for cases and controls*

Employment at Sellafield according to British Nuclear Fuels file	Employment at Sellafield according to:					
	Birth certificate			Questionnaire		
	Yes	No	Not recorded	Yes	No	No response
Cases						
Yes	9	0	1	5	0	5
No	1	75	2	0	36	42
Trace not possible	1	1	7	1	2	6
Controls						
Yes	83	3	7	55	3	35
No	5	759	49	0	224	589
Trace not possible	7	53	35	4	21	70

ately. Although the overall agreement between the sources was reasonable, there were notable discrepancies—for example, out of 35 documented *x* ray examinations 15 (43%) were not recalled by the mother. There was, however, no evidence of any bias between mothers of cases and controls in their recall.

Employment at Sellafield—Table VIII shows findings on fathers' employment at Sellafield at the birth of their children from the three varying sources. There was good general agreement among the different data sets. For example, for the 10 cases identified by computer linkage as having fathers employed at Sellafield this was agreed when suitable data were available from the other two sources. One case of Hodgkin's disease was not linked to Sellafield, although employment there was recorded on the birth certificate. Concordance on Sellafield employment status was also high among controls. Agreement for non-Sellafield occupation and industry data between birth certificates and questionnaires was also high, although results are not shown here.

Conclusions

We recognised at the outset that obtaining complete information on cases diagnosed over a 35 year period and their contemporary controls would be impossible owing to the lack of historical records and the difficulty of tracing parents. This was partly the rationale for taking eight area and eight local controls to allow for some attrition. Cases were ascertained from multiple overlapping sources and their identification was probably as complete as possible. Information on their diagnosis was available almost always from medical records and in over half was subject to independent pathological review. Obstetric records on the mothers of the cases and controls were identified for fewer than half the births and information was necessarily less complete in earlier years.

The level of tracing of vital status and current whereabouts of the parents was quite high, and questionnaires were posted, mainly to mothers, through their general practitioners for 90% of eligible subjects. The response rate for completed questionnaires overall, after one reminder, was 64% but higher for cases than controls. Geographical data on address at birth were coded to grid references with a high degree of accuracy. Occupational and industrial data on most parents were collected from at least one of three sources: birth certificates, questionnaires, and the Sellafield file on the past and present workforce. Annual recordings of the external dose of whole body ionising radiation from personal dose meters worn on the trunk were obtained from an extension of the same databank as used for the follow up study of Sellafield workers.[18 19]

When information was available from more than one source the concordance was generally high—for example, it was high for occupational and social class but less so for exposure to x rays and viral infections. When there was disagreement there were no real indications of biased responses between cases and controls. For data where duplicate sources did not exist it was possible to be more certain of previously documented information, such as parental age, than of questionnaire responses on, for example, shellfish eating habits. Information on a number of factors for some cases and controls was lacking altogether because documents were missing or parents could not be traced or did not respond to the questionnaire. Overall, however, the data were sufficiently reliable for detailed analysis and careful interpretation (see preceding chapter).[20]

We thank the registration division of the Office of Population Censuses and Surveys, the West Cumbria Health Authority, the Cumbrian Family Practitioner Committee, and other sources mentioned in the text for their cooperation in identifying records on subjects included in the study; the National Health Service central register for providing follow up and tracing details and, with the generous collaboration of local general practitioners, for forwarding questionnaires to parents; the parents for completing them; the Ordnance Survey and British Nuclear Fuels for making relevant information available to us; and many staff of the Medical Research Council Environmental Epidemiology Unit for their help, particularly Mick Merwood for computer analyses and Gill Strange for preparing the manuscript. Professor Geoffrey Rose kindly commented on an earlier version of the chapter. The study was approved by the British Medical Association ethical committee and the west Cumbria ethics of research committee and was supported partially by a grant from the Department of Health.

1 Black D for the Independent Advisory Group. *Investigation of the possible increased incidence of cancer in west Cumbria*. London: HMSO, 1984. (Black report.)

2 Gardner MJ, Hall AJ, Downes S, Terrell JD. Follow up study of children born to mothers resident in Seascale, west Cumbria (birth cohort). *BMJ* 1987;**295**:822–7.

3 Gardner MJ, Hall AJ, Downes S, Terrell JD. Follow up study of children born elsewhere but attending schools in Seascale, west Cumbria (schools cohort). *BMJ* 1987;**295**:819–22.

4 Openshaw S, Craft AW, Charlton M, Birch JM. Investigation of leukaemia clusters by use of a geographical analysis machine. *Lancet* 1988;**i**:272–3.

5 Stewart A, Webb J, Hewitt D. A survey of childhood malignancies. *BMJ* 1958;**i**:1495–508.

6 Monson RR, MacMahon B. Prenatal *x* ray exposure and cancer in children. In: *Radiation carcinogenesis, epidemiology and biological significance*. New York: Raven Press, 1984:97–105.

7 Hopton PA, McKinney PA, Cartwright RA, *et al*. X rays in pregnancy and the risk of childhood cancer. *Lancet* 1985;**ii**:773.

8 Knox EG, Stewart AM, Kneale GW, Gilman EA. Prenatal irradiation and childhood cancer. *J Soc Radiol Prot* 1987;**7**:3–15.

9 Doll R. The epidemiology of childhood leukaemia. *Journal of the Royal Statistical Society [Series A]* 1989;**152**:341–51.

10 Adelstein AM, Donovan JW. Malignant disease in children whose mothers had chicken pox, mumps or rubella in pregnancy. *BMJ* 1972;**iv**:629–31.

11 Fedrick J, Alberman ED. Reported influenza in pregnancy and subsequent cancer in the child. *BMJ* 1972;**ii**:485–8.

12 Draper GJ, Birch JM, Bithell JF, *et al*. *Childhood cancer in Britain: incidence, survival and mortality*. London: HMSO, 1982. (Office of Population Censuses and Surveys, Studies on Medical and Population Subjects No 37).

13 Gardner MJ, Winter PD. Cancer in Cumberland during 1959–78 with reference to cancer in young people around Windscale. *Lancet* 1984;**i**:216–7.

14 Urquhart J, Palmer M, Cutler J. Cancer in Cumbria: the Windscale connection. *Lancet* 1984;**i**:217–8.

15 Craft AW, Openshaw S, Birch J. Apparent cluster of childhood malignancies in northern England. *Lancet* 1984;**ii**:96–7.

16 General Register Office. *Classification of occupations, 1966*. London: HMSO, 1966.

17 Central Statistical Office. *Standard industrial classification*. Revised 1968. London: HMSO, 1968.

18 National Radiological Protection Board. *Radiation dose histories at British Nuclear Fuels plc, Sellafield*. Chilton: NRPB, 1986. (NRPB-M136.)

19 Smith PG, Douglas AJ. Mortality of workers at the Sellafield plant of British Nuclear Fuels. *BMJ* 1986;**293**:845–54.

20 Gardner MJ, Snee MP, Hall AJ, Powell CA, Downes S, Terrell JD. Results of case-control study of leukaemia and lymphoma among young people near Sellafield nuclear plant in west Cumbria. *BMJ* 1990;**300**:423–9.

21: Paternal occupations of children with leukaemia

Letter to the *British Medical Journal*

MARTIN J GARDNER

My colleagues and I have found a few small numerical mistakes in tables II and VI of our case-control study of leukaemia and lymphoma among young people near Sellafield nuclear plant in west Cumbria published in the *BMJ* in 1990.[1] These tables related to risks of leukaemia and non-Hodgkin's lymphoma in children with reference to mother's and father's ages at their child's birth and to father's employment and radiation dose during

TABLE I—*Numbers of cases and controls with relative risks for leukaemia and non-Hodgkin's lymphoma in children by parental age at birth*

Parental age (years)	Type of control	Cases Total	Cases Positive (≥25 or ≥40)	Controls Total	Controls Positive (≥25 or ≥40)	Relative risk	95% Confidence interval
			Leukaemia				
Mother	Area	52	34	351	227	1·00	0·54 to 1·86
≥25 v < 25	Local	52	34	344	227	0·94	0·50 to 1·77
Mother	Area	52	5	351	7	5·27	1·39 to 20·05
≥40 v < 25	Local	52	5	344	10	3·54	1·01 to 12·35
Father	Area	46	39	287	225	1·53	0·65 to 3·59
≥25 v < 25	Local	46	39	276	215	1·64	0·68 to 3·96
Father	Area	46	6	287	27	1·99	0·61 to 6·50
≥40 v < 25	Local	46	6	276	24	2·49	0·72 to 8·56
			Leukaemia and lymphoma				
Mother	Area	74	51	492	324	1·11	0·66 to 1·89
≥25 v < 25	Local	74	51	484	326	1·04	0·61 to 1·78
Mother	Area	74	8	492	9	6·65	2·24 to 19·80
≥40 v < 25	Local	74	8	484	14	4·26	1·55 to 11·75
Father	Area	66	53	403	322	0·98	0·51 to 1·90
≥25 v < 25	Local	66	53	389	305	1·08	0·55 to 2·12
Father	Area	66	10	403	32	1·87	0·74 to 4·69
≥40 v < 25	Local	66	10	389	33	1·95	0·76 to 5·05

TABLE II—*Numbers of cases and controls with relative risks for leukaemia and non-Hodgkin's lymphoma in children by timing of paternal employment and external ionising radiation dosimetry at Sellafield*

Father's employment/radiation group	Type of control	Cases	Controls	Relative risk	95% Confidence interval
		Leukaemia			
Total	Area	46	288		
	Local	46	276		
Dose record:					
Before conception	Area	8	34	1·76	0·71 to 4·35
	Local	8	40	1·40	0·50 to 3·94
At conception	Area	8	21	3·71	1·27 to 10·82
	Local	8	27	2·90	0·93 to 9·05
Total dose before conception:					
> 0–49 mSv	Area	3	18	1·20	0·34 to 4·32
	Local	3	26	0·77	0·20 to 3·00
50–99 mSv	Area	1	11	0·69	0·08 to 5·75
	Local	1	11	0·78	0·08 to 7·73
⩾ 100 mSv	Area	4	5	6·30	1·52 to 26·03
	Local	4	3	8·38	1·35 to 51·99
Dose during 6 months before conception:					
> 0–4 mSv	Area	3	14	1·79	0·41 to 7·73
	Local	3	22	1·30	0·28 to 6·07
5–9 mSv	Area	1	3	3·62	0·33 to 39·97
	Local	1	2	4·60	0·37 to 57·83
⩾ 10 mSv	Area	4	5	7·38	1·74 to 31·31
	Local	4	4	6·82	1·46 to 31·86
		Leukaemia and non-Hodgkin's lymphoma			
Total	Area	66	404		
	Local	66	389		
Employed*:					
Before diagnosis	Area	11	73	0·95	0·45 to 1·99
Dose record:					
Before conception	Area	10	44	1·66	0·75 to 3·70
	Local	10	56	1·09	0·45 to 2·66
At conception	Area	10	29	3·09	1·25 to 7·65
	Local	10	40	1·90	0·73 to 4·97
Total dose before conception:					
> 0–49 mSv	Area	4	26	1·11	0·37 to 3·35
	Local	4	39	0·62	0·19 to 1·96
50–99 mSv	Area	2	13	1·16	0·25 to 5·48
	Local	2	14	1·04	0·19 to 5·60
⩾ 100 mSv	Area	4	5	6·45	1·57 to 26·48
	Local	4	3	8·59	1·41 to 52·20
Dose during 6 months before conception:					
> 0–4 mSv	Area	5	18	2·31	0·72 to 7·36
	Local	5	29	1·27	0·37 to 4·35
5–9 mSv	Area	1	4	2·46	0·25 to 23·94
	Local	1	6	1·34	0·15 to 12·14
⩾ 10 mSv	Area	4	8	4·41	1·19 to 16·39
	Local	4	6	4·50	1·08 to 18·78

*Only this amendment has been necessary for paternal employment results in table VI.[1]

employment at the Sellafield nuclear plant. Tables I and II here show the amended results.

The original calculation of parental age was either one year lower or higher than it should have been, depending on whether the parent's birthday was earlier or later in the year than that of the child. The new relative risks in table I are similar to, but generally larger than, the previously published figures. We have revised the estimates of radiation dose to take account of men whose periods of employment in the year of, or before, their child's conception did not cover complete calendar years. No cases and only a few controls were reclassified, and the new relative risks in table II are in general similar to, or a little higher than, the earlier figures.

We regret the changes but believe that they do not alter our interpretation of the study.

1 Gardner MJ, Snee MP, Hall AJ, Powell CA, Downes S, Terrell JD. Results of case-control study of leukaemia and lymphoma among young people near Sellafield nuclear plant in west Cumbria. *BMJ* 1990;**300**:423–9.

22: Leukaemia and radiation

H JOHN EVANS

In 1990, Martin Gardner and colleagues published the results of their study of the apparent excess cases of childhood leukaemia near the nuclear waste reprocessing plant at Sellafield, west Cumbria.[1] Their suggestion is that the excess is due to the increased risk to children of fathers working at the plant. That conclusion, however, is questionable.

The report of Gardner *et al* follows other investigations of leukaemia clusters near nuclear facilities.[2][3] The authors analysed 52 cases of leukaemia, 22 cases of non-Hodgkin's lymphoma, and 23 cases of Hodgkin's lymphoma in people under the age of 25 years born in west Cumbria and diagnosed between 1950 and 1985, and 1001 controls matched for sex and age, and taken from the same birth registers as the cases. The authors focused on the 74 cases of leukaemia and non-Hodgkin's lymphoma and the variables studied that were thought to increase the risks. By cross linking birth certificate entries to British Nuclear Fuels Ltd (BNFL) files on Sellafield, the authors discovered the occupations of the parents of 64 cases; 10 of these cases had fathers who had worked at Sellafield. This compared with 383 local controls, of whom 54 had fathers who had worked at the plant.

Other industries

Most commentators, however, ignored the comparisons between the relative risks of luekaemia and non-Hodgkin's lymphoma for occupations at Sellafield and for those with other industries. Gardner *et al* looked at the main industrial groups in west Cumbria that employed more than 5% of the control fathers. They found that the relative risk of leukaemia and non-Hodgkin's lymphoma was roughly doubled for the children of Sellafield workers, but was also similarly raised for the children of farmers, iron and steelworkers, and chemical workers. There is no information about whether the chemicals in the environs of these workers are leukaemogenic, and no measure of the exposure, so that further analysis of these groups is not possible. But there are some findings that suggest an excess of childhood cancers among offspring of workers exposed to certain organic chemicals such as benzene, a known leukaemogen. For radiation workers, external radiation exposure is measured by a film badge, and it is this that allows a more detailed analysis of the Sellafield workers as opposed to those in the other industries.

Gardner *et al* conclude that the excess of leukaemia and non-Hodgkin's lymphoma near Sellafield is not due to radionuclide contamination of the environment by nuclear waste discharges, or to eating local seafood or vegetables, or to playing on the beach. The authors found that four of the 10 case fathers, but only three of the 54 control fathers, had accumulated exposures of 100 millisieverts (mSv) or more before the conception of their children and that this was associated with a sixfold to eightfold greater risk of leukaemia in the offspring. An association was also noted for those fathers who had received 10 mSv or more in the six months before conception.

The expected (or more than expected) increased risk of leukaemia with the age of the mother (relative risk about 4) or with previous diagnostic antenatal *x* ray exposure (relative risk about 1·5) was observed, but could not account for the excess cases among the offspring of radiation workers. The authors say that their findings indicate an "effect of the radiation exposure on germ cells producing a mutation in sperm that may be leukaemogenic in subsequent offspring". Is there any evidence in support of this suggestion, and is it a realistic possibility?

Shu *et al*, studying childhood leukaemia in Shanghai, reported a roughly four times greater risk to children of fathers who had received 10 or more doses of diagnostic *x* rays preconceptually: the occupation of the fathers or whether they were receiving therapeutic drugs was not noted, and the findings are open to question because of recall bias.[4] Similar increased risks were also found for the offspring of mothers employed in the chemical, metal refining, or agricultural industries, particularly those associated with exposure to benzene and to pesticides. Also relevant is the absence of an excess of leukaemia in offspring of atom bomb survivors at Hiroshima and Nagasaki (five cases observed, 5·2 expected) in a population of 7387 men who had been acutely exposed to a high dose (mean of 492 mSv).[5] Additionally, Nomura showed roughly a doubling of lymphocytic leukaemia in the offspring of mice exposed to high acute doses of *x* rays (360–5040 mSv).[6]

Gardner *et al* refer to the Nomura studies as evidence for heritability of mutational change resulting in leukaemias in offspring of exposed parents, but argue that the absence of such effects in the offspring of survivors at Hiroshima and Nagasaki may be a consequence of their exposure to acute high doses in contrast to the low doses accumulated by the Sellafield workers. But Nomura used doses equivalent to those received by the atom bomb survivors; his studies also showed, as expected, an increased frequency of inherited congenital abnormalities among the offspring. It might be argued, therefore, that if doses of 100 mSv resulted in mutations of workers' sperm that lead to a sixfold to eightfold increase in leukaemia, then a considerable increase in a wide range of heritable diseases or anomalies among their children would also be expected. No such epidemic has been noted in the Sellafield area.

Inherited factors

Is there any evidence for inherited factors that predispose to human leukaemia and lymphoma? Aside from an association with the rare and well characterised syndromes (for example, Bloom's, Fanconi's anaemia, and so on) caused by single gene defects and associated with various physical abnormalities and defects in immune response, there is no unambiguous evidence that childhood leukaemia is associated with an inherited single gene. In those leukaemias in monozygotic twins that have been studied cytogenetically, each member of a pair shares the same abnormal marker chromosome, indicating a single transformation event and the transfer of leukaemia cells from one twin to the other by their shared blood circulation in utero. So twin studies are not helpful. And several consanguinity studies show that most leukaemias are not associated with an inherited predisposing recessive gene. There are, nevertheless, a number of well documented cases of familial childhood leukaemia, but in most of these the possibility of a transmissible infectious agent or of common exposure to a leukaemogenic chemical cannot be ruled out.

Assuming, despite the lack of evidence, that one or more mutations acting within a given genetic background (multifactorially) could predispose to leukaemia, then are the exposures at Sellafield sufficient to produce such mutations and at the frequencies implied? Apart from data on acute x ray induced chromosomal mutations in human spermatozoa (which require a dose of about 4000 mSv to double the background mutation frequency, and $> 20\,000$ mSv to raise it six to eight times)[7] there is no information on viable inherited x ray induced mutations in man. But mouse studies show that the minimum x ray dose to spermatozoa or spermatogonia required to double the spontaneous frequency of a wide range of different single gene defects is about 1500–3000 mSv given as an acute exposure[8]): these doses are at least 15–20 times greater than the dose accumulated by the most heavily exposed Sellafield workers.

Although there is a lack of evidence for heritability of human leukaemias, they are nevertheless genetic diseases; but the genetic changes that characterise them are somatic genetic changes. Even though detailed pathological findings have not been reported, most of the west Cumbrian childhood leukaemias were acute lymphocytic leukaemias, the most common childhood leukaemia. About 50% of acute lymphocytic leukaemias are charac-

terised by the presence of one of several consistent chromosome transloca-
tions, which in many cases results in the activation of proto-oncogenes at
the sites of chromosome exchange.[9 10] These chromosome alterations,
which are clearly causal factors in leukaemogenesis, are confined to the
leukaemic cells and involve genes associated with growth, development,
proliferation, and differentiation. Such chromosome alterations would be
inconsistent with the viability of an early embryo and are not found as
constitutional changes in the normal cells of leukaemia patients. There is
no information on chromosome changes for the Sellafield cases, but the
highly unlikely inheritance of such changes would be associated with
various other abnormalities as well as leukaemia.

Overall therefore, the evidence pointing to an inherited mutational
change induced by low doses of radiation as a cause of the excess leukaemia
among the offspring of radiation workers does not stand up to scrutiny. Are
there other possible explanations apart from various non-specific suggestions such as unusual genetic imprinting or induced suppression of the
immune response resulting in an enhanced response to leukaemia-causing
agents encountered postnatally? There are several. First, we cannot rule
out the possibility of chance, as the main conclusion of the case-control
study rests heavily on four of the cases born to Sellafield fathers. Similar
control studies are in progress for the nuclear plant at Dounreay in
Scotland and at the atomic weapons establishment and ordnance factory at
Aldermaston (Berkshire) and Burghfield (Hampshire); the Dounreay results are soon to be published. Other studies are under way in France,
Canada, and the United States, but preliminary negative published data are
so far insufficient to draw any conclusions. Perhaps the most important
study is that proposed by the National Radiological Protection Board
(NRPB) and the Oxford Childhood Cancer Research Group. The Oxford
group has records on over 10 000 children with leukaemia diagnosed in
Britain since 1962, and the NRPB has a register of over 100 000 radiation
workers with details of film badge doses. Linking these two registers will be
formidable but well worthwhile.

Chemical agents

A second possibility is that the film badge may not measure the relevant
exposure to radiation (or, indeed, to other agents). It is unlikely that the
most heavily exposed workers inadvertently carry radioactive dust home,
but the possibility that these workers have internal gonadal contamination
that could result in sperm being exposed to higher doses, or in radioactivity
being transmitted to the female partner in seminal fluid, still exists. Indeed,
the finding that the risk of prostatic cancer is increased among the
employees most heavily exposed to radiation at Harwell and Aldermaston

has led to the suggestion that some radionuclides are concentrated in the prostate.[11] But radiation workers are exposed to more than radiation. For the four leukaemia cases with fathers in the highest radiation dose group, one of the fathers was an analytical chemist, one a fitter's mate, and the others process workers. Whether these workers all worked in the same building and were exposed to a common chemical leukaemogenic agent is not known. The evidence that preconceptual exposure to chemical agents induces leukaemia in animals, and probably also humans, is at least as strong as the evidence for radiation exposure, and there is no information on what chemicals are in the environs of the Sellafield workers. A possible carry-over of traces of leukaemogenic chemicals, for example, decontaminating chemicals, on the bodies and clothing of such workers cannot therefore be discounted, and neither can the possibility that the leukaemias are induced postnatally and not as a consequence of preconceptual exposure to a mutagen. If these diseases were indeed induced postnatally, and as a secondary consequence of radiation or chemical exposure, then humans may be no different from chickens, mice, cats, cattle, and gibbons, all of which suffer leukaemias as a consequence of viral infection. Studies on mouse strains harbouring a leukaemogenic virus show that activation of latent virus can occur after exposure of animals to radiation or other environmental insults. Human lymphoid cells in culture that harbour the Epstein-Barr virus can be made to release large quantities of replicating virus after exposure to agents that damage DNA; whether a similar phenomenon is involved in clusters of childhood leukaemias is not known.

In view of the public concern about radiation and cancer, it is worth emphasising that childhood leukaemia is a tragic but not a common disease. Its prevalence in the UK is about 1 in 2000, and it is far less common than genetic abnormalities in the newborn that result in other forms of ill health and which are some 70 times more frequent. Although an excess of half a dozen childhood leukaemia cases has been noted over a 35 year period near Sellafield, over 12 000 cases occurred elsewhere in the UK over this interval. Gardner has said that his intriguing findings are "a pointer"; let us hope that they will point the way to a much needed understanding of the causal factors in this disease.

1   Gardner MJ, Snee MP, Hall AJ, Powell CA, Downes S, Terrell JD. Results of case-control study of leukaemia and lymphoma among young people near Sellafield nuclear plant in west Cumbria. *BMJ* 1990;**300**:423–9.

1a Gardner MJ, Hall AJ, Snee MP, Downes S, Powell CA, Terrell JD. Methods and basic data of case-control study of leukaemia among young people near Sellafield nuclear plant in west Cumbria. *BMJ* 1990;**300**:429–34.

2   Black D for the Independent Advisory Group. *Investigation of the possible increased incidence of cancer in west Cumbria.* London: HMSO, 1984. (Black report.)

3   Committee on Medical Aspects of Radiation in the Environment. London: HMSO, 1989.

4   Shu XO, *et al. Cancer* 1988;**62**:635–44.

5 Ishimaru T, Ichimaru M, Mikami M. *Hiroshima Radiation Effects Research Foundation Technical Report 11–81*. Japanese National Institute of Health: Tokyo, 1981:1–10.
6 Nomura T. *Nature* 1982;**296**:575–7.
7 Kamiguchi Y, Tateho H, Mikamo K. *Mutat Res* 1990;**228**:133–40.
8 Nomura T. *Mutat Res* 1988;**198**:309–20.
9 Nourse J, *et al. Cell* 1990;**60**:535–45.
10 Kamps MP, Murre C, Sun X-H, Baltimore D. *Cell* 1990;**60**:547–55.
11 Beral V, Inskip H, Fraser P, Booth M, Coleman D, Rose G. Mortality of employees of the United Kingdom Atomic Energy Authority 1946–1979. *BMJ* 1985;**291**:440–7.

23: Leukaemia and lymphoma among young people near Sellafield

Letters to the *British Medical Journal*

N K NOTANI

Although Dr Martin Gardner and colleagues have done a fine epidemiological study of increased leukaemia cases around nuclear installations;[1] their explanation, that the fathers' occupational exposure to radiation is associated with this increase, does not seem to be congruent with several biological and radiobiological principles.

It is implied in the explanation that a dominant mutation is being induced in the father's sperm and that this then specifically leads to leukaemia on a probabilistic basis.

A very high frequency of this class of mutations inducing leukaemia would have to be imagined. If there are about 4000 male workers and about 10 000 progeny are sampled, then five excess cases of leukaemia would yield an estimated frequency of 0·05% (compared to an average spontaneous frequency of 10^{-5} per locus).

Ionising radiation is considered a "democratic" agent for inducing mutations, and a specific class of mutations would be difficult to explain. If radiation is still "secular" it would induce other mutations as well. A virtual genetic meltdown (to use Bob Haynes's term) would be expected.

Part of the difficulty of inducing a specific class of mutations may be overcome by assuming certain breakage events in the chromosome(s)—for example, a breakage-fusion-bridge cycle—but this is likely to put that sperm at a competitive disadvantage because it then would carry a large deletion.

Valerie Beral has correctly pointed out that increased leukaemia is not detectable in the progeny of the survivors of Hiroshima–Nagasaki bombings. These studies, taken together, would implicate "something else" for the raised incidence for leukaemia in Seascale.

Latent periods for inducing leukaemia (somatically) in bombed populations from Hiroshima and Nagasaki are known. Do the germinally induced leukaemias have similar latent periods? Are they similar to the leukaemias not induced by radiation?

Perhaps there are counterarguments or flaws in the foregoing; I would like to hear these.

1 Gardner MJ, Snee MP, Hall AJ, Powell CA, Downes S, Terrell JD. Results of a case-control study of leukaemia and lymphoma among young people near Sellafield nuclear plant in west Cumbria. *BMJ* 1990;**300**:423–9.
2 Beral V. Leukaemia and nuclear installations. *BMJ* 1990;**300**:411–2.

J W KOTEN, W DenOTTER

In the study of Professor Martin J Gardner and colleagues[1] on leukaemia and lymphoma among young people near Sellafield no attention was given to the paternal age of the radiation workers. In a recent survey of sporadic hereditary retinoblastoma we observed a "paternal age effect"—that is, we noted in the offspring of older fathers a considerably increased risk of hereditary tumours (D J Derkinderen *et al*, unpublished work). So if the incidences of tumours in the offspring of radiation workers are to be compared with those in the general population the effect of the paternal age should be discounted.

1 Gardner MJ, Snee MP, Hall AJ, Powell CA, Downes S, Terrell JD. Results of case-control study of leukaemia and lymphoma among young people near Sellafield nuclear plant in west Cumbria. *BMJ* 1990;**300**:423–9.

R H MOLE

If irradiation can cause leukaemia in a child as a result of radiation damage to the father's sperm—that is, by causing a dominant mutation—the consequences for understanding carcinogenesis in general outweigh any application to a particular occupational hazard. Professor Martin J Gardner and colleagues did no more than claim that paternal irradiation explains statistically the occurrence of four cases of leukaemia.[1] They took the greatest pains to avoid epidemiological biases, but their statistical tests depended on accepting annual records of occupational radiation exposures at face value as if they truly represented radiation doses to parental testes and seminal vesicles.

When trying to relate annual exposure records more closely to conception Professor Gardner and colleagues halved the annual record and called that the radiation dose during the six months before conception. This is valid only if paternal exposures were uniform month by month during the year. Moreover, sperm have a limited lifetime; they continue to be made all the time, and those irradiated four to six months before conception of a child must represent a very small proportion of the sperm in the ejaculate responsible for the conception. Even sperm made between two and three months before the conception will have formed a far smaller proportion than the sperm made during the month before. A much more critical assessment is needed that takes account of the biology of conception to support the claim that it is an irradiated sperm that caused each excess case of childhood leukaemia at Sellafield.

It is obligatory, when reporting annual occupational exposures to radiation, to make an allowance for missing records (for example, loss of a film badge). The missing record must be given the value corresponding to the annual dose limit—that is, one thirteenth of the dose limit for 52 weeks if the film badges are changed every four weeks. In most circumstances now the maximum monthly dose for a radiation worker is such a "nominal dose", a dose it was most unlikely he ever received. It is forbidden by regulation to replace the missing record by any more realistic assessment, such as the average of preceding and succeeding film badge readings. When the annual dose limit is 50 mSv, as it has been recently, and as 150 mSv (as it was in the 1950s), such a four week nominal dose would have been about 4 mSv and 12 mSv respectively. Thus the dose groupings used by Professor Gardner and colleagues to show an increased risk of childhood leukaemia with increase in exposure during the six months before conception (1–4 mSv, 5–9 mSv, and > 10 mSv; table VI) are critically dependent on whether the recorded radiation exposure of the father of a child with leukaemia was inflated by a dose he never had.

Professor Gardner and colleagues now have the detailed occupational dose records and will be able to dispose of these methodological uncertainties. Did no referee draw the authors' attention to uncertainties that deserved mentioning?

1 Gardner MJ, Snee MP, Hall AJ, Powell CA, Downes S, Terrell JD. Results of a case-control study of leukaemia and lymphoma among young people near Sellafield nuclear plant in west Cumbria. *BMJ* 1990;**300**:423–9.

Authors' reply

MARTIN J GARDNER, MICHAEL P SNEE

Dr N K Notani gives an interesting discussion of the genetic aspects associated with our findings, on which we would also be interested in comments from others. We recognise that if our result was causal and occurred through a genetic pathway it would imply greater effects than predicted by previous estimates. We would point out, however, that we did not give "the explanation" but suggested "some explanations" and in our overall conclusions did not specify any preferred mechanism.

We did note, though, as did Dr Valerie Beral, that our findings did not concur with those from Japan. We offered one thought on how the nature of the radiation exposure differed that was related to an interval of time between the bomb and the child's conception, and Dr Beral offered others; we would suggest that these be considered carefully. It would, in addition, be interesting to see an updated analysis from Japan of leukaemia in children of parents exposed to radiation before conception that included the revised lower dose estimates and was by year of birth. Other Japanese findings, of course, also do not concur with a raised incidence of childhood leukaemia after prenatal exposure to x rays.

In relation to latent periods, interestingly, the age distribution at diagnosis of the children with leukaemia born to fathers with a radiation record at Sellafield before their child's conception was lower than that of the other children with leukaemia. For example, five of the eight (62%)

Number of children with leukaemia by age at diagnosis and recorded paternal exposure to ionising radiation at Sellafield before conception

Age (years) at diagnosis	Father with radiation record		
	Yes	No	Unknown
≤4	5	9	3
5–9	2	11	0
10–24	1	18	3

Test for trend in proportions of fathers with radiation record by age gives $\chi^2 = 4.62$, df = 1, p = 0.03.

who were born to fathers who had been exposed to radiation had been diagnosed as having leukaemia when they were under 5 years of age compared with nine of the 38 (24%) children with leukaemia whose fathers had not been exposed. The table gives more detail. This suggested difference in age is in the direction that has been predicted in general if any mechanism involved were to contain a germ line component.[1]

In reply to Drs J W Koten and W DenOtter, we did give in our paper some results on the relative risk of childhood leukaemia in relation to paternal age at birth, showing an increase in children of fathers over the age of 40 years of somewhat more than 50%; but there was an even greater increase with maternal age, which was therefore discussed in more detail. The average age at their children's birth, for example, of the four fathers of children with leukaemia in the highest radiation dose groups that we used (≥ 100 mSv total or ≥ 10 mSv during the six months before conception) was 34 years (mothers 32), with one father (and one mother) being over age 40 compared with the average for their matched control fathers of 30 (mothers 27). The average age of the four fathers exposed to lower doses was 35 (mothers 33), again one father (and one mother) being over age 40; and for the remaining 38 fathers of children with leukaemia in our analysis the average age was 30 (mothers 27).

Dr R H Mole makes some reasonable comments about our estimation of paternal radiation exposure in the six months before conception in terms of the time period considered and the apportioning of annual doses. We accept these and had already planned to revise the analysis to examine a shorter period—probably two months—and to use the original dose records. What was reliably available to us for initial analysis was the annual dose estimates from British Nuclear Fuels, which had been checked by the National Radiological Protection Board,[2] and these were considered appropriate by colleagues whom we consulted. Of course any misclassification suggested by Dr Mole could equally apply to control fathers as much as to fathers of children with leukaemia and would be expected to bias the relative risks towards unity. Moreover, his comments do not affect our analysis of total radiation dose before conception.

1 Wheldon TE, Mairs R, Barrett A. Germ cell injury and childhood leukaemia clusters. *Lancet* 1989;i:792–3.
2 National Radiological Protection Board. *Radiation dose histories at British Nuclear Fuels plc, Sellafield.* Chilton: NRPB, 1986. (NRPB M136.)

24: The Sellafield childhood leukaemia cluster: are germ line mutations responsible?

MELVYN F GREAVES

A recent epidemiological study has provided an important new clue to the enigma of childhood leukaemia clusters associated with nuclear installations in the United Kingdom.[1] The findings, suggesting a possible transmission of radiation induced germ line mutations predisposing the offspring of exposed fathers to leukaemia, may have important medicosocial, legal, and political repercussions as well as implications for leukaemia aetiology in general.

A cause for concern

In 1983, a Yorkshire Television report entitled *Windscale: the Nuclear Laundry* identified an apparent excess or cluster of childhood leukaemias in the village of Seascale, which is next to the nuclear reprocessing plant, Windscale (subsequently renamed Sellafield), in west Cumbria (see figure). The television crew had gone to Sellafield itself to look into the possibility of health effects in workers, but their attention was drawn to what seemed to them to be an excessive number of leukaemias in local children. Seven cases were identified in the report. These were diagnosed between 1956 and 1983, and census data were used to calculate that this was 10 times the national incidence rate.[2 3]

The television programme focused attention on the possible harmful effects of radioactive discharges and prompted a government inquiry, chaired by Sir Douglas Black. The 1984 Black report identified a total of 14 cases of leukaemia, eight cases of lymphoma, and 10 cases of non-hemopoietic cancers, all of this total of 32 being in young people under the age of 25 years.[4] Seven of the leukaemia cases were in children who lived in

214

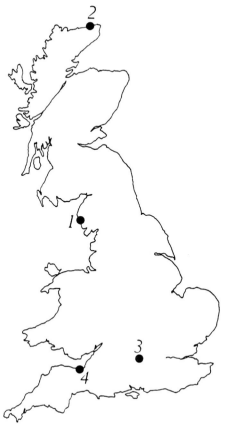

1 = Sellafield nuclear reprocessing plant; 2 = Dounreay nuclear reprocessing plant; 3 = west Berkshire north Hampshire area, Atomic Weapons Research Establishment, Aldermaston, and Royal Ordnance Factory, Burghfield; 4 = Hinkley Point nuclear power station.

the village of Seascale, all of whom had fathers working at the Sellafield plant operated by British Nuclear Fuels Ltd (BNFL). The Black report concluded that there was a roughly fourfold higher rate of leukaemia mortality (in people aged under 25) in the district (Millom) around Sellafield during the period 1968–78 and a 10-fold higher rate of *incidence* of leukaemia (mostly lymphoid) in the population of Seascale village aged under 10, thus largely corroborating the television report.

These findings fuelled public alarm about the safety of nuclear plants and appeared to endorse the concerns of environmental groups such as Greenpeace who had long been campaigning against what they believed to be unacceptable discharge levels of radionuclides. Certainly the nuclear industry, and Sellafield (as Windscale) in particular, had already acquired a suspect safety record, derived in the main from a major fire and radioactivity release in 1957 which, until Chernobyl, represented the worst nuclear plant accident, but also from other substantial leakages.[5] Local concern over the apparent excess of leukaemias has culminated in four families with leukaemic children suing BNFL for compensation. BFNL has vigorously denied negligence or culpability. The case has yet to go to court and could well be influenced by recent events. (Writs were served on BNFL on 6 March this year (1990).)

Following a recommendation of the Black report, a group named the Committee on Medical Aspects of Radiation in the Environment (COMARE) was established in 1985 to look further into the health consequences of man-made and natural radiation and to advise the UK government. In 1988, COMARE, following up an earlier report of the Scottish Health Service, documented a roughly 10-fold excess ($p = <0.0002$) of childhood leukaemia within a 12 km radius of the Dounreay nuclear establishment on the north coast of Scotland (see figure).[7] COMARE concluded that the similar observations at Sellafield and Dounreay were unlikely to be coincidental but emphasised that the calculated exposure doses of the population to radiation released from the plants was far too low to account for the observed effect, being in the case of Dounreay only around 1% of the natural or background exposure. Nevertheless, some association with the proximity of the nuclear plants seemed likely. Many uncertainties surrounded these studies, including statistical problems associated with the small number of cases involved, the lack of information on both possible routes of exposure to radiation (seafood and milk were considered among others) and the actual received dose to the bone marrow of infants or fetuses.

Several other independent studies were conducted to investigate the possible association of leukaemia with nuclear plants, which gave somewhat divergent results and interpretations. Childhood leukaemia mortality appeared to be only marginally in excess (1.1–1.2 times for lymphoid leukaemia) in association with proximity to nuclear installations in general,[8–10] but some modest excess in incidence (1.4 times) was reported in proximity to atomic weapons establishments in Berkshire (see figure),[11] and this was confirmed by a subsequent COMARE report.[12] A more substantial increase in risk (up to fourfold) was suggested for children living near Hinkley Point nuclear power station in Somerset (see figure) during the period 1969–73.[13] The picture was further complicated by the reports of small excesses of leukaemia in areas that were simply chosen as sites for nuclear plant development but which did not actually go ahead,[14] coupled with the suggestion that these relatively isolated sites tended to be rich in bracken which might itself be leukaemogenic.[15] It was further suggested that even the much more impressive extra risk at Sellafield and Dounreay might have nothing to do with radiation but reflect leukaemic consequences of viral infections arising in isolated communities[16]—an idea akin to a hypothesis suggested for childhood common acute lymphoblastic leukaemia in general.[17] All of these studies were plagued with numerical and other difficulties and, as emphasised in the COMARE reports, were difficult, if not impossible, to interpret in the absence of any detailed information on the distribution of childhood leukaemia throughout the country. COMARE strongly recommended that such studies be undertaken, and they have now (1990) been started. In addition, the British nuclear industry initiated a major sponsorship of research into basic radiobiology with some emphasis on the biological effects of low level high lineal energy transfer radionuclides such as plutonium or radon.

By the time the COMARE report on Dounreay was published, a study by Gardner and colleagues had produced evidence that the extra risk of leukaemia around Sellafield might be restricted to children who were born in the locality, as opposed to those who moved there later.[18] This finding, though again based on very small numbers, focused attention on early life events—that is, in infancy or pregnancy—and also raised the possibility of germ line preconceptual mutations in parents.[7] Analogies were drawn with x ray induced inherited predisposition to cancer in mice as shown in one large study by Nomura[19 20] and with the inheritance of paternal Rb gene mutations in retinoblastoma.[21] At the same time, it was recognised that there was no evidence for radiation induced germ line leukaemogenic mutations in humans and, in particular, no evidence for an increased risk of leukaemia in the offspring of parents who were exposed to the atomic bomb in Japan (see further below).

The "Gardner" report

The recent study by Gardner et al[1] was commissioned and funded by the UK government Department of Health following the recommendations of the Black report. The paper was published in the *British Medical Journal* on Saturday 17 February 1990, but was preceded on Thursday 15 February with a press conference. The latter precipitated an avalanche of media coverage which, true to British newspaper traditions, varied from the sombre to the sensational or macabre.

The study itself is something of an epidemiological tour de force; and, paradoxically perhaps, its key observation depends on the good record-keeping habits of BNFL at Sellafield. The case-control study involved 52 patients with acute leukaemia, 22 with non-Hodgkin's lymphoma, and 23 with Hodgkin's disease, all under 25 years of age and diagnosed between 1950 and 1985. Just over 1000 age-matched controls were chosen from birth registers for the same west Cumbria area. The investigating team used an extensive questionnaire that inquired into the children's residence at birth in relation to the Sellafield plant, their eating and play habits, mother's age and exposure to x rays and infections during pregnancy, and paternal occupation. The factors that came out as being significantly associated with leukaemia or leukaemia and non-Hodgkin's lymphoma combined (but not Hodgkin's disease) were: residence close to Sellafield, paternal occupation, radiation dose received (for Sellafield workers) and parental (especially maternal) age. If those living < 4 km from Sellafield were given a relative risk of 1·0, then for those living further away the risk fell from 0·35 to 0·14, depending on distance. It should be stressed that this remarkable result had very wide confidence limits and hinged on five patients who were resident in Seascale village—that is, the previously recognised Seascale "cluster". Several paternal occupations were associated with an increased relative risk, again with very wide confidence limits, including iron and steel working and farming. The most striking result was, however, that concerning employment at the Sellafield plant itself. Nine of 46 people with leukaemia had (as indicated by birth certificates) a father employed at the plant, compared with a smaller proportion of controls, which gave a relative risk of 2·82. Cases and controls were next compared for paternal radiation dose (for those working at Sellafield), considering either the total accumulative dose recorded by external monitors (while in BNFL employment for 6–13 years) up until the time of conception of the case or control child or the corresponding inferred dose received during the six months immediately prior to conception. Of the nine case fathers, four had received a total recorded preconceptual dose of ≥ 100 milliseivert (mSv; radiation dose equivalent, given as dose in text) (maximum 188 mSv) compared with only three of 276 or five of 288 control fathers (depending upon particular geographical definition of control group), with the same numbers (and presumably individuals) in each group having a 6 months preconceptual dose of ≥ 10 mSv, giving relative risk in the range of 6·24–8·38. Roughly translated into absolute risk, this means that children of fathers exposed at this level may have a one in 300 chance of developing leukaemia compared with the national average of a 1 in 2000 chance. Quite extraordinarily, three of these four case fathers with relatively high exposure levels were among the five case fathers identified in Seascale village, suggesting that the local cluster itself was associated with occupational exposure. (Of these four cases, three were acute lymphoblastic anaemia and one was unspecified leukaemia). Occupational exposures may not be the whole story, however, as there is no obvious reason why workers exposed to higher levels of radiation at the plant should live close to the plant in Seascale village (most workers at the plant do not), and proximity to the plant or living in Seascale might itself be a risk factor. Indeed, it now becomes apparent that if three of the case fathers exposed to ≥ 100 mSv had not all lived in Seascale village, the association of Sellafield with increased risk of leukaemia might not have come to light. The association with living close to Sellafield has not been explained but provides at least a hint of additional exposure of either the father, mother, or child.

The number of cases involved in the study and, in particular, in the Seascale clusters is obviously very small, so much so that the editor of *Nature* states that "no logical conclusions can be drawn".[23] Nevertheless, many people have drawn what must be the obvious and most likely correct conclusion, which is that there is an *association* between childhood leukaemia and occupational exposure to a mutagenic agent. Mutation of germ cells induced by radiation is considered the most likely pathway, but much more work needs to be done to establish the direct causal mechanism with some certainty.

The Gardner study has major implications for working practices at nuclear plants, for genetic counselling of workers and their families, for the current litigation by some of these families, and for the continuing political debate on the future of nuclear establishments, be they power generators, reprocessing plants, or weapons factories. In addition, if the favoured interpretation is correct, then there would be other important implications for leukaemia and cancer in the general population. It is therefore crucial that the uncertainties surrounding the Sellafield data and its interpretation be thoroughly examined and clarified as quickly as possible.

What is the mutagen?

One crucial question is whether the monitored exposure to radiation (presumably mostly γ rays) is a surrogate measure for something else, obvious candidates being ingested α-emitting radionuclides such as plutonium, which can be concentrated near sites of spermatogenesis in testes,[24] or a non-radioactive mutagen—for example, a chemical solvent, plenty of which is used in such plants. Data on ingested radioactivity in the same workers is apparently being analysed, along with details of their precise work schedules. A similar study to that of Gardner *et al* is expected to be completed soon on workers at the Dounreay nuclear plant in Scotland, and a national survey of the children of nuclear industry workers is being initiated. Other national epidemiological studies of childhood leukaemia in relation to possible parental exposure to mutagenic substances are currently being set up in the USA and UK. These additional studies should help establish whether exposure to radioactive substances (or other non-ionising mutagenic substances) are consistently associated with leukaemia in offspring.

A lack of precedent?

Epidemiologists interested in health effects of radiation have relied heavily on the precedent of the Japanese atomic bomb and have been surprised by the implication of the Sellafield data as there was no recorded increase in leukaemia in the offspring of exposed fathers (or pregnant mothers). The situation in Japan was quite different, however, with a single large dose of γ radiation (individuals grouped as receiving 10–490 mSv or $\geqslant$ 500 mSv). Interpretation of the Japanese data is further compromised by the possible importance of the time interval between exposure and conception, by the competing effects of dominant lethal mutations in sperm precursors, and by the possibility of deficient recording of childhood leukaemia before 1950. The extraordinary study by Nomura using 12 000 mice analysed over a 15 year period does provide a precedent in so far as it showed x ray induced germinal (male) mutations manifested as congenital abnormalities and a high incidence (about 10%) of cancers, mostly in the lung but including some lymphocytic leukaemias.[19][20] This mode of induction of congenital abnormalities has been confirmed elsewhere.[25] Other, earlier, studies have shown the germ line transmission of x ray induced (6 Gy (600 rad)) skeletal abnormalities in offspring.[26][27] Irradiation of animal testes with internal radionuclides has also been shown to transmit damage to offspring.[28] In these studies, fractionated doses seemed to be more mutagenic to spermatogonia (the stem cells of the sperm lineage) than a single dose; Nomura's data indicated no difference in response to variation in dose scheduling except in the case where the timing of the radiation dose in relation to mating was lengthened to assay mutation in spermatogonia; here the opposite effect emerged—that is, a single dose was more potent. Note that the dose of radiation is much greater (0·36–5·04 Gy (36–504 rad)) in these mouse experiments than in the Sellafield fathers.

The frequency of transmitted "cancer" mutations in sperm in the Nomura study (about 3% per Sv) would seem to be high compared with that for defined specific genetic changes, which is estimated to be about 1% per Sv for all relevant loci together and about 0·01% per Sv for a single gene (D Goodhead, personal communication). Thus, both the Nomura study and that of Gardner *et al* appear not to conform to the expectations of conventional radiation genetics.

Risk and target cell

If a minimum of two mutations is required for leukaemogenesis, then any risk factor calculated—for example, 1:2000 for "normal" children, 1:300 for children of fathers most exposed to radiation at Sellafield—represents the sum of probabilities of each independent mutation occurring. The individual risk for each of a pair of mutations could, however, be very different depending on the nature of the mutation and the number of cells carrying it and probably a host of other cofactors. For example, if a leukaemogenic mutation is deliberately inserted into the germ line in transgenic mice up to 100% of offspring can develop leukaemia even though a second, independent spontaneous mutation appears to be required in this particular model.[29][30] In this situation every blood cell has the first mutation, and therefore an enormous number of cells are at risk. In contrast with acquired somatic mutations (as presumed in most childhood leukaemias), a single cell plus its descendants are at risk, and the probability of the second event (after birth) is likely to be more limiting. This line of reasoning is only helpful in the Sellafield case in so far as it predicts that an infant inheriting a mutation in a gene relevant to leukaemia via the germ line may be more at risk than an infant who acquires the same or similar mutation in a hemopoietic cell.

Other indicators of germ line mutations?

If leukaemia in the offspring of Sellafield workers is due to the inheritance of mutations, whatever the inducing agent and dose, then we would certainly expect to see an increased incidence of fetal deaths, other paediatric cancers, and congenital malformations; indeed, the latter should be more common than the leukaemias as they can arise by single dominant mutations. Acute leukaemia in children, in contrast, probably requires a minimum of two independent mutations in most cases.[17] There are unsubstantiated, anecdotal reports of more than expected cases of spontaneous abortions, malformations, and Down's syndrome in west Cumbria, but no systematic study has been conducted. A survey now proposed of the study of offspring of all workers exposed to ionising radiation should help clarify this important point. The Japanese precedent is not helpful here as, unexpectedly, no increase in congenital abnormalities was recorded.

Risks from other natural sources of radiation?

Accepting the uncertainties surrounding the precise nature of occupational exposure at Sellafield and its causal link to leukaemogenesis in workers' offspring, there are nevertheless implications for the aetiology of leukaemia in general. This is especially the case if one accepts the possibility that an accumulative dose of around 100 mSv over several years (rather than an acute dose of 10–20 mSv prior to conception) can cause leukaemogenic mutations. A 25 year old in the UK accumulates, on average, about 25 mSv to testes and bone marrow from natural sources. It is therefore difficult to avoid the conclusion that natural radiation may be a significant cause of childhood leukaemia. Indeed, Knox et al have suggested that a substantial proportion of all childhood cancers and leukaemias may be caused by natural radiation, particularly that received during pregnancy, and claim that there is a correlation between levels of indoor (terrestrial) γ radiation and childhood cancer.[31] The case for α emitting radon gas and its daughter products is even more intriguing. The average annual dose of ionising radiation in the UK is calculated at about 1 mSv to most organs and about 10 times this to the lung from radon decay, which is present at an *average* level in UK homes of 20 Bq/m³. There are parts of the UK, USA and Scandinavia where levels are considerably higher by up to two orders of magnitude, because of the release of radon gas from underlying rocks (especially granite) into homes and, to a lesser extent, from the materials used to build homes (such as pumice stone, alum shales, and phosphogypsum).[32 33] Additional exposure may come from radon or radium in water. Potentially, the occupants of such homes have a higher exposure to radiation than most nuclear workers at Sellafield, as can workers at radon spas, some of whom may receive over 2500 mSv a year to lung.[33] Radon²²² is an α emitting nuclide that decays to produce a polonium daughter nuclide which can be absorbed on dust particles into the lungs. Radon inhalation has been associated with lung cancer in uranium miners, and radon exposure may be responsible for around 6% of all lung cancers in the UK.[32] Until recently, little serious consideration has been given to the possibility that exposure to natural radon might cause leukaemia, either by mutagenesis of bone marrow stem cells or via germ line mutations, presumably because the route of uptake appeared to preclude significant direct exposure of either target tissue: α emitters have a very short path length of about 50 µm and therefore would have to enter the bloodstream to damage DNA effectively in most organs. Recent observations indicate that this presumption needs reappraisal. Henshaw and colleagues at Bristol have calculated that the solubility of radon in the fat content of blood and marrow is likely to be such that individuals living in "high radon" households could be receiving a marrow dose (and a gonad dose?) of 1–7 mSv a year for exposure levels of 1000 Bq/m³.[34] Other indirect clues that radon might contribute to leukaemogenesis come from geographical analyses of leukaemia incidence rates. Lucie has recently suggested that there might be a correlation between indoor radon levels and the incidence of acute myeloblastic leukaemia.[35] An atlas of leukaemia distribution in England and Wales recently published in the UK[36] documents significant excesses (of around 1·4 times) of childhood leukaemias (acute lymphoblastic leukaemia) in three areas—south west England (Cornwall, Devon, Somerset), Derbyshire, and Cumbria. These areas are to some extent coincident with regions having above average natural radon levels. A number of case-control studies are planned to see if there is indeed a correlation between radon exposure in the house and childhood cancer.

If any leukaemogenic effects of natural ionising radiation operated primarily via cumulative dose to the *germ line* and these leukaemias represent a significant fraction of total childhood leukaemia cases, then two other predictions can be made. Firstly, there should be an increased rate of congenital abnormalities in areas of high exposure. Secondly, increasing parental age at conception should constitute a significant risk factor for leukaemia. Several studies have documented an increasing risk with *maternal* age (independent of those cases of Down's syndrome) but not for paternal age.[37-40] In the study of Gardner *et al* maternal age ($\geqslant 40$ *v* < 25 years) was a significant risk factor (3·38–4·94 times for leukaemias alone) with a more marginal but possible increased risk with increased paternal age (1·87–2·27 times). Unfortunately, the Gardner study does not identify the ages of the fathers involved in the Seascale cluster itself or in the case of the fathers exposed at the plant. Only one of the four mothers of the crucial case children (those with high exposure level fathers) was over 40 years old.

These speculations all serve to reinforce the point that it is crucial that the actual dosage and mutagen to which the Sellafield workers were exposed be identified.

Identifying germ line mutations

Finally, it is likely that epidemiological studies will continue to be frustrated by small or modest numbers of cases with wide confidence limits restraining whatever increased risks are observed. Some consideration should therefore be given to laboratory investigations that would support or refute a germ line route of leukaemogenesis. Certainly, Nomura's rodent experiments should be repeated,[19] perhaps with α particle exposure. More definitive evidence for germ line transmission might come from recent developments in molecular biology. The accurate measure of clonal mutation frequencies in marker genes, including *hprt*[41] or HLA,[42] provides a quantitative approach to detecting higher than normal levels of mutations in long lived cells such as T cells and, indeed, has been used to detect high mutant frequencies in Japanese individuals 40 years after their single exposure.[43] Detection of mutant blood cells in exposed individuals would be a surrogate for sperm cell precursors, but some measurements of sperm might also be possible, at least if the mutations arose in spermatogonia and were thus preserved for some time. Another prediction is that surviving children who may have acquired their leukaemia via germ line inheritance of the first mutation in their leukaemogenic sequence should obviously retain this same mutation in all cells of the body. Although we have an incomplete list of genes whose alteration can contribute to the development of leukaemia, a screen for constitutive mutation in those that we can currently identify might prove informative.

I am grateful to Dr D Goodhead for critical comments and suggestions and to Barbara Deverson for preparation of the manuscript. The views expressed in this article are my own and do not necessarily reflect those of COMARE of which I am a member. This work was supported by the Leukaemia Research Fund of Great Britain.

1 Gardner MJ, Snee MP, Hall AJ, Powell CA, Downes S, Terrell JD. Results of case-control study of leukaemia and lymphoma among young people near Sellafield nuclear plant in west Cumbria. *BMJ* 1990;**300**:423–9.

2 Urquhart J, Palmer M, Cutler J. Cancer in Cumbria: the Windscale connection. *Lancet* 1984;**i**:217–8.

3 Gardner MJ, Winter PD. Mortality in Cumberland during 1959–78 with reference to cancer in young people around Windscale. *Lancet* 1984;**i**:216–7.

4 Black D for the Independent Advisory Group. *Investigation of the possible increased incidence of cancer in west Cumbria.* London: HMSO, 1984. (Black report.)

5 Committee on Medical Aspects of Radiation in the Environment. *The implications of the new data on the releases from Sellafield in the 1950s for the conclusions of the report on the investigation of the possible increased incidence of cancer in west Cumbria.* London: HMSO, 1986. (COMARE 1st report.)

6 Heasman MA, Kemp IW, Urquhart JD, Black R. Childhood leukaemia in northern Scotland. *Lancet* 1986;**i**:266.

7 Committee on Medical Aspects of Radiation in the Environment. *Investigation of the possible increased incidence of leukaemia in young people near the Dounreay nuclear establishment, Caithness, Scotland.* London: HMSO, 1988. (COMARE 2nd report.)

8 Cook-Mozaffari PJ, Darby SC, Doll R, Forman D, Herman C, Pike MC, et al. Geographical variation in mortality from leukaemia and other cancers in England and Wales in relation to proximity to nuclear installations, 1969–78. *Br J Cancer* 1989;**59**:476–85.

9 Forman D, Cook-Mozaffari P, Darby S, Davey G, Stratton I, Doll R, et al. Cancer near nuclear installations. *Nature* 1987;**329**:499–505.

10 Wakeford R, Binks K, Wilkie D. Childhood leukaemia and nuclear installations. *J R Statist Soc A* 1989;**152**:61–86.

11 Roman E, Beral V, Carpenter L, Watson A, Barton C, Ryder H, et al. Childhood leukaemia in the West Berkshire and Basingstoke and North Hampshire District Health Authorities in relation to nuclear establishments in the vicinity. *BMJ* 1987;**294**:597–602.

12 Committee on Medical Aspects of Radiation in the Environment. *Investigation of the possible increased incidence of childhood cancer in the west Berkshire and north Hampshire area, in which are situated the Atomic Weapons Research Establishment, Aldermaston and the Royal Ordnance Factory, Burghfield.* London: HMSO, 1989. (COMARE 3rd report.)

13 Ewings PD, Bowie C, Phillips MJ, Johnson SAN. Incidence of leukaemia in young people in the vicinity of Hinkley Point nuclear power station, 1959–86. *BMJ* 1989;**299**:289–93.

14 Cook-Mozaffari P, Darby S, Doll R. Cancer near potential sites of nuclear installations. *Lancet* 1989;**ii**:1145–7.

15 Evans IA, Galpin OP. Bracken and leukaemia. *Lancet* 1990;**i**:231.

16 Kinlen L. Evidence for an infective cause of childhood leukaemia: comparison of a Scottish new town with nuclear reprocessing sites in Britain. *Lancet* 1988;**ii**:1323–26.

17 Greaves MF. Speculations on the cause of childhood acute lymphoblastic leukaemia. *Leukemia* 1988;**2**:120–5.

18 Gardner MJ, Hall AJ, Downes S, Terrell JD. Follow up study of children born to mothers resident in Seascale, west Cumbria (birth cohort). *BMJ* 1987;**295**:822–7.

19 Nomura T. Parental exposure to x-rays and chemicals induces heritable tumours and anomalies in mice. *Nature* 1982;**296**:575–7.

20 Nomura T. Further studies on x-ray and chemically induced germ-line alterations causing tumors and malformations in mice. In: Ramel C, Lambert B, Magnusson J, eds. *Genetic toxicology of environment chemicals, part B: genetic effects and applied mutagenesis.* New York: Alan R Liss, 1986:13–20.

21 Greaves MF. Letters to the editor. *Lancet* 1989;**i**:95.

22 Ishimaru T, Ichimaru M, Mikami M. Leukemia incidence among individuals exposed in utero, children of atomic bomb survivors, and their controls: Hiroshima and Nagasaki, 1945–79. *Radiat Effects Res Foundation* 1982; Technical Report 11-81:1–10.

23 Maddox J. Sellafield makes news again. *Nature* 1990;**343**:690.

24 Ash P, Parker T. The ultrastructure of mouse testicular interstitial tissue containing plutonium-239 and its significance in explaining the observed distribution of plutonium in the testis. *Int J Radiat Biol* 1978;**34**:523–36.

25 Kirk KM, Lyon MF. Induction of congenital malformations in the offspring of male mice treated with x-rays at premeiotic and postmeiotic stages. *Mutat Res* 1984;**125**:75–85.

26 Ehling UH. Dominant mutations affecting the skeleton in offspring of X-irradiated male mice. *Genetics* 1966;**54**:1381–9.

27 Russell WL. An augmenting effect of dose fractionation on radiation-induced mutation rate in mice. *Proc Natl Acad Sci USA* 1962;**48**:1724–7.

28 Searle AG. Cytogenic effects of incorporated radionuclides on mammalian germ cells. In: Ishihara T, Sasaki MS, eds. *Radiation-induced chromosome damage in man.* New York: Alan R Liss, 1983;347–67.

29 Adams JM, Harris AW, Pinkert CA, Corcoran LM, Alexander WS, Cory S, *et al.* The c-myc oncogene driven by immunoglobulin enhancers induces lymphoid malignancy in transgenic mice. *Nature* 1985;**318**:533.

30 Langdon WY, Harris AW, Cory S, Adams JM. The c-myc oncogene perturbs B lymphocyte development in Eμ-myc transgenic mice. *Cell* 1986;**47**:11.

31 Knox EG, Stewart AM, Gilman EA, Kneale GW. Background radiation and childhood cancers. *J Radiol Prot* 1988;**8**:9–18.

32 Clarke RH, Southwood TRE. Risks from ionizing radiation. *Nature* 1989;**338**:197–8.

33 *Radiation. Doses, effects, risks.* United Nations Publication, 1985.

34 Richardson RB, Eatough JP, Henshaw DL. *The contribution of radon exposure to the radiation dose received by the red bone marrow and the fetus.* Proceedings of the UK Association for Radiation Research Meeting 20–22 September 1989, Bristol, 1989.

35 Lucie NP. Radon exposure and leukaemia. *Lancet* 1989;**ii**:99–100.

36 Cartwright RA, Alexander FE, McKinney PA, Rubetts TJ. *Leukaemia and lymphoma: atlas of distribution within areas of England and Wales, 1984–1988.* London: Leukaemia Research Fund of Great Britain, 1990.

37 Stark CR, Mantel N. Maternal-age and birth-order effects in childhood leukemia: age of child and type of leukemia. *J Natl Cancer Inst* 1969;**42**:857–66.

38 MacMahon B, Newill VA. Birth characteristics of children dying of malignant neoplasms. *J Natl Cancer Inst* 1962;**28**:231–44.

39 Stewart A, Webb J, Hewitt D. A survey of childhood malignancies. *BMJ* 1958;**i**:1495–508.

40 Manning MD, Carroll BE. Some epidemiological aspects of leukemia in children. *J Natl Cancer Inst* 1957;**19**:1087–94.

41 Nicklas JA, Hunter TC, O'Neill JP, Albertini RJ. Molecular analyses of in vivo *hprt* mutations in human T lymphocytes. III. Longitudinal study of *hprt* gene structural alterations and T cell clonal origins. *Mutat Res* 1989;**215**:147–60.

42 McCarron MA, Kutlaca A, Morley AA. The HLA-A mutation assay: improved technique and normal results. *Mutat Res* 1989;**225**:189–93.

43 Hakoda M, Akiyama M, Kyoizumi S, Awa AA, Yamakido M, Otake M. Increased somatic cell mutant frequency in atomic bomb survivors. *Mutat Res* 1988;**201**:39–48.

25: Of mice and men?

Letter to *Nature*

TAISEI NOMURA

Is it true that parents' exposure to radiation and chemicals causes tumours in their children?[1] Although my experiments with mice anticipated the suggestion that parental exposure to radiation and chemicals could induce heritable tumours in the next generation,[2-4] this finding has not been supported by the large scale epidemiological survey[5] of the children of atom bomb survivors in Hiroshima and Nagasaki.[5 6] Gardner *et al* recorded a risk of leukaemias (mostly acute lymphatic leukaemia) six to eight times higher than normal in the children of fathers who were employed at the Sellafield nuclear reprocessing plant and who had been exposed to more than 100 millisieverts (mSv) (as external doses) before conception,[1] although total doses were about a quarter of that in Hiroshima and Nagasaki (see table).

The most puzzling problem is the difference in the epidemiological surveys between Sellafield and Hiroshima/Nagasaki. I believe that my mouse experiments can help to reconcile the difference between the two population studies, assuming that the Sellafield results are in fact correct and not simply due to statistical artefacts. I propose three main reasons for the difference in the human studies: different germ cell susceptibility to leukaemia-causing mutations in Japanese and English people; different germ cell stages exposed in the two populations; and different postnatal tumour-promoting environments.

In the first case, I have shown that there is no increase of leukaemia in offspring of the ICR strain of mouse derived from spermatogonia that had been acutely dosed with *x* radiation (see table).[3 4] On the other hand, in the N5 strain, single acute irradiation to the spermatogonia induces about a 10 times greater incidence of acute lymphocytic leukaemia in the offspring than in unirradiated controls, and a high incidence of leukaemias persists in subsequent generations.[7] The large difference in leukaemia incidence in the offspring between the two strains reflects the difference in genetic predisposition to leukaemia induction by radiation. Such a difference could account for the different population responses of Sellafield and Hiroshima/ Nagasaki. Lung cancer, for example, developed at a seven times higher

Leukaemia in the F_1 offsrping after paternal exposure to radiation in man and mice

	Dose (mSv)	Relative risk	Doubling dose (mSv)	Rate mSv^{-1} ($\times 10^6$)
Sellafield				
All stages of spermatogenesis	$\geqslant 100$	3	$\geqslant 33$	
Postgonia*	$\geqslant 10$	4	$\geqslant 2\cdot5$	
Hiroshima				
Spermatogonia	435	1	—	
Mouse				
ICR				
Spermatogonia	360–5040	1	—	0
Spermatozoa and spermatids	360–5040	1·9–3·2	450	2·3
N5				
Spermatogonia	5040	9·6	260	7·0

Relative risk of leukaemia at Sellafield was estimated by subtracting the risk value at conception from those before conception.[1] Doubling doses of mice were calculated as a dominant trait.[7 15] For humans, doses were simply divided by relative risk to estimate doubling doses, because the mothers could also have been exposed to radionuclides via house dust and through their partners.[1 11]

* Fathers' exposure during the six months before conception indicates mainly post-spermatogonial exposure, but includes some spermatogonial exposure.

incidence in white uranium miners than in non-white miners in the United States at equal doses, although not by germinal exposure.[8] Nevertheless, there is a surprisingly large (10 times or more) difference in the doubling doses in the mouse and Sellafield human studies. (The lower the doubling dose, the greater the radiosensitivity, see table.) This disparity could result from undetermined doses of either neutron exposure or internally incorporated radionuclides and chemicals in the Sellafield study, which should be taken into account in the estimation of genetic risk.

Secondly, the extremely high risk of childhood leukaemia from the father's exposure during the six months before conception[1] suggests that the postmeiotic sperm is more sensitive to radiation than spermatogonia. This finding is well supported by the mouse experiments; although leukaemia was not induced in ICR mouse offspring by spermatogonial exposure of males, a twofold to threefold increase in the incidence of leukaemia was induced by the x ray exposure of the spermatozoa and spermatids. Similarly, higher mutational sensitivity of postmeiotic sperm has been observed in mice by the specific loci method[9] and chromosome rearrangement studies.[10] The negative results in Hiroshima and Nagasaki, which involved both spermatogonial exposure (in males) and immature oocytes exposure (of females), can be explained by the reduced sensitivities to radiation of these stages compared with sperm and spermatids, in addition to the possible difference in genetic predisposition in the two populations.

Thirdly, some studies at Sellafield have revealed an unusually high contamination of workers' homes with radioactive materials.[11] Children of irradiated fathers might be sensitive to leukaemia induction by postnatal radiation exposure and other environmental factors. The mouse studies have shown that preconceptually irradiated ICR mice show persistent hypersensitivity to tumorigenesis and, when subsequently exposed postnatally to tumour promoting agents, develop clusters of tumours.[12 13]

Although leukaemia and other childhood cancers have not increased in the children of atom bomb survivors in Hiroshima and Nagasaki, other types of cancers, especially adult type cancers, could increase as this population reaches cancer-prone age. A recent epidemiological survey in Hiroshima and Nagasaki revealed a higher risk of adult type cancers (but not leukaemia) in individuals of 40 years and older, exposed in utero to atomic radiation.[14] This was also anticipated by the mouse experiments.[13 15 16] Parental exposure to radiation does not necessarily increase the incidence of specific childhood human cancers such as retinoblastoma and Wilms' tumour.

There are no similar childhood tumours in mice, and radiation-induced germ line alteration (mutation) causing tumours suggests that heritable changes raise (for the most part) the incidence of various kinds of tumours commonly observed in mice.[3 4 7 13] Such changes might be concerned with an array of genes modifying immunological, biochemical, and physiological conditions which can lead to the increase in tumour incidence. Thus, it will be important to follow up all the human subjects throughout their lives to decide whether the mouse studies can predict the human response.

1 Gardner MJ et al. BMJ 1990;**300**:423–9.
2 Nomura T. Cancer Res 1975;**35**:264–6.
3 Nomura T. In: L Severi, ed. Tumors of early life in man and animals. Perugia, Italy: Perugia University Press, 1978:873–91.
4 Nomura T. Nature 1982;**296**:575–7.
5 Yoshimoto T, et al. RERF Tech Rep 1990 (TR 4–90).
6 Evans HJ. Nature 1990;**345**:16–7.
7 Nomura T. In: Ramel C, Lambert B, Magnusson J, eds. Genetic toxicology of environmental chemicals. New York: Liss, 1986:13-20.
8 Genetic and somatic effects of ionizing radiation. UNSCEAR Report, 1986.
9 Russell WL. In: Hollaender A, ed. Radiation biology. New York: McGraw-Hill, 1954:825–59.
10 Russell LB, Saylors CL. In: Sobels FH, ed. Repair from genetic radiation. Oxford: Pergamon, 1963:313–42.
11 Beral V. BMJ 1990;**300**:411–2.
12 Nomura T. Mutat Res 1983;**121**:59–65.
13 Nomura T. IARC Sci Publ 1989;**96**:375–87.
14 Kato H, Yoshimoto Y, Schull WJ. IARC Sci Publ 1989;**96**:365–74.
15 Nomura T. Environ Mol Mutagen 1984;**6**:33–40.
16 Nomura T, Nakajima H, Hatanaka T, Kinuta M, Hongyo T. Cancer Res 1990;**50**:2135–8.

26: Retinoblastoma in grandchildren of workers at Sellafield nuclear plant

J A MORRIS, JANE M EDWARDS,
JENNIFER BUCKLER

Evidence indicates that exposure of workers to radiation at Sellafield nuclear reprocessing plant increases the risk of acute lymphoblastic leukaemia in the next generation.[1] This could be due to a germinal mutation occurring in the workers or to an increased rate of somatic mutation occurring in their children during intrauterine or early extrauterine life.[2] One way to investigate this is to study the incidence of retinoblastoma in the offspring of those who work in the nuclear industry. This is because more is known about the genetic basis of retinoblastoma than of leukaemia[3] and it is often possible to work out the stage at which mutation has occurred. For instance, if there is an increased rate of germinal mutation this would lead to an increased frequency of bilateral retinoblastoma, and an increased rate of somatic mutation would lead to an increased incidence of unilateral retinoblastoma.

We report three cases of retinoblastoma that are relevant to this debate. These cases were recognised not as a result of a systematic study but because the mother of the index child knew of the two other cases and brought them to our attention.

Case reports

The maternal grandfathers of all three children worked at Sellafield, and the mothers had lived in Seascale, a small village less than 3 km from

Sellafield, during part of their childhood: one mother had been born there and the two others had moved there at the age of 6 months and 11 years of age. None of the children, however, had been born in Seascale. One child (case 1) developed a unilateral retinoblastoma at 6 months of age, which was treated by enucleation of the eye. At the age of 5 years she was well and had no evidence of tumour in the remaining eye. The constitution of her chromosomes was 46,XX. The second child (case 2) developed a unilateral retinoblastoma at 12 months of age, which was treated by enucleation. The other eye was still free of tumour when she was seen at the age of 3. The constitution of her chromosomes was 46,XX. The third child (case 3) developed retinoblastoma in one eye at 3 months of age, which was treated by enucleation, and a tumour in the other eye at 8 months, which was treated with a cobalt plaque. At the age of 12 she is well. The constitution of her chromosomes was 46,XX with a partial deletion of one chromosome 13 (del 13 [q12–q21]); this defect was not present in the cells of either parent.

The diagnosis of retinoblastoma was confirmed by histological examination of the enucleated eyes in all three cases. There was no history of retinoblastoma in any other member of these families. In addition, the fundi of the parents of the three children showed no evidence of a healed retinoblastoma. The fathers of the children had not had any contact with the nuclear industry and had never worked in Cumbria.

Comment

There was no evidence of a germinal mutation derived from the maternal grandfather in any of the three cases. In case 3 there was evidence of a germinal mutation derived from one of the parents. In the two other cases the evidence pointed to somatic mutation, although the possibility of germinal mutation derived from the parents cannot be completely excluded.

It is, of course, possible that this cluster of cases is a chance occurrence unrelated to exposure to radiation. Retinoblastoma, however, is extremely rare, occurring with a frequency of 1 in 20 000 live births and being 10 times less common than acute lymphoblastic leukaemia. To calculate the probability of a cluster of cases reliably it is necessary to define in advance the total population from which the cases have arisen. This is not possible if the cluster is observed in retrospect. In 1987, however, Gardner *et al* calculated that roughly 2600 children had been resident in Seascale at some time between 1950 and 1983.[45] This cohort is unlikely to have produced more than 5000 children. The expected number of cases of retinoblastoma in 5000 children is 0·25 and the chance of three occurring is 0·002.

If these cases are related to exposure to radiation then one possible explanation is that the mothers, who had spent part of their childhood in Seascale, had accumulated radionuclides and had an increased rate of cell mutation. This could then lead to an increased risk of a germinal mutation being passed on to the next generation and to an increased rate of somatic mutation affecting their children during intrauterine life. The mothers could have been exposed to radiation in the general environment or in contaminated homes. If this is the correct explanation it has important implications for the pathogenesis of other childhood tumours in this locality, and possible ways in which nuclear power workers contaminate their homes need urgent investigation. A large scale study of the incidence of retinoblastoma in the offspring of those who work in the nuclear industry is also required. This study will need to include not only the workers' children but also their children's children.

1 Gardner MJ, Snee MP, Hall AJ, Powell CA, Downes S, Terrell D. Results of a case-control study of leukaemia and lymphoma among young people near Sellafield nuclear plant in west Cumbria. *BMJ* 1990;**300**:423–9.
2 Morris JA. Leukaemia and lymphoma among young people near Sellafield. *BMJ* 1990;**300**:676.
3 Goudie RB. What are antioncogenes? *J Pathol* 1988;**154**:297–8.
4 Gardner MJ, Hall AJ, Downes S, Terrell JD. Follow up study of children born elsewhere but attending schools in Seascale, west Cumbria (schools cohort). *BMJ* 1987;**295**:819–22.
5 Gardner MJ, Hall AJ, Downes S, Terrell JD. Follow up study of children born to mothers resident in Seascale, west Cumbria (birth cohort). *BMJ* 1987;**295**:822–7.

27: Comments on the case-control study of Gardner *et al* of leukaemia and lymphoma among young people in west Cumbria

Independent assessment requested by British Nuclear Fuels Limited (BNFL)

P G SMITH

The case-control study of Gardner *et al* (chapters 19 and 20) included all known cases of leukaemia and lymphoma that were diagnosed in people aged under 25 at some time during the 36 year period 1950–85 while resident in the area served by West Cumbria Regional Health Authority and who were also born in the same area. The cases were ascertained using a variety of medical and other records. An attempt was made to select eight "area" controls and eight "local" controls for each case from the birth register in which a case's birth was entered. Those selected were those of the same sex as the case whose entries in the register were closest to that of the case (in time) and whose mothers were resident in west Cumbria at the time of the birth (area controls), or whose mothers were resident in the same civil parish as the case (local controls). Some controls fell into both groups. Controls who had died or who were not resident in west Cumbria at the date of diagnosis of the matched case were subsequently excluded.

As all known cases in a defined time period were included in the study it was appropriate to conduct a "population based" case-control study and, for this purpose, the method of selecting controls and for excluding some of them, as described in the papers and summarised above, was appropriate.

The cases eligible for inclusion in analyses consisted of 52 with leuk-

TABLE I—*Success rates for obtained risk factor and related data from various sources*

	Cases	Controls	p Value
Antenatal data obtained from obstetric records	35/97 (36%)	446/1001 (45%)	0·13
Completed questionnaire obtained from parents/No for whom blank questionnaire was sent to GP to be forwarded to parents	64/86 (74%)	403/727 (55%)	0·001
Completed questionnaire obtained from parents to whom GP sent a questionnaire	64/76 (84%)	403/654 (62%)	<0·001
Birth certificates (father's occupation)	91/97 (94%)	969/1001 (97%)	0·21
Birth date of father (for matching with name and initials to Sellafield records)	88/97 (91%)	906/1001 (91%)	0·91

aemia, 22 with non-Hodgkin's lymphoma, and 23 with Hodgkin's disease. For these cases there were 1001 controls remaining after exclusions, of whom 248 served as both area and local controls.

Attempts were made to obtain data for cases and controls on possible risk factors from various sources, including obstetric records, birth certificates, questionnaires to the mother or father, and from Sellafield employment records.

The success rates using these various sources varied (see table I). Father's occupation was recorded on most birth certificates but obstetric notes were located for only about 40% of cases and controls. Attempts were made to obtain questionnaire responses from parents by asking general practitioners to forward the questionnaires to them. This was not done if both parents were known to be dead, and no attempt was made to contact the parents of controls if the parents of the matched case were known to be dead. Blank questionnaires were sent to general practitioners for 86 cases and 727 controls. Of the questionnaires sent to the general practitioners to forward, completed questionnaires were obtained from 74% of the parents of cases but only 55% of the parents of controls. General practitioners actually sent questionnaires to the parents of 76 cases and 654 controls, and completed questionnaires were returned from 84% of those sent to the parents of cases and from 62% of those sent to the parents of controls. The differences are highly significant but this is not an unexpected finding in such a study (as it is a general finding that the parents of a child with a serious disease are more likely to respond than those with a healthy child). This could have been a potentially serious source of bias had any important differences emerged between cases and controls based on the questionnaire data. There would have been similar concerns about comparisons based on the obstetric notes, not because of differences in the success rates in

233

obtaining these notes for case and controls, but because the notes were obtained only for the minority of cases and controls. Information on the occupation of the father, recorded on the birth certificates of cases and controls, was obtained for most children and information on the parental date of birth (necessary for linkage with Sellafield employment and radiation records) was obtained for 91% of cases and the same percentage of controls.

Before considering the results of the study it is perhaps worth discussing what the results of the study might have been predicted to be at its outset, based on knowledge of the epidemiology of leukaemia and on experience in conducting case-control studies of a similar kind.

Firstly, it was clear that it would be a difficult study to conduct. Inclusion of cases diagnosed over a 36 year period meant that information would have to be sought on events and exposures that occurred, in many instances, 20 or more years previously, in some cases about persons who will have died many years ago. It would be expected, therefore, that it would be difficult both to trace obstetric notes (in the circumstances 40% seems to be a creditable achievement) and to achieve a high level of success in tracing parents and getting them to complete a questionnaire.

Secondly, a study including about 50 cases of leukaemia and 20 each of non-Hodgkin's and Hodgkin's lymphoma would be unlikely to detect any risk factors as statistically significant unless their association with disease was very much stronger than any currently known associations for these cancers. For example, although a positive association was found with in utero x rays, this was far from statistically significant and it would not have been surprising to find a relative risk less than unity due to chance even if the true relative risk was in the range 1·5–2·0.

Thirdly, it is important to bear in mind the observation that prompted the investigation—that is, an unusually high incidence of leukaemia in the village of Seascale next to the Sellafield plant during the study period. It would be expected, therefore, that in the case-control study comparison of cases with area controls would indicate a relatively high risk of leukaemia in the immediate vicinity of Sellafield. Furthermore, as those who live near to Sellafield are probably more likely to work in the plant than those who live further away, it would not be surprising if there was an association found with employment at Sellafield. Both of these findings were apparent in the case-control study. The analyses on distances away from Sellafield at which cases and controls were born indicated an excess risk within 5 km but no convincing gradient in risk at greater distances. Also, a significant excess of cases of leukaemia whose fathers worked at Sellafield was found in comparison to the "area" controls. Selecting "local" controls would have been expected to remove the confounding effect of residence close to Sellafield on assessing the effect of employment at the plant. Using local controls did reduce the relative risk associated with employment at

Sellafield from 2·8 to 2·0, the latter number being not significantly different from unity, but some association remained.

Thus some of the findings that would have been predicted for the case-control study were, in fact, observed. Furthermore, no convincing evidence was found of an increased risk associated with several postulated risk factors, including playing on beaches, eating fish or shellfish, growing own vegetables, or using seaweed as fertiliser, but the confidence limits on the relative risks associated with many of those factors were wide (because of the small number of cases included in the study).

The success rates in obtaining obstetric notes were low (36% for cases and 45% for controls) and completed questionnaires were obtained for only about 60% of all surviving parents, with a higher percentage for the parents of cases (74%) than of controls (55%). Although these success rates were probably as high as it would be reasonable to expect in a study including cases diagnosed over such a long period (36 years), by conventional standards they would be judged as unsatisfactory in a case-control study to assess risk factors for disease. In any such study in which risk factor information is not obtained from the great majority of cases and controls, there is concern that the information obtained on possible risk factors may not be representative of that for all cases and controls. Furthermore, the comparison of information from cases and controls may be subject to bias if different factors influence the probability of obtaining risk factor data for cases and for controls, and this is of special concern if the success in obtaining information is different for cases and controls, as was so for the questionnaires to parents. Thus, even if statistically significant associations had been found using the data derived from obstetric notes or from questionnaires to parents, there would have been considerable difficulties of interpretation. Non-significant findings are also difficult to interpret, both for the reasons just discussed and because of the wide confidence intervals on many of the risk estimates given. These deficiencies were acknowledged by the authors.

The data on risk factors which are least susceptible to bias are those which have been obtained for a high proportion of cases and controls and which are "objective" (that is, do not depend on the recall of individuals). The occupational data from birth certificates and the information from the linkage of parental names to the Sellafield employment and radiation records are in this category and it is from the analyses of these data that the most interesting and important results are derived, especially from the comparison of the names of case and control fathers with the Sellafield records. This aspect of the study is much less susceptible to criticism than aspects related to comparisons of obstetric records or questionnaire data for which the ascertainment of information was incomplete and, in some instances, contradictory (for example, different information from clinical notes than from questionnaire responses with respect to in utero x rays).

TABLE II—*Preconceptual radiation doses of case and control fathers who had ever been exposed to external radiation at Sellafield*

	Fathers of:		
Total dose before conception	Leukaemia cases	Local controls	Area controls
1–49 mSv	3	26	19
50–99 mSv	1	11	11
> 100 mSv	4	3	5

χ^2 Test for trend; 5·92 (p = 0·015) 2·78 (p = 0·10).
(This test is not strictly valid but should give a reasonable indication of significance.)

We know from the study on the mortality of Sellafield workers that there exists a near complete list of all those who have ever worked at the plant. Furthermore, as identification information on case and control fathers was supplied in identical format for computer matching with Sellafield records it is very unlikely that any systematic bias could have occurred.

The findings derived from information on paternal occupation extracted from birth certificates show increased risks of leukaemia associated with employment at Sellafield (relative risk = 2·0), in iron and steel (2·4), in farming (2·6) and in chemical (1·6) industries (based on a comparison of cases with local controls, which I consider most appropriate for the reasons outlined above). None of these relative risks are significantly in excess of unity but that for employment in the iron and steel industry becomes so if leukaemia and non-Hodgkin's are considered together (relative risk = 3·2; 95% confidence limits 1·2 to 8·3). These findings are compatible with the children of workers at Sellafield, and those in several other industries, being at increased risk of leukaemia but do not provide strong evidence for or against such an hypothesis.

Most convincing evidence that employment at Sellafield is associated with a raised risk of leukaemia in the children of workers is provided by the linkage of case and control fathers to the Sellafield employment and radiation records. These analyses showed that the fathers of cases who had worked at Sellafield had accumulated higher external radiation doses before the conception of the affected child than had the fathers of controls for the corresponding period. The differences between case and control fathers in this respect were highly significant. Even if the analyses are restricted to those who had been recorded as ever having had a "positive" external radiation dose, despite the small number of cases (eight), there is a marked difference in the exposure histories between cases and controls (see table II). (For this comparison it might be argued that both area and local controls would be equally appropriate as the analysis is conditional on working at the plant.) There is a similar difference between cases and controls in the distribution of radiation doses estimated to have been accumulated in the six months before conception, though it appears there may be quite a high correlation between the doses accumulated in this shorter period and those accumulated in the entire period before conception, which makes it impossible to sort out in this small dataset which is the most relevant exposure period (and this is clearly an issue of considerable importance with respect both to possible biological mechanisms and to issues of radiation protection).

How should these findings be interpreted? A large number of different possible risk factors were examined and thus it might be expected that some correlations might be found that would be "statistically significant" by chance alone. This is a possible explanation for the association found with external radiation dose. Further analysis of the existing dataset is unlikely, however, to enable such an explanation to be either substantiated or refuted. There is an urgent need for further evidence derived from studies of other groups of men who have been exposed to radiation before conceiving a child. The children of men exposed to the atomic bomb explosions in Japan show no excess risk of cancer but there do not appear to be many other relevant studies. Further information should be provided by the ongoing case-control studies of children with cancer around other nuclear sites. It will be important to identify other potentially informative groups. Among these might be the children of patients cured by radiotherapy for malignant disease (for example, Hodgkin's disease) and of other groups of workers occupationally exposed to radiation (for example, radiologists). The Department of Health has also solicited for studies of the children of nuclear workers, and these should be a priority, but careful planning is essential as there will be substantial overlap with ongoing work (such as the case-control investigation already conducted in west Cumbria). Until there is confirmatory evidence of the association represented by Gardner *et al* I think it likely that many scientists may keep an open mind on the causal nature of the association reported. In terms of radiation protection it would be prudent to assume the association is causal unless greater evidence accumulates against such an hypothesis.

Prior to the Gardner *et al* study there was not much evidence to suggest a preconceptual oncogenic effect for exposure to radiation. Workers exposed to relatively high external radiation doses may also have unusual exposures to other agents (for example, internal radiation or chemicals). Further information on the cases and controls employed at Sellafield in these respects may assist in the interpretation of the observations in the paper and Dr Gardner might be encouraged to explore the possibility of such an extension to the study. Also, the method used to estimate radiation exposure in the six months prior to conception was cruder that it could have been, because only cumulated *annual* exposure data was used in the analyses, and it would be worthwhile to analyse the data again using the more accurate dose estimates that could be made available by BFNL.

In summary, the study of Gardner *et al* appears to have been well planned, well executed, and well analysed. There are several aspects of the study that are unsatisfactory, as might have been expected in an investigation including cases diagnosed over a 36 year period. These relate to the relatively low proportions of cases and controls for which it was possible to obtain obstetric notes and interview data from parents. However, the comparison of Sellafield radiation histories between cases and controls is not subject to these criticisms, and the association of leukaemia risk with accumulated radiation exposure before conception is an important finding which may indicate a cause-effect relation. The data presented are consistent with such an interpretation but other explanations are possible. It may have been a chance association, though the significance level is quite strong. Evidence for or against this is likely to be provided by independent studies on other groups.

28: Childhood cancer and nuclear installations

Eighth Duncan Memorial Lecture
University of Liverpool, 1990

M J GARDNER

Dr William Henry Duncan was the first man in the country to be given the title of medical officer of health and Liverpool was the first city to have such a post. Dr Duncan was of course a remarkable man and the fact of his appointment as medical officer of health was a realisation of much that he had done before that date in 1847 to consider the reasons why the health of some people living in Liverpool was less satisfactory than others.

The first Duncan memorial lecturer seven years ago in 1983 was the late Dr Sidney Chave and he described very adeptly in his lecture the life and activities of Dr Duncan—I would suggest that it is recommended reading for anybody who has not yet read it.[1] One of the subsequent lectures was given by Sir George Godber, a former chief medical officer, and he traced the history of medical officers of health from the time of Duncan onwards.[2] Another more recent Duncan memorial lecture was given by the present chief medical officer, Sir Donald Acheson, who examined the state of public health in this country.[3] My topic is somewhat narrower than either of these but addresses a problem that has emerged in the past few years and which has been the cause of some anxiety and much activity. My plan is to try to describe the picture to you and put the current view in some perspective.

However, I thought that I would start off by staying with the time of Duncan for a short while. Soon after Dr Duncan became medical officer of health for Liverpool in 1847, it became a legal requirement that each death in this country had to be registered and for the cause of death to be certified—this took place in 1850. One of the things that emerged as a consequence was the ability to look at public health on a geographical basis around the country in a way that had not been possible before, and in the 1870s there became available maps for England and Wales showing the picture of fatal disease by area.

Cancer in the 1850s

The first maps that I know of were produced by a surgeon at St Bartholomew's Hospital in London called Alfred Haviland and, to consider one example, he produced a map of mortality from cancer of all types in women for the years 1851–60.[4] The general picture that he commented on was of lower cancer death rates in the west of the country with higher rates in the east. His explanations for these differences were nearly all in terms of geophysical factors. He mentioned, for example, that on the west side of the country there are elevated hilly and mountainous areas, with geologically old formations of hard rock, which are well drained by rivers flowing down to the sea. On the east side of the country, however, the landscape is different. It is low lying, with more recent geological formations of chalk and other soft rock, where the rivers tend to flow in valleys and flood.

To quote from Haviland's text, he commented that: "The maps teach us that the high, dry sites on the older rocks are the places where cancer does not thrive, and that it does thrive in the vales by the sides of large rivers which overflow their banks, and in the neighbourhood of which are to be found the drifts of ages of washing from the inhabited country above. When there is a tendency to cancer let the patient be removed to the high dry sites; and perchance if whole families were thus to emigrate, we should not hear so much of the hereditary character of this and many other diseases." This paragraph is just a short abstract from a remarkable book. The point that comes over is that almost his total explanation of the geographical distribution of cancer was in relation to the geophysical environment. However, as you will have noticed, Haviland was also thinking ahead from causation to prevention, through the idea of moving people to the areas with low rates from those with high cancer mortality. Appropriately, in the context of the Duncan lecture, Haviland was also one of the first medical officers of health—for Northamptonshire, Leicestershire, Rutland, and Buckinghamshire.

It is interesting to reflect that in 1875, when writing the text, Haviland remarked that he thought it worthwhile to produce a map of cancer for women, but not for men, because the number of deaths from cancer among men was far fewer than among women. During the 1850s, in fact, the number of cancer deaths among women was about three times that among men. Of course, the sex ratio has reversed since then—not to the same degree—so that cancer death rates are now higher in men than women. There are two main reasons why this change has happened. First, ever since 1850, the principal cancer in women has remained cancer of the breast. This dominated the cancers that were diagnosed during 1851–60, and is why cancer mortality was higher in women than men. Secondly, the fact that cancer death rates in men are now higher than in women is because they are dominated by cigarette related lung cancer cases. Without these the death rates from cancer in women would still be 25% higher than in men. It is an interesting change that has taken place over a period of just over 100 years, from cancer reporting being far more common among women to cancer being slightly more common among men.

Cancer in the 1970s

As far as the Merseyside area goes, cancer rates in women in the 1850s were among the lowest in the country. Has the pattern changed since then? A more recent map gave cancer death rates among women during 1968–78 by local authority areas such as county boroughs and rural districts, and showed that areas with high cancer death rates and those with low cancer death rates were spread around the country.[5] However, Merseyside had rates during the 1970s that were among the highest in the country. In particular, the overall cancer rates in Liverpool and surrounding areas were some 10–30% above the national average. Why is this? What has changed? Well, to consider specifically first cancer of the breast, rates are low in this part of the country and the high rates are, just as they were in Haviland's days, mainly in the southern and eastern parts of the country. Thus it does not seem that the geographical distribution of breast cancer has changed much at all in over 100 years' time span. In fact, the Merseyside area as a whole had a death rate from breast cancer some 10% below the national average during the 1970s. So why is overall cancer high now among local women if breast cancer is low? The answer is because of high lung cancer rates, which are concentrated very much in London and its surrounding areas but also on Merseyside and Tyneside in particular. Specifically, lung cancer rates during the 1970s among women in this area were as much as 50% above the national figure—in Liverpool itself exactly 50% above the average for England and Wales. It is, of course, well known that this area also has one of the highest lung cancer rates among men. As part of the World Health Organisation's "Healthy Cities" project there is a major move to remedy this situation.

Cholera and disease clusters

I want to stay with historical maps for a moment and consider a map of a different kind that was partially responsible for the discovery of the cause and prevention of one of the diseases that ravaged the country during the time of Duncan. In the Soho area of London during the month of August 1854—seven years after Dr Duncan had been installed as medical officer of health for Liverpool—there was a cholera epidemic that has been described as the most terrible outbreak which ever occurred in this kingdom. An anaesthetist called Dr John Snow, who lived about half a mile from this area, had already taken an interest in why, where, and which people cholera struck.[6] His suspicions quickly fell on a well in Broad Street, and were strengthened when he discovered that "nearly all the deaths had taken place within a short distance of the pump". He soon established that almost all the people who had died in this particular epidemic had consumed water from the same pump. As a consequence of Snow's enquiry the pump handle was removed to stop any further people drinking water from that particular source. This was one of the first important observations which led finally to proof that cholera was a waterborne disease and, among other things, led to the sanitary revolution that later followed. So this was a success story of a cluster of disease being observed, the source being identified, and later leading to the elucidation of the cause and subsequent prevention of this illness.

I have discussed this bit of medical history, contemporary with Duncan's time as Liverpool's medical officer of health, because the issue as to whether clusters can lead to the elucidation of new causes of disease is still one which is the subject of much discussion and debate. One does not have to listen too hard or often to hear allegations that some disease or other is being produced in the area of a source of contamination of some nature—for example, around an incinerator, a toxic waste dump, a polluted river, or, in the case of what I want to talk about now, around a nuclear installation.

Childhood leukaemia around Sellafield

There are a number of nuclear installations within the United Kingdom, including research establishments, power generating stations, and waste reprocessing centres. In particular Windscale and Calder Hall, collectively known as Sellafield, is on the west coast of Cumbria just under 100 miles to the north of Liverpool. My own involvement with this subject started towards the end of 1983 when the Yorkshire Television programme called *Windscale: the Nuclear Laundry* was screened. The television producer approached the management of Sellafield with a request for their cooperation in producing a documentary on the health of the radiation workforce at Sellafield, to be told that there were no definite indications of any long term ill health effects of radiation exposure on their workers—which was justified and in accord with both a study that had been carried out by the company itself[7 8] and also one independently.[9] However, while in the area negotiating for the programme the producer heard incidentally of some cases of childhood leukaemia near the installation, and decided to switch the thrust of his programme to describing and discussing these childhood leukaemia cases. He finally presented a programme that suggested that there was a cluster of childhood leukaemia cases in the area near Sellafield—in particular the village of Seascale, some three kilometres to the south—and alleged that these cases were linked to the discharges of radioactive liquids from the plant to the Irish Sea, which subsequently polluted the beaches, fish, and seafood. The government set up an independent inquiry under the Chairmanship of Sir Douglas Black to investigate the suggestion and allegation. I was asked to be a member of this team, not because of any detailed knowledge of childhood leukaemia or radiation biology but because of the work on cancer mapping which we were then undertaking.

Is there an excess?

A major question is: how to tackle such an allegation? Because this has become a fairly common occurrence there are now emerging quite clear guidelines for how to go about such an investigation—and a lot of these owe much to the methods of John Snow back in the 1850s. One of the first things that needs to be done is to investigate the cases that are alleged to have occurred and to confirm that they exist in medical records—either hospital or cancer registration records—or on death certificates. If the cases are not genuine and not known to the medical profession then the allegation can effectively be discounted at that stage. On the other hand, as in this instance, if the cases are shown to be genuine then the investigation needs to go further. One of the next questions needs to be "is there an excess?", given that the cases suggested have been confirmed. In this situation the question was addressed by carrying out geographical studies of childhood cancer in districts in the neighbourhood of Sellafield and other parts of the country.

The location of Sellafield is on the coast of west Cumbria with the village

243

of Seascale some three kilometres to the south. Sellafield is in what was called the rural district of Ennerdale and Seascale in the rural district of Millom—in what follows I will consider some statistics for these areas.[10] Deaths from leukaemia under 25 years of age during 1968–78 in Ennerdale were very much the same as expected on the basis of the size and age distribution of its population considering the rates for leukaemia in England and Wales as a whole. However, in Millom there were six deaths compared with 1·4 expected, an excess of just over fourfold.

Dr Alan Craft and his colleagues from Newcastle looked at childhood leukaemia in the 675 electoral wards of the Northern region for which they had cancer registration details in under 15 year olds for the years 1968–1982. Among these 675 electoral wards there were 19 that were statistically considered to have raised rates. Seascale was one of these and in a direct statistical sense could be considered to have the most extreme rate of childhood leukaemia among all the 675 wards.

It is helpful to try to put the fourfold excess that was found in Millom rural district into context by comparing it with the other 151 rural districts around England and Wales of similar population size. It was not, in fact, the most extreme as one other rural district had a slightly higher excess, but the fact that it was very near the top did indicate that the rate in that area was at least somewhat unusual. As a consequence of this evidence the conclusion of the Black report was that the suggestion of the Yorkshire Television programme could not be rejected. There did seem to be an excess of childhood leukaemia in this area around Sellafield although it was based on a small number of cases and seemed to be particularly focused in the village of Seascale.

Why is there an excess?

This then leads on to the question: "what is the suggested cause of the excess?" I have already mentioned that the Yorkshire Television programme suggested that it was related to the level of radioactive discharges from Windscale. The liquid discharges from Windscale have been substantially greater than those from any other nuclear establishment in Britain, and this is also true for airborne discharges.

The next question has to be: "is the suggestion plausible?" It is worth looking at the evidence that suggests there is a causal relation between exposure to ionising radiation and some cancers.[11] First of all, as examples among occupationally exposed groups of workers, it is accepted that leukaemia was caused among early radiologists, that uranium miners inhaling radon gas have had up to a fivefold increase of lung cancer, and that workers who painted luminous dials on watches, using paint containing radium isotopes, developed bone cancers. It is also known that leukaemia and other cancers developed among survivors of the atomic bombs that were dropped on Hiroshima and Nagasaki during the second world war with the leukaemias following relatively soon after the bomb and the other cancers somewhat later. As well it is clear that some patients who have had x rays or radiotherapy have subsequently developed cancers. Examples include women developing breast cancer after x ray of the chest as treatment for pulmonary tuberculosis, leukaemia among patients given radiation therapy for ankylosing spondylitis, and leukaemia again among patients with cervical cancer also treated by radiotherapy. Additionally, it is now generally accepted that antenatal x rays of the abdomen of pregnant mothers can produce about a 50% excess risk among their children of developing leukaemia after birth. This final example is clearly a relevant one in the context of the problem being discussed. So the plausibility of the excess of childhood leukaemia in Seascale being related to radiation at Sellafield cannot be totally rejected, as we know that radiation figures quite high on the list of candidates for causing cancer—leukaemia in particular.

Other nuclear sites

One of the next obvious questions is to ask: "what about near other nuclear sites?" Thus it is sensible to look at childhood leukaemia and cancer around other nuclear installations in this country.[12] First, let us consider the Scottish sites for the reason that they include Dounreay, which is the only other nuclear waste reprocessing site, apart from Sellafield, in Britain. Part of the evidence produced by the Scottish group researching this problem showed that during the years 1968–84 there were five cases of leukaemia under age 25 years within 12·5 kilometres of Dounreay compared with about 1·5 expected. Thus, as for Sellafield, there was an excess—although it was smaller if a 25 kilometre radius was used instead of 12·5—but apparent excesses around Hunterston and Chapel Cross were much smaller. In England and Wales during 1961–80 leukaemia registrations, again under age 25 years, were found to be somewhat higher in areas near the nuclear installations contrasted with control areas that were taken for comparison. The installation areas were higher than the control areas, apart from Sellafield, by a figure of between 10% and 20%. As a final example consider the figures for leukaemia and also other cancers in areas around Aldermaston, Burghfield, and Harwell, which are nuclear installations that have specifically been looked at by a research group based in Oxford. There appears to be a 64% increase in leukaemia among under 5 year olds in a 10 kilometre radius around these installations compared with further away, and also an apparent 24% increase in other cancers within the 10 kilometre radius. Thus I think it is possible to make a general statement that there does appear to have been an excess of childhood leukaemia around nuclear installations in the UK, although apart from at Sellafield and Dounreay the excess is relatively small.

Seascale cohort study

I would now like to discuss in further detail the next steps that can be taken in investigating such a cluster by reference to what has taken place around Sellafield. One of the further studies that was recommended by the Black report and which has now been completed was a cohort study. This was essentially a study of all the children who were born or attended schools in Seascale during 1950–83, which at the time of study covered most of the period of operation of the Sellafield plant. Using access to local birth registers we identified just over 1000 children who had been born in the village during these years, and with access to school registers through the local Cumbria education committee and headmistresses of the schools we were able to identify just over 1500 other children who had been born since 1950 and moved into Seascale subsequently to attend one of the three schools up to 1984. It was found that cases of leukaemia had occurred only among children born in the village with none occurring in children who moved in after birth. For other cancers there was no suggestion of any excess among the schoolchildren but a slight suggestion of a possible raised number among those born in the village. Our conclusion at this time was that there was a genuine excess of childhood leukaemia in Seascale and if there was a genuine local factor causing this excess then it appeared to operate either very early in life or before birth.[13 14] The next step, having established that an excess exists—and the cohort study was carried out partly because of potential deficiencies in geographical analysis—is to look at individual factors on these cases to assess whether or not any can be established that help to explain why they have occurred.

West Cumbria case-control study

This can be done by a case-control study, in which children with a disease are compared with healthy children who have not developed the illness. So we carried out such a case-control study that had very specific objectives, which were to examine whether or not the excess was related to the causal factor that I have already mentioned, that is prenatal abdominal x ray of the mother; whether it is related to suggested risk factors for childhood leukaemia such as viral infections or social class; or whether it is related to exposure to radiation as a result of the Sellafield nuclear site either, firstly, through habits which potentially enhance exposure to the radioactive discharges to sea such as playing on the beach or eating fresh fish or shellfish or, secondly, whether exposure to radiation through working at the plant is relevant. To carry out this study we ascertained all the case children with leukaemia and lymphoma (both non-Hodgkin's lymphoma and Hodgkin's disease) who had been born and diagnosed in west Cumbria during the years 1950–85 and diagnosed aged under 25. We then identified, from the same birth registers as where the cases had been entered, control children of the same sex and roughly the same date of birth and who had either been born in any town within the birth registration district or had more specifically been born in the same village or town as the case to whom they were matched.

Without going into all the details of the results of this study,[15][16] I can say that we found similar risks for prenatal x rays to those identified earlier, no important risks in relation to the suggested risk factors that I mentioned, and no apparent risks in relation to exposure to radiation through the discharges. However, we did find that, among the five cases of childhood leukaemia in Seascale, the four fathers whom we fully identified and obtained radiation records for had higher exposures before their child's conception than the fathers of the comparison children who were also born in Seascale. This led to the suggestion that in some way the father's exposure to radiation during his employment at Sellafield before the conception of his child may be relevant to the subsequent development of leukaemia. When we looked at the results for non-Hodgkin's lymphoma, which were based on fewer cases, the findings were not dissimilar to those for leukaemia whereas for Hodgkin's disease, which has never been associated with ionising radiation in medical publications, there was no relation to father's employment at Sellafield as a radiation worker. At this stage we feel that the perspective has changed from that of a suggested childhood leukaemia excess in Seascale which is possibly related to environmental radiation contamination, as proposed by the Yorkshire Television programme, to a confirmed childhood leukaemia excess in the village which is statistically related to father's occupational radiation exposure during his work at Sellafield before the child's conception.

Lowering exposures to radiation

This finding clearly needs, and is receiving, more attention and detail to try to understand whether it is caused by radiation and if so quite how it might operate. In the meantime it is appropriate to consider, as did Haviland and Snow—and indeed Duncan—last century, the issue of what if anything should be done to lead to "prevention". I think that this can be taken in two steps. Firstly, if our results are confirmed then I think we can make a general statement that there would not seem to be a major public health problem in relation to the radiation contamination of the environment that has undoubtedly taken place. This is a minimal statement and it is not in any way meant to imply that contamination therefore is not important. Secondly, the comment can be made that the problem would seem to be one of taking preventive measures among the workforce if anywhere.

So what has happened over the years in terms of radiation exposure levels of the workers and discharges at Sellafield? Average yearly radiation doses among workers at Sellafield were at their highest during the 1950s and have decreased since then through the 1970s and 1980s. So worker exposure to radiation has been declining. Average yearly radioactive liquid discharges to the Irish Sea from Sellafield were relatively low until the early 1970s, when they peaked, and have declined during the 1980s. So again, as for worker exposure, discharges to the sea have declined and are continuing to do so.

What else can be done? As a consequence of our case-control study there has been discussion at British Nuclear Fuels about how radiation exposures of workers can be even further reduced, in particular now among those who are contemplating having children. This has resulted in dose reduction working groups, with representatives of various sections of the workforce and management, aimed at reducing exposure throughout the plant as much as is possible without jeopardising the work environment. In addition, contour maps for each part of the plant have been and are being produced which show the dose rate of ionising radiation that applies to each area in which workers may find themselves operating. Thus there are certainly intentions to lower the exposure levels to as low as reasonably achievable within the context of appropriate working practices.

Summary

So where are we now? I think the first thing to say is that there is a well established excess around Sellafield of childhood leukaemia, although excesses around other nuclear sites are of a lower magnitude. The excess near Sellafield is strongly associated with fathers having high exposure to external whole-body penetrating radiation while working at the installation before their child's conception. But is this association pointing towards a causal mechanism? One possibility is genetic damage, but most geneticists and radiobiologists would consider that the levels of occupational exposure, even at Sellafield, are too low for this to be a plausible pathway on current knowledge. This is based to some extent on the lack of any similar effect among children born subsequently to Japanese survivors of the atomic bombs—however, the scenario is somewhat different, contrasting a high short term exposure with a lower long term exposure. As well, some workers at Sellafield will also be exposed to radionuclides, such as plutonium, which we have not yet been able to analyse for. In addition, there are other exposures in a complex environment, which may or may not be relevant. One experimental study in the laboratory using animals supports the idea that a pathway through irradiation of the parents is plausible, although this one result needs replication.[17] Other causes have been suggested for the excess childhood leukaemia levels in particular around nuclear establishments—these include population movement,[18] implicating viruses that have long been considered to be associated with childhood leukaemia, high rates in isolated communities,[19] and also selection of areas for nuclear sites that have a natural propensity to high rates.[10]

Geographical studies have now been carried out in some other countries, such as France[21] and the United States,[22] where excesses like those seen around nuclear establishments in the UK have not been observed. It may be that they genuinely do not occur but it is also possible that the geographical areas used, particularly in the United States, are too large to identify any localised effect. A similar study in Canada is less negative and is currently being extended in its coverage. There are currently two other case-control studies in the United Kingdom under way and nearing completion. The first of these is around Dounreay, the other nuclear waste reprocessing site, and the other is around the Aldermaston and Burghfield installations. The results of these studies will be of interest, of course, but how much they can be considered to be reproductions of the circumstances at Sellafield is less clear. As well, there are preliminary plans to do detailed studies around several of the oldest nuclear installations in the United States and France.

Finally, I would mention that there are advanced intentions to carry out two major studies in an attempt to take the position further. One of these is to do a follow up study of all the children, maybe also grandchildren, of radiation workers at Sellafield both past and present—this will give a much wider coverage than the studies that we have been able to carry out thus far. Secondly, there is a proposal to look for cases of cancer among children of all registered radiation workers in the UK regardless of their place of employment. By the nature of this kind of work these studies will take three or more years to complete, but they will both be part of exploring further the linkage of the various pieces of this jigsaw.

I would like to express my appreciation at being invited to be the Duncan Memorial Lecturer for 1990.

1 Chave S. Duncan of Liverpool—and some lessons for today. *Community Med* 1984;6:61–71.
3 Godber GE. Medical officers of health and health services. *Community Med* 1986;8:1–14.
3 Acheson ED. On the state of the public health. *Public Health* 1988;5:431–8.
4 Haviland A. *The geographical distribution of heart disease and dropsy, cancer in females and phthisis in females in England and Wales.* London: Smith Elder & Co, 1875.
5 Gardner MJ, Winter PD, Taylor CP, Acheson ED. *Atlas of cancer mortality in England and Wales, 1968–1978.* Chichester: Wiley, 1983.

6 Snow J. *On the mode of communication of cholera.* New York: The Commonwealth Fund, 1855. (2nd ed. reprinted 1936, with Appendix of 1856).

7 Clough EA. The BNFL radiation-mortality study. *Journal of the Society for Radiological Protection* 1983;3(1):24–7.

8 Clough EA. Further report on the BNFL radiation-mortality study. *Journal of the Society for Radiological Protection* 1983;3(3):18–20.

9 Smith PG, Douglas AJ. Mortality of workers at the Sellafield plant of British Nuclear Fuels. *BMJ* 1986;293:845–54.

10 Black D for the Independent Advisory Group. *Investigation of the possible increased incidence of cancer in west Cumbria.* London: HMSO, 1984. (Black report.)

11 Boice JD, Land CE. Ionising radiation. In: Schottenfeld D, Fraumeni JF, eds. *Cancer epidemiology and prevention.* Philadelphia: Saunders, 1982:231–53.

12 Gardner MJ. Review of reported increases of childhood cancer rates in the vicinity of nuclear installations in the UK. *Journal of the Royal Statistical Society [Series A, Statistics in Society]* 1989;152:307–25.

13 Gardner MJ, Hall AJ, Downes S, Terrell JD. A follow up study of children born to mothers resident in Seascale, west Cumbria (birth cohort). *BMJ* 1987;295:822–7.

14 Gardner MJ, Hall AJ, Downes S, Terrell JD. A follow up study of children born elsewhere but attending schools in Seascale, west Cumbria (schools cohort). *BMJ* 1987;295:819–22.

15 Gardner MJ, Hall AJ, Snee MP, Downes S, Powell CA, Terrell JD. Methods and basic data of case-control study of leukaemia and lymphoma among young people near Sellafield nuclear plant in west Cumbria. *BMJ* 1990;300:429–34.

16 Gardner MJ, Snee MP, Hall AJ, Powell CA, Downes S, Terrell JD. Results of case-control study of leukaemia and lymphoma among young people near Sellafield nuclear plant in west Cumbria. *Br Med J* 1990;300:423–9.

17 Nomura T. Parental exposure to X-rays and chemicals induces heritable tumours and anomalies in mice. *Nature* 1982;296:575–7.

18 Kinlen LJ, Clarke K, Hudson C. Evidence from population mixing in British new towns 1946–85 of an infective basis for childhood leukaemia. *Medical Science* 1990;336:577–82.

19 Alexander FE, Ricketts TJ, McKinney PA, Cartwright RA. Community lifestyle characteristics and risk of acute lymphoblastic leukaemia in children. *Lancet* 1990;336:1461–5.

20 Cook-Mozaffari P, Darby SC, Doll R. Cancer near potential sites of nuclear installations. *Lancet* 1989;ii:1145–7.

21 Hill C, Laplanche A. Overall mortality and cancer mortality around French nuclear sites. *Nature* 1990;347:755–7.

22 Jablon S, Hrubec Z, Boice JD, Stone BJ. *Cancer in populations living near nuclear facilities.* Volumes I, II and III. Washington: National Institutes of Health, 1990. (NIH Publication No 90–874.)

29: Fathers' occupational exposure to radiation and the raised level of childhood leukaemia near the Sellafield nuclear plant

MARTIN J GARDNER

The first indications that childhood leukaemia rates could be high near the Sellafield nuclear plant in west Cumbria, England, came from largely anecdotal evidence in a television programme *Windscale: the Nuclear Laundry* shown during 1983. During subsequent years, various epidemiological studies have investigated the claim in more detail. Geographical analyses of childhood leukaemia incidence in the northern region and mortality in England and Wales using routinely available data made the first contribution. As a result, it was confirmed that leukaemia rates in the area, particularly the neighbouring village of Seascale, were high compared with other districts, although not totally extreme.

Cohort studies of children born in Seascale or attending schools in Seascale were carried out to resolve some of the difficulties of interpretation of geographical analysis. Cohort studies indicated that the excess of leukaemia was concentrated among children born in Seascale and was not found among those moving in after birth and suggested that any causal factors may be acting before birth or very early in life. A case-control study of leukaemia (and lymphoma) among young people in west Cumbria has examined potentially important individual factors in detail. The study showed a relation between the raised incidence of leukaemia in children and fathers' recorded external radiation dose during work at Sellafield before their children's conception. The association can effectively explain statistically the observed geographical excess.

Introduction

Some concern that radioactive emissions from nuclear installations could be a health hazard to local communities had existed for many years, but substantial interest in the United Kingdom was raised only with the airing on national network of the Yorkshire Television documentary, *Windscale: the Nuclear Laundry*, in 1983. The programme had originally intended to discuss the health effects of occupational exposure to radiation on workers in the nuclear industry but was reorientated to the local children when the producer was told by residents in the area near Sellafield (previously named Windscale) of cases of childhood leukaemia and other cancers that seemed to them to occur at an unusually high rate for a rare disease. The suggested excess was said to be concentrated in the village of Seascale, which is on the coast about 3 km south of Sellafield.

Awareness of the scale of radioactive discharges from the nuclear waste reprocessing operation at Sellafield resulted in the possible linkage by the television programme of the childhood cancer cases with environmental contamination from the site. The screening of the programme resulted the following day in an announcement by the British government of an independent inquiry into the allegations to be chaired by Sir Douglas Black. A report was subsequently published.[1]

Geographical studies

Because of the nature of the medical evidence produced by the television programme, one of the first concerns of the Black inquiry was to establish whether the alleged increase in childhood leukaemia could be supported by using routinely available sources (death certificates and cancer registrations). This was examined in two analyses.

Firstly, it was shown (table I) that in Millom rural district (the administrative area containing Seascale) there had been a raised leukaemia mortality rate among persons under 25 years of age during 1968–78 but not during 1959–67, and not in the adjacent area of Ennerdale rural district (containing Sellafield) for either period.[2] These years cover the seventh and eighth revisions of the International Classification of Diseases and are

TABLE I—*Mortality from leukaemia in persons under 25 years of age during 1959–78 in rural districts of England and Wales: Millom and Ennerdale (containing Sellafield area)*

Rural district	1959–67		1968–78	
	Observed	Expected*	Observed	Expected*
Millom	1	1·6	6	1·4
Ennerdale	3	3·3	4	3·3

* At age, sex, and calendar period specific rates for England and Wales.

relevant as Sellafield started operations around 1950. When examined in the context of the 151 other similar rural districts of England and Wales, to adjust for population size and urban or rural status, it was found (table II) that during 1968–78, Millom had the second highest standardised mortality ratio (435). This was second from top, but not extreme,[1] and overall the mortality distribution was not exceptionally different from that expected by chance.

Secondly, data from the children's malignant disease register for the northern region of England and Wales were examined.[3] Cancer registration started for under 15 year olds in 1968, and analyses covered 675 electoral wards for the years 1968–82. Seascale had four cases of lymphoid malignancy compared with 0·25 expected at registration rates for the region overall. This put it third highest in the ranking of registration rates, although in terms of associated Poisson probability (p = 0·0001), it was the most extreme.[1]

These two investigations thus tended to support the allegations of the television programme in terms of a raised childhood leukaemia rate near the nuclear plant, although making no contribution to examination of the effects, if any, of radioactive discharges. Geographical analyses of this nature have a number of limitations: for example, the scale of areas used,

TABLE II—*Mortality from leukaemia in persons under 25 years of age during 1959–78 in England and Wales: 152 rural districts similar in size to Millom*

Standardised mortality ratio	Number of rural districts	
	Observed	Predicted*
0–99	78	85·9
100–199	52	48·4
200–299	19	14·6
300–399	1	2·7
400+	2	0·4

* On the basis of the Poisson distribution.

TABLE III—*Leukaemia and other cancer cases during 1950–86 in Seascale birth and school cohorts*

Diagnosis	Cohort	Number of cases	
		Observed	Expected*
Leukaemia	Birth	6	0·6
	Schools	0	0·6
Other cancer	Birth	6	2·2
	Schools	4	3·4

* At age, sex, and calendar period specific rates for England and Wales.

the potential inclusion of cases after only a short residential period and exclusion of cases diagnosed soon after moving away, and the use of census enumerated populations as denominators when high levels of population change are possible. Thus, other epidemiological methods have their place in elucidating further the nature of the observed area excess and were recommended in the Black report.[1]

Cohort studies

Cohort studies have been carried out on, as far as possible, all children born since 1950 who have at some age lived in Seascale village.[45] Their names and other particulars were identified from birth and school registers, and the cohorts comprised 1068 children born in Seascale and 1546 more children who attended schools in Seascale after having been born elsewhere. The records of mortality and cancer registration on these children, including after moving away from Seascale, were obtained by the usual follow up methods incorporating the National Health Service central register.

The findings of these studies confirmed the geographical analyses, indicating a raised level of leukaemia among Seascale children. However, the excess appeared to be concentrated among children born in Seascale in contrast to those attending the local schools (table III). Thus, there was a 10-fold excess for leukaemia and a twofold or threefold excess of other cancers among the births. There was also a suggestion that this excess was found after the children had left Seascale, alsthough the numbers involved are small.[4] The conclusion of these studies suggested that one or more factors may be acting on a locality-specific basis before birth or early in life to produce the contrasting outcomes.

Case-control study

A case-control study has been carried out including all cases of leukaemia

TABLE IV—*Relative risks for childhood leukaemia by father's external ionising radiation dosimetry during employment at Sellafield before child's conception*

Radiation dose, mSv	Cases	Local controls	Odds ratio	95% confidence interval
0	38	236	1	
>0–49	3	26	0·8	0·2 to 3·0
50–99	1	11	0·8	0·1 to 7·7
≥100	4	3	8·4	1·4 to 52·0

and lymphoma diagnosed at under 25 years of age in the West Cumbria District Health Authority area between 1950 and 1985.[67] This area was chosen to include coastal and inland areas where concern had been raised about potential risks from radiation contamination due to discharges from the nuclear plant to sea or air and also to cover the places of residence of the Sellafield workforce.

The aim was to obtain information on individual cases and controls that might help to explain the excesses found in the anecdotal, geographical, and cohort studies. Factors examined included prenatal x ray exposure as the known risk factor for childhood leukaemia; various other suspected risk factors such as viral illnesses, social class, and maternal age; behavioural habits such as eating fresh seafood and playing on the beach that might have enhanced exposure to radionuclides released from Sellafield; and parental occupation and radiation exposure at Sellafield. The control children for the study were taken from the same birth registers into which the cases' births were entered. For each case, two sets of eight controls were identified, taken to be of the same sex and adjacent in date of birth, with one set covering the total birth registration area (area controls) and the other set confined to the same local village where the case was born (local controls).

The identifying details on the parents of the cases and controls were cross linked with the past and present Sellafield workforce file, and, where matches were found, individual external radiation exposure records were obtained from the company (internal radiation exposure data are not yet available). It was in this respect that the most important result was found, although the expected geographical distribution of leukaemia and association with prenatal x rays were also identified.[6]

The relation between accumulated preconceptual external radiation dose of the fathers during their employment and leukaemia in their children is shown in table IV for local controls, where a high relative risk is found for exposures over 100 mSv, albeit based on small numbers. Three of the four case children in this range were born in Seascale, and each of the four fathers had higher radiation doses than all their matched control fathers. Of the remaining three Seascale children with leukaemia shown in table III, the father of one had an accumulated preconceptual radiation dose of 96 mSv and another has not yet been linked to the Sellafield workforce file, whereas the third case child was diagnosed after leaving west Cumbria and hence excluded from this case-control study. Comparable findings were shown for area controls and for estimated external radiation dose during the six months before conception. Data from questionnaires to parents did not suggest any relation of childhood leukaemia to potential sources of enhanced exposure to radionuclides discharged from the nuclear site. Similar results were also found for non-Hodgkin's lymphoma, although the number of cases was smaller, but not for Hodgkin's disease, which is as would be expected for a non-radiation related condition.

Conclusions

Epidemiological methods have been used to examine a media-suggested excess of childhood leukaemia near a nuclear waste reprocessing plant. Geographical, cohort, and case-control studies have contributed to confirming the excess and showing a strong statistical association with father's exposure to external radiation at work in the plant before their child's conception sufficient to explain the excess cases. Thus, what was perceived as possibly an environmental health problem has resolved into what is probably an occupational health matter.

1 Black D for the Independent Advisory Group. *Investigation of the possible increased incidence of cancer in west Cumbria.* London: HMSO, 1984. (Black report.)
2 Gardner MJ, Winter PD. Cancer in Cumberland during 1959–78 with reference to cancer in young people around Windscale. *Lancet* 1984;i:216–7.
3 Craft AW, Openshaw S, Birch J. Apparent cluster of childhood malignancies in northern England. *Lancet* 1984;ii:96–7.
4 Gardner MJ, Hall AJ, Downes S, Terrell JD. Follow up study of children born to mothers resident in Seascale, west Cumbria (birth cohort). *BMJ* 1987;295:822–7.
5 Gardner MJ, Hall AJ, Downes S, Terrell JD. Follow up study of children born elsewhere but attending schools in Seascale, west Cumbria (schools cohort). *BMJ* 1987;295:819–22.
6 Gardner MJ, Snee MP, Hall AJ, Powell CA, Downes S, Terrell JD. Results of the case-control study of leukaemia and lymphoma among young people near Sellafield nuclear plant in west Cumbria. *BMJ* 1990;300:423–9.
7 Gardner MJ, Hall AJ, Snee MP, Downes S, Powell CA, Terrell JD. Methods and basic data of case-control study of leukaemia and lymphoma among young people near Sellafield nuclear plant in west Cumbria. *BMJ* 1990;300:429–34.

30: Case-control study of leukaemia and non-Hodgkin's lymphoma in children in Caithness near the Dounreay nuclear installation

JAMES D URQUHART, ROGER J BLACK,
MICHAEL J MUIRHEAD, LINDA SHARP,
MARGARET MAXWELL, O B EDEN,
DAVID ADAMS JONES

An excess of childhood leukaemia and non-Hodgkin's lymphoma near the Dounreay nuclear installation has been observed. To examine whether the excess is associated with established risk factors, factors related to the installation, or parental occupation in the nuclear industry, a case-control study was undertaken of 12 children aged under 15 living in Caithness local government district and diagnosed during 1970–86 as having leukaemia or non-Hodgkin's lymphoma compared with 55 controls matched for sex, date of birth, and area of residence within Caithness at time of birth. Factors studied included antenatal abdominal x ray examinations, drugs taken and viral infections during pregnancy, father's occupation, father's employment at Dounreay and radiation dose, distance of usual residence from path of microwave beams, preconceptual exposure to non-ionising radiation in the father, and other lifestyle factors.

No raised relative risks were found for prenatal exposure to *x* rays, social class of parents, employment at Dounreay before conception or diagnosis, father's dose of ionising radiation before conception, or child's residence within 50 metres of the path of microwave transmission beams. Results also proved negative for all lifestyle factors except an apparent association with use of beaches within 25 km of Dounreay—though this result was based on small numbers, arose in the context of multiple hypothesis testing, and is certainly vulnerable to possible systematic bias.

It was concluded that the raised incidence of childhood leukaemia and non-Hodgkin's lymphoma around Dounreay cannot be explained by paternal occupation at the installation or by paternal exposure to external ionising radiation before conception. The observation of an apparent association between the use of beaches around Dounreay and the development of childhood leukaemia and non-Hodgkin's lymphoma might be an artefact of multiple testing and influenced by recall bias.

Introduction

In 1988 the Committee on the Medical Aspects of Radiation in the Environment (COMARE) published the report of its investigation into the incidence of leukaemia and non-Hodgkin's lymphoma in young people in the area around the Dounreay nuclear installation in Caithness during 1968–84.[1] The committee concluded that the apparent excess incidence within the area 25 km from the plant during 1979–84 justified further study. The case-control study of all cases of leukaemia and non-Hodgkin's lymphoma occurring in children aged under 15 in Caithness during 1968–86 reported in this chapter forms one part of the series of investigations recommended by the committee. A follow up study of incidence of cancer in birth and school cohorts in the Dounreay area will be reported later.

Because of the small number of cases the study was not expected to provide insights into the general aetiology of childhood leukaemia; the primary objective was to decide the extent to which the excess incidence of leukaemia and non-Hodgkin's lymphoma occurring within 25 km of the plant might be explained by risk factors suggested by earlier studies. These factors include maternal exposure to *x* rays during pregnancy[2] and aspects of parental occupation, including paternal exposure to relatively small doses of ionising radiation before conception of the child.[3] Other risk factors examined, such as patterns of viral infection in the mother and certain aspects of lifestyle, are necessarily somewhat speculative.

Although the main emphasis of the study was to use case-control methods to investigate cases of leukaemia and non-Hodgkin's lymphoma occurring within 25 km of Dounreay, it was recognised that possible risk factors relating to employment in particular would be present among people living in a wider area of Caithness. For this reason the study was extended to include all cases of childhood leukaemia and non-Hodgkin's lymphoma occurring within Caithness from 1968 to 1986. Results are presented separately for the 25 km zone and for the whole of Caithness.

Subjects and methods

All registered cases of leukaemia and non-Hodgkin's lymphoma in children resident in Caithness during 1968–86 were included in the study, and we selected controls who were matched with case children for sex and date of birth. The controls werr also matched by mother's area of residence at birth, and for this purpose Caithness was divided into two zones: (a) the area lying within 25 km of the Dounreay nuclear installation and (b) the remainder of Caithness. For each case the birth register was used to select four controls for whom the mother's zone of residence at birth corresponded with that of the case child. The controls selected were those meeting the matching criteria with dates of birth closest to the dates of birth of the index cases.

Two cases in children who were resident within 25 km of the Dounreay nuclear installation at the time of diagnosis were born outwith Caithness. To permit analysis of risk factors relating to the period before birth, four controls were selected for these two cases from the registration districts of birth. An additional four matched controls with mothers who were resident in the inner 25 km zone at the time of birth were also selected for these two cases. These further controls were used only in the analysis of those risk factors that related to the period after birth. The names and dates of birth of the parents of each case and control were found by a search of the public marriage and birth records held by the General Register Office for Scotland and the Office of Population Censuses and Surveys. The current addresses of each control and his or her parents were found from the records of health boards' primary care divisions after a search of the NHS central register. If, and only if, their family practitioner agreed to an approach, these parents were asked by letter if they wished to participate in the study. Control children who had died before the date of diagnosis for the index case were omitted from the study. If a control child had left the Caithness area before the date of diagnosis for the matched case all results for that control relating to the period after birth were excluded from the analysis.

Information was collected from each parent by experienced interviewers with a detailed and structured questionnaire. Respondents were asked for signed permissions for access to their medical records and to data (including information on external radiation dose) held by current and former employers. Detailed information was collected for the child and for each parent on all places of residence, on their medical history with particular reference to exposure to x rays, and on any viral infections. A detailed pregnancy history was collected in respect of the index child, and all vaccinations and immunisations were recorded. An exhaustive occupational history was obtained for each parent, which included information on parental exposures to radiation and particular chemicals. When possible, information relating to the period of pregnancy with the index child was extracted from medical records. It included maternal exposure to x rays, viral infections, drug treatments, and complications of pregnancy. All parents included in the study were cross matched against the occupational records held by the United Kingdom Atomic Energy Authority at Dounreay and Harwell and by HMS Vulcan, Caithness, to estimate periods of employment at nuclear installations in Caithness and elsewhere in the United Kingdom. We obtained records of annual radiation dose for the parents who were so employed. In addition, records of monthly radiation dose were obtained in respect of the two years preceding the birth of the child. Information provided by the United States naval authorities permitted the shortest distances from the place of residence at the time of diagnosis to the path of transmission beams of the microwave transmitters in the Thurso area to be calculated from grid references. Information was also collected on aspects of lifestyle of both the child and the parents, including diet and the use of local beaches up to the date of diagnosis in the cases.

Some parents of control children were not approached for an interview at the specific request of their general practitioner, and other parents subsequently refused to be interviewed after an authorised approach had been made. When fewer than two original controls were available for a particular case substitute controls were selected according to the same procedure as before. Interviews were performed with parents of the substitute controls but, to guard against the possibility of systematic bias, information on external radiation doses and employment history before the birth of the child was obtained for all cases and all original controls, irrespective of whether an interview subsequently took place. No substitute controls were required for cases in children living within 25 km of Dounreay at the time of diagnosis.

The study should therefore be regarded as two separate studies with overlapping controls—the first based on birth certificates and the employment records of the nuclear industry and the second on questionnaire information and medical records.

Estimates of odds ratios,[4] which approximate closely to relative risks, were calculated with the conditional logistic regression module of the EGRET computer package.[5] Because of the small numbers eligible for inclusion in the study, problems of analysis existed when there was concordance between cases and controls within the matched sets. When as a consequence the number of cases contributing to the estimation of the relative risk was three or fewer Fisher's exact test was used to test a null hypothesis of homogeneity and the result of this is shown as a p value. The conditional logistic regression was carried out within matched sets of cases and controls and Fisher's exact test on unmatched cases and controls. Reported relative risk estimates are for the presence of each factor compared with its absence.

The cases included in the study have been the subject of intensive investigation by the Committee on the Medical Aspects of Radiation in the Environment in respect both of completeness of recording and of accuracy of diagnosis. One conclusion in the committee's report was that with time and with changes in diagnostic practice uncertainties existed in discriminating between leukaemia and non-Hodgkin's lymphoma. For this reason the results of this study are shown for leukaemia and non-Hodgkin's lymphoma combined. The results of the study based on birth certificates and employment records of the nuclear industry are shown separately from those of the study based on information from the questionnaire and medical records.

COMPLETENESS OF RESPONSE

Fifteen cases of leukaemia and non-Hodgkin's lymphoma were registered in Caithness during 1968–86 in young people aged below 25; one case registered within the 25 km zone around Dounreay was in a subject aged 23 years at diagnosis. The subject was born in 1960 and was excluded from the study because of difficulties in obtaining reliable information about the preconceptual and early childhood periods after such an extended time interval. The 14 other cases were all aged under 15 at the time of diagnosis.

Eight cases were in children resident within the 25 km zone around Dounreay at the time of diagnosis. In one the diagnosis was in 1970 and in the remaining seven during 1979–86. These seven cases provided the focus of concern in the committee's report.[1] Two of these seven cases were in children born outwith the Caithness area and the remaining five were in children born within the 25 km zone.

In four of the six cases in children resident in the area of Caithness outwith the 25 km zone, diagnosis was during 1968–78. One of these was in a child born outwith Caithness. To respect the specific wishes of parents no information about this case has been included in the study.

Thirteen cases were therefore admitted to the study; table I shows for each the areas of birth and diagnosis, the year of diagnosis, and whether the

TABLE I—*Cases eligible for inclusion in study*

Case No	Place of birth*	Place of diagnosis*	Year of diagnosis	Included in employment record and birth certificate study	Included in questionnaire and medical record study
1	$\geqslant$ 25 km	$\geqslant$ 25 km	1969	Yes	Yes
2	$\geqslant$ 25 km	$\geqslant$ 25 km	1969	Yes	Yes
3	< 25 km	< 25 km	1970	Yes	No
4	Outwith Caithness	$\geqslant$ 25 km	1970	No	No
5	$\geqslant$ 25 km	$\geqslant$ 25 km	1974	Yes	Yes
6	$\geqslant$ 25 km	$\geqslant$ 25 km	1979	Yes	Yes
7	$\geqslant$ 25 km	$\geqslant$ 25 km	1979	Yes	Yes
8	< 25 km	< 25 km	1980	Yes	Yes
9	< 25 km	< 25 km	1980	Yes	Yes
10	< 25 km	< 25 km	1980	Yes	Yes
11	< 25 km	< 25 km	1981	Yes	Yes
12	< 25 km	< 25 km	1983	Yes	No
13	Outwith Caithness	< 25 km	1983	Yes	Yes
14	Outwith Caithness	< 25 km	1986	Yes	Yes

* < 25 km or $\geqslant$ 25 km from Dounreay or outwith Caithness.

case was included in the employment record and with certificate study and the questionnaire study. Table II shows the response rates for the two parts of the study.

Information on parental occupation, age of parents at the time of the child's birth, and place of birth of mother was obtained for all 13 cases. For one case in a child born within Caithness but outwith the 25 km area around Dounreay the father could not be traced. Information from questionnaires was available for six of the eight cases in children resident within the 25 km zone at the time of diagnosis and for all five in children resident in the remainder of Caithness. In one of the two cases for which no information was available the parents declined to participate in the study, and in the other no approach was made to the parents, at the specific request of the family practitioner. Information from questionnaires was obtained for 20 controls matched to the six cases in children resident in the 25 km zone around Dounreay at time of diagnosis and for 16 controls matched to the five cases in children resident in the remainder of Caithness. No replacement controls were required for any of the cases in children resident within 25 km of Dounreay at the time of diagnosis. Ten of the controls selected for cases resident in the remainder of Caithness were replacements.

Results

EMPLOYMENT RECORD AND BIRTH CERTIFICATE STUDY

Paternal occupation and employment at Dounreay

Information on parental occupation was obtained from birth certificates and from the computer files of workers employed at Dounreay and elsewhere in the nuclear industry. Information available from questionnaires was used as confirmation. Table III shows the paternal occupation for cases and controls at the time of birth of the child for the main industrial groups found in the Caithness area. For three cases the fathers were employed in the nuclear industry at the time of the birth of the child (odds ratio 0·58, 95% confidence interval 0·13 to 2·59). One of them was described as an electrician, one as a process worker, and one as a charge hand. All these fathers were employed at Dounreay at the time of conception of the child and two were fathers of cases resident within 25 km of Dounreay at the time of diagnosis (odds ratio 0·38, 0·06 to 2·34). No significantly raised risk was associated with employment in farming or fishing (table III). Information derived from the occupational records was used to identify periods of employment in the nuclear industry of fathers of cases and controls before conception of their children. No raised risks were observed in respect of these periods of employment (table IV). None of the fathers of cases had an accumulated external ionising radiation dose

TABLE II—*Numbers of cases and controls included in study*

	No of cases eligible for inclusion	No included in employment record and birth certificate study		No included in questionnaire and medical record study			
		Cases	Controls	Cases	Original controls	Replacement controls	Total controls
Total	13	13	47	11	26	10	36
Diagnosis and birth within 25 km zone	6	6	23	4	14	0	14
Diagnosis within 25 km zone and birth outwith Caithness	2	2	4	2	6	0	6
Diagnosis outwith 25 km zone and birth within Caithness	5	5	20	5	6	10	16

TABLE III—*Numbers of cases and controls and odds ratio or Fisher's exact p value, by paternal occupation recorded on birth certificate*

Father's occupation or industry	Cases		Controls		Odds ratio	95% Confidence interval	Fisher's exact p value
	Total	Positive	Total	Positive			
Resident <25 km from Dounreay at diagnosis							
Dounreay	8	2	25	12	0·38	0·06 to 2·34	*
Farming	8	0	25	3	0	*	0·42
Fishing	8	1	25	2	2·45	0·14 to 42·59	*
Resident anywhere in Caithness at diagnosis							
Dounreay	12	3	41	15	0·58	0·13 to 2·59	*
Farming	12	0	45	5	0	*	0·29
Fishing	12	2	41	5	2·03	0·25 to 16·46	*

* Not calculated.

>100 mSv before conception of the child (table V); the fathers of three cases who were employed in the nuclear industry each had a lifetime dose <50 mSv (40 mSv, 29 mSv, and 17·4 mSv respectively). One father of a case had a dose >10 mSv (13·6 mSv) in the six months before conception; the two other fathers had doses of 3·7 mSv and 0·7 mSv respectively. No

TABLE IV—*Numbers of cases and controls and odds ratio or Fisher's exact p value by paternal employment in nuclear industry at conception of child and estimated ionising radiation doses before conception*

	Cases		Controls		Odds ratio	95% Confidence interval	Fisher's exact p value
	Total	Positive	Total	Positive			
Resident <25 km from Dounreay at diagnosis							
Father employed in nuclear industry at conception	8*	2	25†	12	0·38	0·06 to 2·34	‡
Father's radiation dose (mSv):							
Lifetime dose (≥100 *v* <100)	8	0	25	1	0	‡	0·76
Six months before conception (≥10 *v* <10)	8	1	25	0	∞	‡	0·24
Resident anywhere in Caithness at diagnosis							
Father employed in nuclear industry at conception	12*	3	41†	15	0·58	0·13 to 2·59	‡
Father's radiation dose (mSv):							
Lifetime dose (≥100 *v* <100)	12	0	45	1	0	‡	0·79
Six months before conception (≥10 *v* <10)	12	1	45	0	∞	‡	0·21

* Fathers of three cases who were not employed in the nuclear industry before birth of child were employed before diagnosis.
† Fathers of three controls who were not employed in the nuclear industry before birth of child were employed before diagnosis of matched case.
‡ Not calculated.

TABLE V—*Numbers of cases and controls by estimated ionising radiation dose before conception*

Father's radiation dose before conception	Resident <25 km from Dounreay at diagnosis		Resident anywhere in Caithness at diagnosis	
	Cases	Controls	Cases	Controls
Total lifetime dose (mSv):				
None	6	17	9	33
1–49	2	6	3	9
50–99	0	1	0	2
⩾100	0	1	0	1
Total	8	25	12	45
Dose six months before (mSv):				
None	6	19	9	35
0·1–4·9	1	5	2	8
5·0–9·9	0	1	0	1
⩾10·0	1	0	1	1
Total	8	25	12	45

significant differences were reserved between cases and controls with respect to these external radiation doses.

Exposure to non-ionising radiation

Table VI shows, for the 25 km zone alone, the shortest distance between

TABLE VI—*Numbers of cases and controls resident < 25 km from Dounreay at time of diagnosis by distance from place of residence to transmission path of microwave beams from United States naval communications transmitters in Thurso area*

Distance to transmission path (m)	Cases	Controls
<100	0	0
100 –	0	0
200 –	0	0
300 –	1	0
400 –	2	1
500 –	0	1
600 –	1	1
700 –	0	2
800 –	0	0
900 –	1	3
⩾1000	3	19

Kolmogorov-Smirnov $D = 0.39$, $p > 0.10$.

the place of residence of cases at diagnosis and of their controls and the transmission paths of United States naval communications transmitters situated at Murkle, Cairnmore Hillock, and Forss. These transmitters emit a line of sight beam in the frequency range 7735·5–8340·0 mHz and have a reported beam width of 2°, giving a maximum area of putative risk of 50 m on either side of the transmission path. In neither cases nor controls was the place of residence within this area. A Kolmogorov-Smirnov test showed no significant difference between cases and controls in their cumulative distributions of distance from the place of residence to the pathway of the beam.

Place of birth of mother, age of parents, social class

No significantly raised risks were observed in relation to the mother's or father's age at time of birth of the child or to the mother's place of birth outwith Caithness (table VII). For the cases in the 25 km zone and for those in Caithness as a whole there was a non-significant excess of cases in children whose parents were classified as being in social classes III manual, IV, or V at the time of the child's birth.

QUESTIONNAIRE AND MEDICAL RECORDS STUDY

Antenatal exposure to x rays

Information on antenatal exposure to *x* rays was derived from the questionnaire and verified when possible from the antenatal medical records. No mother of a case was recorded as having received *x* rays antenatally according to either the questionnaire or the medical records. *x* Rays were received antenatally by the mothers of two controls according to the antenatal records (table VIII).

In three of the five cases in children resident in the 25 km zone for whom information was available from medical records, drugs had been prescribed during their mother's pregnancy compared with none in the controls for whom equivalent information was available ($p = 0·01$). There was no consistent pattern in the drugs that were prescribed; one mother had received lactulose and co-phenotrope, one penicillin, and one flurazepam and cimetidine.

Aspects of lifestyle

No raised risks were observed in either those resident within the 25 km zone or in the study group taken as a whole in respect of consumption of locally grown vegetables, fish, game, or shellfish (table IX). Parents were asked detailed information about their children's use of local beaches. Information was recorded on which beaches were visited and on the years in which the child had played there. The results reported are for the use of beaches within 25 km of Dounreay. Of the five cases in children resident in

TABLE VII—*Numbers of cases and controls and odds ratio or Fisher's exact p value by parental age (years), mother's place of birth, and social class*

Suspected risk factor	Cases		Controls		Odds ratio	95% Confidence interval	Fisher's exact p value
	Total	Positive	Total	Positive			
Resident <25 km from Dounreay at diagnosis							
Mother born outwith Caithness	8	5	27	16	0·95	0·13 to 6·77	*
Mother's age (≥25 v <25)	8	4	25	14	0·78	0·16 to 3·81	*
Father's age (≥25 v <25)	8	6	24	21	0·26	0·02 to 3·26	*
Social class†	8	0	26	7	0	*	0·12
Resident anywhere in Caithness at diagnosis							
Mother born outwith Caithness	13	7	46	19	1·70	0·35 to 8·20	*
Mother's age (≥25 v <25)	13	7	42	19	1·40	0·40 to 4·89	*
Father's age (≥25 x <25)	12	9	38	28	0·96	0·20 to 4·49	*
Social class†	13	0	46	7	0	*	0·16

* Not calculated.
† Of father at child's birth (I, II, III non-manual v III manual, IV, V).

TABLE VIII—Numbers of cases and controls and odds ratio or Fisher's exact p value by abdominal x ray exposure and drugs received during mother's pregnancy

Suspected risk factor	Cases		Controls		Odds ratio	95% Confidence interval	Fisher's exact p value
	Total	Positive	Total	Positive			
Resident <25 km from Dounreay at diagnosis							
Abdominal x rays during pregnancy	5	0	19	1	0	*	0·79
Drugs received during pregnancy	5	3†	15	0	∞	*	0·01
Drugs received during labour	4	3	16	15	*	*	0·37
Pethidine received during labour	4	3	16	12	*	*	0·72
Resident anywhere in Caithness at diagnosis							
Abdominal x rays during pregnancy	7	0	31	2	0	†	0·66
Drugs received during pregnancy	7	3†	18	1	7·42	0·77 to 72·00	*
Drugs received during labour	6	4	28	22	*	*	0·44
Pethidine received during labour	6	4	16	11	1·14	0·10 to 13·27	*

* Not calculated.
† One mother received lactulose and co-phenotrope, one penicillin, and one flurazepam and cimetidine.

TABLE IX—*Numbers of cases and controls and odds ratio or Fisher's exact p value by eating habits and use of local beaches*

Habit factor	Cases		Controls		Odds ratio	95% Confidence interval	Fisher's exact p value
	Total	Positive	Total	Positive			
Resident <25 km from Dounreay at diagnosis							
Eating:							
Locally grown vegetables or fruit	6	2	18	11	0·38	0·06 to 2·28	*
Locally caught fish	6	3	18	12	0·50	0·07 to 3·37	*
Locally caught shellfish	6	0	18	4	0	*	0·29
Locally caught game	6	0	18	1	0	*	0·75
Playing on beach†	5	5	16	7	∞	*	0·04
Resident anywhere in Caithness at diagnosis							
Eating:							
Locally grown vegetables or fruit	11	6	31	16	1·16	0·32 to 4·16	*
Locally caught fish	11	6	31	14	1·46	0·32 to 6·72	*
Locally caught shellfish	11	1	31	5	0·42	0·04 to 4·60	*
Locally caught game	11	0	31	1	0	*	0·74
Playing on beach†	9	5	30	8	∞	*	0·12

* Not calculated. † Within 25 km of Dounreay.

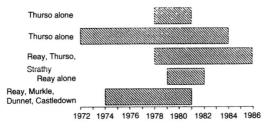

Use of beaches within 25 km of Dounreay in five cases of leukaemia and non-Hodgkin's lymphoma diagnosed within the 25 km zone, 1972–86.

the 25 km zone at the time of diagnosis for whom information was available, all were reported by both the mother and the father as using these beaches before diagnosis, both in 1979 and in 1980 (figure). When cases and controls were compared there was an excess incidence of use of the beaches by cases resident in the 25 km zone (p = 0·04).

Other risk factors

No viral infections during pregnancy were recorded in the medical records in respect of the mothers of any of the cases included in the study. In one case and nine controls the mothers were recorded on the questionnaire as having had a viral infection during pregnancy (p = 0·26); the case was in a child resident outside the 25 km zone (table X). No significantly raised risks were observed in either the group resident in the 25 km zone or the study group taken as a whole in respect of caesarean section, breast feeding, high birth weight (> 3500 g), or smoking during pregnancy.

Discussion

In their case-control study of leukaemia and lymphoma among young people in west Cumbria Gardner *et al* observed higher relative risks in children whose fathers were employed at the Sellafield plant and, in particular, in those whose fathers had had high radiation dose recordings before their conception.[3] The Dounreay and Sellafield installations are the only nuclear reprocessing plants in Britain, and both have a reported excess of childhood leukaemia in their immediate surrounding areas,[6-10] which, in the view of the Committee on the Medical Aspects of Radiation in the Environment, seem unlikely to be the result of chance.[1] In view of the findings of Gardner *et al* there seems to be a prior hypothesis of a possible association between paternal employment at Dounreay and the development of leukaemia by their children, but no raised relative risks associated with such employment were observed in this study.

A particular focus of concern in the committee's report was the seven

271

TABLE X—*Numbers of cases and controls and odds ratio or Fisher's exact p value by suspected prenatal and postnatal risk factors and vaccination of child*

Suspected risk factor	Cases		Controls		Odds ratio	95% Confidence interval	Fisher's exact p value
	Total	Positive	Total	Positive			
Resident <25 km from Dounreay at diagnosis							
Smoking during pregnancy	6	3	20	8	1·41	0·23 to 8·51	*
Caesarean delivery	6	0	20	2	0	*	0·58
Breast feeding	6	1	20	12	0·17	0·02 to 1·52	*
Birth weight (≥3500 v <3500 g)	6	0	20	4	0	*	0·32
Maternal viral infection in pregnancy	6	0	20	5	0	*	0·24
Child vaccinated before diagnosis	5	5	18	18	*	*	1·00
Resident anywhere in Caithness at diagnosis							
Smoking during pregnancy	11	5	35	16	1·03	0·26 to 4·12	*
Caesarean delivery	11	2	35	3	2·30	0·31 to 17·24	*
Breast feeding	11	2	35	14	0·33	0·06 to 1·76	*
Birth weight (≥3500 v <3500 g)	11	1	35	11	0·22	0·03 to 1·91	*
Maternal viral infection in pregnancy	10	1	30	9	0·35	0·04 to 3·09	*
Child vaccinated before diagnosis	9	9	30	30	*	*	1·00

* Not calculated.

cases occurring between 1979 and 1986 in children resident in the 25 km zone around Dounreay. A primary objective of this study was to assess whether any of these cases could be explained by possible risk factors identified in earlier studies. Six of the fathers of these cases were not employed in the nuclear industry before conception of the child. Thus, although the results of the current study do not contradict the hypothesis developed by Gardner et al, this particular hypothesis clearly does not explain the excess incidence of childhood leukaemia and non-Hodgkin's lymphoma observed in the 25 km radius circle around Dounreay from 1979 to 1986. For example, the exclusion of the case occurring after 1979 in a child whose father was employed in the nuclear industry still leaves a significant excess incidence of childhood leukaemia and non-Hodgkin's lymphoma for 1979–86 (observed 6, expected $1 \cdot 2$; $p = 0 \cdot 002$). Speculation in the press that the microwave transmitters in the Thurso area might be a source of risk in the development of childhood leukaemia was based on inconclusive results of studies in the United States.[11 12] The results of our study do not provide evidence to support this hypothesis as in none of the cases was the child resident in the reported area of putative risk at the time of diagnosis.

The results of this study suggest a possible association between the children's use of beaches and risk of leukaemia. This result differs from that found by Gardner et al, who reported no raised relative risk for children using beaches in Cumbria.[3] However, the results of the two studies in this respect are not comparable. In this study interviewers were able to identify the particular beaches used by the children. In contrast, the west Cumbria study did not attempt to differentiate between beaches close to the Sellafield plant and other beaches in Cumbria. In interpreting the result, consideration must be given to possible confounding factors and sources of bias. Residence in the immediate vicinity of one of the beaches within 25 km of Dounreay might be postulated as increasing the likelihood of a child visiting a beach to play. If the cases and controls differed in this respect then the higher proportion of cases reported to have used the beaches might simply reflect the geographical distribution of their places of residence. However, the proportion of cases and controls living within 1 km of a beach were similar (four of five cases and 12 of 16 controls). The potential for interviewer bias was reduced in this study by using trained interviewers and a structured questionnaire, but recall of the parents of children with leukaemia or non-Hodgkin's lymphoma may have been influenced by media speculation about the role of local beaches as a potential route of exposure of children to radiation. It should also be noted that reliable information on the use of the beaches was not available for three of the eight cases in children resident within 25 km of Dounreay at the time of diagnosis. Furthermore, there was no prior reason for selecting use of beaches as a factor for testing in preference to any other possible risk factors relating to lifestyle. Thus the observation of a possible association between use of beaches and risk of leukaemia arose in the context of multiple testing. The observation that all five cases for whom information was available had used the beaches in the same two years may be of interest, but without other evidence of possible sources of risk is inconclusive.

The main conclusion from this study is that the observed excess incidence of childhood leukaemia and non-Hodgkin's lymphoma in the area within 25 km of the Dounreay nuclear installation cannot be explained by any of the risk factors for which evidence has been adduced from earlier studies. In addition to paternal occupation, raised risk was previously found to be associated with maternal exposure to x rays during pregnancy[2] and with higher social class.[13] In this study in none of the cases had mothers received x rays during pregnancy and in all the cases the fathers were of social class III manual or below.

It must be emphasised that the results from such a small study cannot be used to refute claims of association with risk factors that have been based on studies carried out in other geographical areas. Thus the results of this study do not provide evidence that contradicts observations for west Cumbria of an association between the employment of fathers in the nuclear industry and the development of leukaemia or lymphoma in their children; they simply show that the excess incidence around Dounreay is not explained by such an association. Nor, on the other hand, should apparent disparities between the results of the west Cumbria study and those of this study be assumed to indicate that different explanations exist for the two observations of excess incidence. The causes of the excess incidence of leukaemia in children in the two areas might be the result of a complex multifactorial aetiology in which the effects of individual risk factors are multiplicative. Thus, for example, the excess incidence observed in the Sellafield area might be the result of the multiplicative effects of preconceptual exposure to radiation in fathers and some hitherto unrecognised risk factor or factors that are also present in the area around Dounreay. If preconceptual exposure to radiation in the father increased predisposition to developing childhood leukaemia then differences in the levels of exposure to other risk factors might be the crucial determinant of the extent to which leukaemia occurred in the respective populations of children.

We thank the United Kingdom Atomic Energy Authority, the General Register Office for Scotland, and the primary care units of health boards for their help in providing data; the general practitioners for their cooperation; Anne Macarthur for her help in this study; Jean Connor for preparing the manuscript; and Maria Barrett and Ann Crearie, who were involved in the interviews.

1 Committee on the Medical Aspects of Radiation in the Environment. *Investigation of the possible increased incidence of leukaemia in young people near the Dounreay nuclear establishment, Caithness, Scotland.* London: HMSO, 1988. (COMARE, 2nd report.)

2 Stewart A, Webb J, Hewitt D. A survey of childhood malignancies. *BMJ* 1958;i:1495.
3 Gardner MJ, Snee MP, Hall A, *et al*. Results of a case-control study of leukaemia and lymphoma among young people near the Sellafield nuclear plant in west Cumbria. *BMJ* 1990;**300**:423–9.
4 Breslow NE, Day NE. *Statistical methods in cancer research (vol I). The analysis of case-control studies*. Lyons: International Agency for Research on Cancer, 1980.
5 Anonymous. *EGRET*. Seattle: Statistics and Epidemiology Research Corporation, 1989.
6 Heasman MA, Urquhart JD, Kemp IW, Black RJ. Childhood leukaemia in northern Scotland. *Lancet* 1986;i:266.
7 Heasman MA, Kemp IW, Urquhart JD, Black RJ. Leukaemia and lymphatic cancer in young people near nuclear installations. *Lancet* 1986;i:385.
8 Heasman MA, Urquhart JD, Kemp IW, *et al*. Leukaemia in young persons in Scotland: a study of its geographical distribution and relationship to nuclear installations. *Health Bull (Edinb)* 1987;**45**:147–51.
9 Black D for the Independent Advisory Group. *Investigation of the possible increased incidence of cancer in west Cumbria*. London: HMSO, 1984. (Black report.)
10 Gardner MJ, Winter PD. Mortality in Cumberland during 1959–78 with reference to cancer in young people around Windscale. *Lancet* 1984;i:216–7.
11 Savitz DA, Wachtel H, Barnes FA, *et al*. Case-control study of childhood cancer and exposure to 60 Hz magnetic fields. *Am J Epidemiol* 1988;**128**:21–38.
12 Severson RK, Stevens RG, Kaune WT, *et al*. Acute non-lymphocytic leukaemia and residential exposure to power frequency fields. *Am J Epidemiol* 1988;**128**:10–20.
13 McWhirter WR. The relationship of incidence of childhood lymphoblastic leukaemia to social class. *Br J Cancer* 1982;**46**:640–5.

31: Case-control studies of leukaemia clusters

Children of parents receiving higher doses of radiation than most nuclear workers should be studied now

P G SMITH

Exposure to ionising radiations either in utero or when young increases the risk of childhood leukaemia, but such exposures are estimated to account for only a small proportion of all cases. The causes of most cases are unknown. Recent work on the aetiology of childhood leukaemia has been stimulated by finding geographical clusters of the disease associated with nuclear plants. The most notable cluster was in the village of Seascale, adjacent to the Sellafield nuclear reprocessing plant in Cumbria.[1] Conventional radiobiological explanations are inadequate to explain this and other clusters around Dounreay[2] and Aldermaston and Burghfield,[3] because of the very low doses of radiation to which the populations are estimated to have been exposed. There has been a search for other explanations using case-control studies that compare possible aetiological factors for cases and matched control children in areas where an apparent excess of cases has occurred.

Case-control studies of this kind are difficult both to conduct and to interpret. Some of the cases may have been diagnosed years before a study is done, and parents have to be located and asked to recall events in the distant past. Parents of a child who has been seriously ill and may have died may respond to questions differently from the parents of a healthy child— potentially a serious source of bias, especially when the case is one of a cluster that has attracted media interest and public speculation about possible causes.

The first of these studies, based on cases of childhood leukaemia and lymphoma in west Cumbria, produced unexpected findings.[4] Comparison of the questionnaire responses from parents of cases and controls did not provide evidence of appreciable differences between the two groups with respect to the exposures examined. But even if differences had been shown the findings may have been difficult to evaluate because responses had been obtained from only about 74% of the parents of cases and 55% of the parents of controls.[56] Perhaps the most reliable information in the study, for which bias was unlikely, was on parental occupational exposure to radiation. This was obtained by linking case and control records to employment and radiation records at the Sellafield plant and did not depend on tracing parents and receiving correct answers to a questionnaire. About 91% of both cases and controls were included in this analysis, and a striking association was uncovered between paternal exposure to radiation before conception and the risk of leukaemia in offspring. The association was strong enough to explain the cluster of cases in Seascale and was strongest with exposure to radiation just before conception. No evidence exists in humans that germ cell mutations induced by radiation increase susceptibility to leukaemia, so many people will want further evidence before accepting the causative explanation.[7]

Two more case-control studies have been reported. Urquhart et al included 14 cases of leukaemia and non-Hodgkin's lymphoma diagnosed under the age of 15 years between 1970 and 1986 in Caithness.[8] At diagnosis eight had been living within 25 km of the Dounreay nuclear installation, where an appreciable excess of leukaemia (seven of the eight cases) had been reported between 1979 and 1984. The authors checked the names of case and control fathers against the employment records of the Dounreay nuclear plant and found that the fathers of only two of the eight cases resident within 25 km of the nuclear establishment had been employed in the nuclear industry before conception of the child (compared with 12 of 25 controls); and none had accumulated preconceptual doses of more than 100 mSv (the exposure level that the west Cumbria study found was associated with an increased risk) compared with one of 25 controls. Thus paternal occupational radiation exposure did not explain the observed excess of leukaemia. The study's only significant finding was that all five cases with data available had used beaches within 25 km of Dounreay before their diagnosis, compared with only seven of 16 controls. This apparent excess must be interpreted with caution, however, and could be due to bias or be a chance finding. It is based on small numbers and no corresponding association was found in west Cumbria.

McKinney and colleagues also studied cases of leukaemia in areas where "clusters" had been reported and an environmental exposure was suspected as the cause.[9] Only one of the clusters, in west Cumbria, was near a nuclear plant. Many possible aetiological factors to which parents might have been exposed were investigated. Much interest will focus on the authors' conclusion that their findings support the hypothesis, generated by the study of Gardner et al, that fathers' exposure to radiation before conception is causal. Unfortunately, in this new study few of the reported radiation exposures have been verified, and no information on dose is available. Also, three of the six fathers of cases who reported prenatal radiation exposures were included in the study of Gardner et al.[4] If these cases are excluded, as would be appropriate for an independent assessment, the evidence suggesting an effect for preconceptual irradiation is much weaker.

Although the findings from both the above studies are not incompatible with an effect of paternal preconceptual radiation exposure of the size described by Gardner et al,[4] neither offers strong confirmatory evidence. Indeed, the findings in the Scottish study indicate that if the cluster of cases around Dounreay truly results from reasons other than chance the excess cannot be explained by paternal exposure to radiation while working at the Dounreay nuclear plant.

As well as radiation, McKinney et al examined many possible causative exposures. If exposure to ionising radiations before conception really does increase the risk of leukaemia then other mutagenic agents might be expected to have a similar effect, and McKinney et al examined exposures before, during, and after pregnancy. They report increased risks associated with several exposures at different periods, including paternal exposure to wood dust, carbon tetrachloride, trichloroethylene, benzene, coal, or graphite and maternal exposure to wood dust. Unfortunately, for none of these is the exposure verified or the amount of exposure measured. The strongest link is reported to be with exposure to wood dust before conception in both mothers and fathers. At least some of these findings may be due to chance. The authors made 480 comparisons and a significant result ($p < 0.05$) could be expected in about 10 to 20 by chance alone. At this stage it would therefore be prudent to regard the study of McKinney et al as having generated some interesting hypotheses rather than providing strong evidence of new aetiological factors.

The most persuasive evidence that factors before conception influence the risk of childhood leukaemia is provided by the finding of a 20-fold increased risk of luekaemia in children with Down's syndrome. How may we assess the leukaemogenic potential of radiation exposure before conception? The findings from the study of Gardner et al[4] suggesting an effect of paternal preconceptual radiation may be an important new lead, but it is important to seek verification of the findings shown in other populations.

Studies are already under way of the children of nuclear workers, but investigation is needed of people who may have conceived children after having been exposed to higher radiation doses than nuclear workers are typically exposed to—in such populations larger effects might be expected. A group of special interest in this respect would be children conceived after their parents had been successfully treated with radiotherapy for malignant or other disease (for example, the children of patients treated with x rays for Hodgkin's disease). This would allow the assessment of the effects of a high radiation dose delivered over a short period. (Relevant to this assessment is the finding that the children of the survivors of the atomic bomb explosions in Japan do not show an increased risk of cancer.[10]) If exposure to radiation must occur shortly before conception for leukaemogenesis, as was suggested by the findings of Gardner et al, the studies of the children of people exposed to a high radiation dose in a short period are less relevant. A more informative group would be the children of radiologists, especially of those radiologists who were in practice when radiation exposure levels were comparatively high.

1 Black D for the Independent Advisory Group. *Investigation of the possible increased evidence of cancer in west Cumbria.* London: HMSO, 1984. (Black report.)
2 Committee on Medical Aspects of Radiation in the Environment. *Investigation of the possible increased incidence of leukaemia in young persons near the Dounreay nuclear establishment, Caithness, Scotland.* London: HMSO, 1988. (COMARE 2nd report.)
3 Committee on Medical Aspects of Radiation in the Environment. *Report on the incidence of childhood cancer in the west Berkshire and north Hampshire area, in which are situated the Atomic Weapons Research Establishment, Aldermaston, and the Royal Ordnance Factory, Burghfield.* London: HMSO, 1989. (COMARE 3rd report.)
4 Gardner MJ, Snee MP, Hall AJ, Powell CA, Downes S, Terrell JD. Results of case-control study of leukaemia and lymphoma among young people near Sellafield nuclear plant in west Cumbria. *BMJ* 1990;**300**:423–9.
5 Gardner MJ, Hall AJ, Snee MP, Downes S, Powell CA, Terrell JD. Methods and basic data of case-control study of leukaemia and lymphoma among young people near Sellafield nuclear plant in west Cumbria. *BMJ* 1990;**300**:429–34.
6 Smith PG. Comments on the case-control study of Gardner et al of leukaemia and lymphoma among young people in west Cumbria. *Trop Dis Bull* 1990;**65**:R1–6.
7 Beral V. Leukaemia and nuclear installations. *BMJ* 1990;**300**:411–2.
8 Urquhart JD, Black RJ, Muirhead MJ, *et al.* Case-control study of leukaemia and non-Hodgkin's lymphoma in children in Caithness near the Dounreay nuclear installaton. *BMJ* 1991;**302**:687–92.
9 McKinney PA, Alexander FE, Cartwright RA, Parker L. Parental occupations of children with leukaemia in west Cumbria, north Humberside, and Gateshead. *BMJ* 1991;**302**:681–7.
10 Yoshimoto Y, Neel JV, Schull WJ, *et al. Frequency of malignant tumors during the first two decades of life in the offspring (F1) of atomic bomb survivors.* Hiroshima: Radiation Effects Research Foundation, 1990. (RERF technical report 4-90.)

32: Contacts between adults as evidence for an infective origin of childhood leukaemia: an explanation for the excess near nuclear establishments in west Berkshire?

L J KINLEN, C M HUDSON, C A STILLER

The increasing tendency for people to work outside their home community—one of the most striking of modern demographic changes—has relevance to a recent aetiological hypothesis about childhood leukaemia: that a community's immune response to an underlying infection can be disturbed by increases in new social contacts. This was tested in the only 28 former county boroughs in which accurate comparisons of workplace data from the 1971 and 1981 censuses are possible—because their boundaries were left unaltered by the major reorganisation in 1974. After ranking the districts according to extent of commuting *increase*, a significant trend in leukaemia incidence was found at ages 0–14 (p < 0·05) and a suggestive one at ages 0–4 (p = 0·055). Among 10 similar sized groups of county districts ranked by commuting increase, the only significant increases (p < 0·001) of leukaemia in 1972–85 at ages 0–4 and 0–14 were in the highest tenth for commuting increase. These excesses persisted after excluding Reading, a major part of an area where an excess of leukaemia has been linked to the nearby nuclear establishments at Aldermaston and Burghfield. This whole area has experienced greater commuting increases than 90% of county districts in England and Wales. The findings are consistent with other evidence supporting the above hypothesis; they also suggest that contacts between adults may influence the incidence of leukaemia in children.

Introduction

A recent hypothesis about childhood leukaemia holds that the transmission of an underlying but unrecognised infection (or infections) may be facilitated by pronounced increases in levels of new social contacts. This can happen when large numbers of people move into new towns, particularly under conditions of high density and from a variety of origins.[1,2] A notable feature of modern life in Britain is the increasing tendency for people to work in communities away from where they live: commuting has become commonplace. Indeed in certain cities, the number of daily boundary crossings by people travelling to, or from, work is equivalent to the total population of those cities. Such journeys and the area of work itself provide opportunities for new contacts that may be relevant to the above infective-based hypothesis. This possibility has therefore been investigated in all the former county boroughs of England and Wales that were left unchanged by the 1974 reorganisations of local authority districts. Only in such areas can comparisons be made of commuting levels across town boundaries in 1981 with those in 1971, using census data for those years. These boroughs include Reading, part of an area of Berkshire and Hampshire where an increased incidence of childhood leukaemia in the period 1972–85 has been reported and had been linked by some to the nearby nuclear establishments at Aldermaston and Burghfield.[3,4]

Methods

In consequence of the major reorganisation of administrative areas in 1974, the local authority areas in the 1971 and 1981 censuses were generally dissimilar. However, 28 county boroughs became county districts without any boundary change.

For these 28 county boroughs (later county districts) details were abstracted from the census publications of (a) the numbers of residents who worked outside the borough and (b) the numbers of residents of other areas who worked within the borough. The sum of outward and inward movements has been used in census publications for over 50 years and can be regarded as a measure of commuting for the area in question. What seems most relevant to the present hypothesis, however, is the extent of any *increase* in commuting level between 1971 and 1981 and its possible association with the corresponding local incidence of childhood leukaemia. For each county district, the change in commuting level has been calculated as the level in 1981 minus that in 1971, related to the baseline total population (1971) and expressed as a percentage. Changes in commuting level were also calculated using the mean of the 1971 and 1981 total population.

It could be argued that the measure of commuting change should be related to the group among whom its possible effects are being investigated, namely children. Another set of values was therefore calculated using as the denominator the total person-years of children below age 15 over the period 1972–85 for each district.

The national registry of childhood tumours at the Childhood Cancer Research Group includes children resident in Great Britain and aged under 15 at the time of diagnosis of a malignant neoplasm. The principal sources of ascertainment are the national cancer registration schemes which cover the whole of Britain through a network of regional registries. Children are also ascertained from entries to the Medical Research Council leukaemia trials, from the register of patients treated by members of the United Kingdom Children's Cancer Study Group since 1977, and from death certificates. Over 90% of childhood leukaemias are notified to cancer registries,[5] and when notifications from other sources are added the ascertainment rate of cases is believed to exceed 95%.

Details were obtained from the national registry of the numbers of cases of leukaemia at ages 0–4, 5–9 and 10–14 in each of the 28 districts during the periods 1972–75, 1976–80, and 1981–85. Expected numbers were calculated by applying the corresponding registration rates for these malignancies for England. The denominators for these rates were the population estimates for England for the relevant age groups for each of the years 1972–85, provided by the Office of Population Censuses and Surveys (Wales was excluded because registration is known to be less complete there than in England, and because none of the districts under study is in Wales).

Results

Table I gives the 1971 total population and the extent of its change by 1981 for each of the 28 county districts. Also shown are the numbers of residents in 1971 and 1981 working outside the district combined with the numbers of non-residents working within the district (the commuting level), together with the change in commuting level (1981 minus 1971) divided by the 1971 population, expressed as a percentage (termed the "total commuting change"). Table II shows the observed numbers of leukaemias in the period 1972–85 at ages 0–4, 5–9, 10–14, and 0–14 together with the ratios of observed to expected numbers for each of the 28 districts, ranked in ascending order of total commuting change. It is striking that the only two (Gloucester and Lincoln) with significant excesses of childhood leukaemia in any age group are among those with the greatest commuting increases, ranking 2nd and 3rd highest respectively. A significant trend with respect to commuting increase (p = 0·05) was found at ages 0–14, and a suggestive trend (p = 0·055) at ages 0–4.

In table III we have attempted to simplify the above findings. In the absence of any a priori basis for grouping the county districts, we have chosen (for reasons of sensitivity) the maximum number of similar sized groups (in terms of child-years under age 15). That the number of groups was 10 was determined by Liverpool which happens to have both the lowest rank of commuting increase and the largest population. In the category with the greatest increase in commuting level, highly significant excesses (p < 0·001) of leukaemia are present at ages 0–4 and 0–14 (observed to expected ratios 1·76 based on 46 cases, and 1·50, based on 79 cases). There is also a significant excess at ages 10–14 (p = 0·05), but not at ages 5–9.

The district with the greatest increase in commuting is Reading, which forms part of an area of Berkshire and north Hampshire in which an excess of childhood leukaemia had already been recorded. However this district is not solely responsible for the significant excesses in the highest tenth, for they persist after excluding Reading, the observed to expected ratios being as follows: at ages 0–4, 1·77 (p < 0·01); at ages 10–14, 2·36 (p < 0·01), and at ages 0–14, 1·6 (p < 0·001). No other group showed a significant excess either at ages 0–4 or 0–14, but the 2nd, 5th, and 7th tenths showed less pronounced excesses (p < 0·05) at ages 10–14. Given the many categories examined, some significant differences would be expected by chance alone. When the groupings were based on ranking the two alternative commuting measures, increases with similar levels of statistical significance were again found in (only) the highest tenth for commuting increase. These used as denominators respectively, the mean of the 1971 and 1981 populations, and the total children-years at ages 0–14 over the period 1972–85. In each case, the significant excess persisted after exclusion of Reading.

Several other analyses were carried out to investigate further the reliability of the above relation. Thus it might be argued that the high incidence of childhood leukaemia in the districts within the highest tenth, far from being related to the recent commuting changes in the 1970s, might be typical of those districts over a longer period. Leukaemia incidence in the study period 1972–85 was therefore compared within each district to the

TABLE I—*Population and "commuting" details of 28 county districts 1971 and 1981*

County district	1971 Total population	Population change in 1981	Commuting level (out + in)		Commuting increase %	Commuting level (in only)	
			1971	1981		1971	1981
Bath	84 670	−6711	15 120	20 890	6·82	9 750	13 630
Blackpool	151 860	−6084	24 220	26 620	1·58	10 090	11 280
Bournemouth	153 870	−13666	29 050	33 230	2·72	16 800	19 150
Brighton	161 350	−18016	37 600	40 140	1·57	21 840	24 780
Bristol	426 655	−41780	79 420	97 460	4·23	53 590	70 530
Derby	219 580	−5150	31 160	39 400	3·75	23 720	28 460
Eastbourne	70 920	+3178	9 070	11 320	3·17	6 240	7 590
Exeter	95 730	−3095	14 810	21 650	7·15	12 200	16 290
Gloucester	90 230	+610	22 000	29 700	8·53	13 360	18 600
Great Grimsby	95 540	−3999	23 120	25 360	2·35	16 610	17 970
Hastings	72 410	+1212	7 400	9 130	2·39	3 200	4 600
Ipswich	123 310	−3810	19 040	28 020	7·28	12 970	18 560
Kingston upon Hull	285 970	−19210	39 260	44 520	1·84	25 910	30 330
Leicester	284 210	−7965	71 870	84 700	4·51	57 900	67 530
Lincoln	74 270	+1347	17 010	23 160	8·28	13 860	18 500
Liverpool	610 115	−106393	166 570	142 460	−3·95	119 080	105 480
Luton	161 405	+1804	34 410	42 540	5·04	20 590	24 160
Nottingham	300 630	−32373	90 420	100 150	3·24	66 180	77 290
Oxford	108 805	−15305	42 050	47 270	4·80	38 570	41 480
Plymouth	239 450	+1202	18 210	24 970	2·82	13 240	18 200
Portsmouth	197 430	−22048	42 950	53 900	5·55	33 340	43 250
Reading	132 940	−2049	40 000	52 560	9·45	26 440	36 150
Southampton	215 120	−13131	45 780	56 350	4·91	31 950	39 810
Southend-on-Sea	162 770	−6955	36 370	38 450	1·28	13 150	16 470
Stoke-on-Trent	265 260	−15422	53 550	58 020	1·69	36 500	41 360
Torbay	109 255	+1450	7 900	9 870	1·80	3 440	3 930
Wolverhampton	269 110	−16648	62 410	64 010	0·60	38 090	39 470
York	104 780	−7540	24 690	31 660	6·65	18 140	23 750

TABLE II—*Leukaemia 1972–85 by age group: observed numbers (Obs) and observed to expected ratios (O/E), commuting increase (%), and cumulative person years (PYs)*

County district*	Commuting increase	Cumulative PYs	0–4		5–9		10–14		0–14	
			Obs	O/E	Obs	O/E	Obs	O/E	Obs	O/E
Liverpool	−3·95	1 582 709	25	0·87	18	1·10	9	0·68	52	0·89
Wolverhampton	0·60	2 435 318	23	1·46	9	1·00	5	0·72	37	1·17
Southend-on-Sea	1·28	2 847 440	7	0·90	7	1·62	4	1·20	18	1·17
Brighton	1·57	3 213 123	6	0·90	4	1·05	1	0·33	11	0·81
Blackpool	1·58	3 567 867	3	0·48	3	0·81	2	0·66	8	0·62
Stoke-on-Trent	1·69	4 325 857	13	0·91	10	1·26	7	1·14	30	1·06
Torbay	1·80	4 592 989	5	1·05	1	0·36	1	0·44	7	0·71
Kingston upon Hull	1·84	5 484 549	16	0·95	6	0·64	10	1·40	32	0·96
Great Grimsby	2·35	5 790 368	5	0·88	2	0·62	4	1·61	11	0·96
Hastings	2·39	5 985 506	2	0·53	3	1·47	2	1·31	7	0·95
Bournemouth	2·72	6 292 117	7	1·29	2	0·62	1	0·39	10	0·89
Plymouth	2·82	7 037 875	15	1·04	9	1·15	4	0·68	23	0·82
Eastbourne	3·17	7 196 413	2	0·67	1	0·60	2	1·59	5	0·84
Nottingham	3·24	8 064 638	11	0·69	7	0·76	8	1·12	26	0·81
Derby	3·75	8 753 931	10	0·77	7	0·96	6	1·09	23	0·89
Bristol	4·23	9 875 713	24	1·14	11	0·94	11	1·21	46	1·10
Leicester	4·51	10 763 154	14	0·80	8	0·88	5	0·71	27	0·80
Oxford	4·80	11 032 440	2	0·40	3	1·10	1	0·44	6	0·60
Southampton	4·91	11 650 019	8	0·68	5	0·78	6	1·20	19	0·82
Luton	5·04	12 214 044	12	1·07	5	0·84	3	0·69	20	0·93
Portsmouth	5·55	12 700 099	8	0·86	4	0·81	4	1·01	16	0·88
York	6·65	12 976 745	8	0·98	3	1·04	1	0·44	9	0·88
Bath	6·82	13 185 727	5	0·82	5	2·30	1	0·55	9	1·18
Exeter	7·15	13 452 575	7	1·41	3	1·08	2	0·91	12	1·21
Ipswich	7·28	13 824 800	6	0·84	4	1·03	3	1·01	13	0·93
Lincoln	8·28	14 051 936	12	2·70‡	3	1·27	4	2·22	19	2·22‡
Gloucester	8·53	14 348 518	9	1·62	3	0·96	6	2·49†	18	1·63†
Reading	9·45	14 759 034	12	1·51	4	0·93	1	0·31	17	1·10
Test for trend (p value)				0·055		NS		NS		0·037†

* County districts are in ascending order of commuting increase. † p<0·05; ‡ p<0·01; NS = not significant.

TABLE III—*Adjusted observed to expected (O/E) ratios (and observed (Obs) numbers) of leukaemia by age group and 10 county district groups (tenths) ranked by commuting increase*

Tenth	County district	0–4		5–9		10–14		0–14	
		O/E	Obs	O/E	Obs	O/E	Obs	O/E	Obs
I	Liverpool	1·00	(25)	1·00	(18)	1·00	(9)	1·00	(52)
II	Wolverhampton, Southend-on-Sea	1·46	(30)*	1·09	(16)	1·28	(9)	1·30	(55)
III	Brighton, Blackpool, Stoke-on-Trent	0·93	(22)	1·00	(17)	1·21	(10)	1·00	(49)
IV	Torbay, Hull, Grimsby, Hastings	1·04	(28)	0·63	(12)	1·87	(17)*	1·04	(57)
V	Bournemouth, Plymouth, Eastbourne	1·21	(24)	0·50	(7)	1·06	(7)	0·94	(38)
VI	Nottingham, Derby	0·84	(21)	0·78	(14)	1·63	(14)	0·95	(49)
VII	Bristol, Leicester	1·14	(38)	0·83	(19)	1·46	(16)	1·07	(73)
VIII	Oxford, Southampton	0·69	(10)	0·79	(8)	1·43	(7)	0·85	(25)
IX	Luton, Portsmouth, York, Bath	1·11	(28)	0·97	(17)	1·08	(9)	1·06	(54)
X	Exeter, Ipswich, Lincoln, Gloucester, Reading	1·76	(46)†	1·03	(17)	1·87	(16)*	1·50	(79)‡
[X	Excluding Reading	1·77	(34)†	0·98	(13)	2·36	(15)†	1·60	(62)‡]

* p < 0·05; † p < 0·01; ‡ p < 0·001.

rates in the preceding period, 1962–71. By this method the excesses in group X were greater than previously, being around twofold at ages 0–4 and 0–14, as shown in table IV, B. On the other hand, and as expected, there was no relation between commuting change in 1971–81 and leukaemia in the preceding period, 1962–71 (table IV, A). However, leukaemia at ages 0–4 in the period 1962–71 did show a significant excess (ratio of observed to expected cases 1·49 based on 36 cases) in the group of county boroughs with the greatest contemporary (1961–71) commuting increase, though not in the entire age group 0–14 (O/E ratio 1·10). The fact that these effects were less striking than the main study period (1972–85) is in keeping with the smaller commuting changes and the shorter period of observation (1962–71).

Any effect of commuting increase in the 1970s on leukaemia incidence would presumably be greatest in the later part of the study period. The relation was therefore examined using leukaemia data for the decade 1976–85 and, as predicted, the observed to expected ratios were more pronounced, being 2·0 at ages 0–4 and 1·7 at 0–14 (p < 0·001, table IV, C). This also applied to Reading and indeed here there was no excess in any childhood age group in the early period, 1972–75.

When (as in table IV) leukaemia at ages 0–4 and 0–14 was examined in the groups of districts with the greatest increases in commuting-*out* (D) separately from commuting-*in* (E), an excess was found only with the

TABLE IV—*Adjusted*† *observed to expected (O/E) ratios of cases of leukaemia in the highest tenth for different measures of commuting and population change (observed numbers in parentheses)*

Measure	Period (leukaemias)	Age: 0–4 O/E	Obs	Age: 0–14 O/E	Obs
A Total commuting change 1971–81	1962–71	0·82	(21)	0·75	(32)
B Measure as A‡	1972–85	2·15***	(46)	1·99***	(79)
Excluding Reading‡	1972–85	2·38***	(34)	1·97***	(62)
C Measure as A	1976–85	2·00***	(34)	1·72***	(54)
Excluding Reading	1976–85	1·91**	(24)	1·72**	(40)
D Commuting-out change 1971–81	1972–85	1·36	(34)	1·25	(63)
E Commuting-in change 1971–81	1972–85	1·64**	(46)	1·45**	(79)
Excluding Reading	1972–85	1·60*	(34)	1·44**	(62)
F Total commuting level 1971	1972–85	0·94	(25)	0·93	(49)
Excluding Reading	1972–85	0·67	(13)	0·83	(32)
G Total commuting level 1981	1972–85	0·94	(25)	0·93	(49)
Excluding Reading	1972–85	0·67	(13)	0·83	(32)
H Population change 1971–81	1972–85	1·40	(33)	1·22	(58)

† Adjusted to the lowest group of the relevant measure as reference.
‡ Expected numbers based on county borough specific rates in 1962–71.
* $p < 0.05$, ** $p < 0.01$, *** $p < 0.001$.
Composition of the above highest (and lowest, the reference) groups are as follows:
A, B, and C—as in X (and I) of table III.
D—Gloucester, Ipswich, Luton, Exeter (Liverpool).
E—Portsmouth, York, Gloucester, Lincoln, Reading (Liverpool).
F—Nottingham, Reading, Oxford (Torbay, Plymouth, Hastings, Eastbourne).
G—Nottingham, Reading, Oxford (Torbay, Plymouth, Hastings, Eastbourne).
H—Luton, Torbay, Hastings, Lincoln, Eastbourne (Liverpool).

latter. No relation was found with the absolute levels of commuting, either in 1971 (F) or 1981 (G).

The data for ages 0–4 are shown in table V, analysed both by change in commuting and change in population. Four similar sized groups of person-years were formed from a ranking of districts in terms of commuting increase (the rows) and similarly four groups by population increase 1971 to 1981 (the columns). (If smaller fractions than quarters are used, the proportion of empty cells rises markedly.) A significant excess of leukaemia is present only in the group of county districts forming the highest category for both measures.

Discussion

An infective basis for childhood leukaemia is a longstanding hypothesis[9] and indeed a specific viral cause is established in adult T cell leukaemia (HTLV-1), as well as in certain animal leukaemias. The absence of notable space-time clustering suggests that, if the disease is infective in origin, leukaemic children cannot be important in spreading the underlying infection, which must mainly be done by symptomless or trivially affected

TABLE V—*Leukaemia at ages 0–4: observed to expected ratios* by quarters of population increase and of commuting increase 1971–81 (Observed numbers in parentheses)*

Quarters of relative population increase	Quarters of commuting increase			
	1	2	3	4 (Highest)
1	1·00 (31)		0·71 (13)	0·98 (8)
2		1·18 (23)	1·30 (24)	0·89 (16)
3	1·27 (33)	1·03 (18)	0·92 (14)	1·23 (13)
4 (Highest)		1·06 (24)	0·88 (10)	1·77 (45)† ‡

*Adjusted to the lowest quartile for both measures (Liverpool and Brighton: unadjusted 0·87). † Includes Reading, Gloucester, Luton, Lincoln. ‡ p < 0·001 (p < 0·01 after exclusion of Reading). Quarters of population increase: (1) Liverpool, Oxford, Brighton, Portsmouth, Nottingham; (2) Bristol, Bournemouth, Bath, York, Kingston upon Hull, Southampton; (3) Wolverhampton, Stoke-on-Trent, Southend, Grimsby, Blackpool, Exeter, Ipswich, Leicester; (4) Derby, Reading, Plymouth, Gloucester, Luton, Torbay, Hastings, Lincoln, Eastbourne. Quarters of commuting increase: (1) Liverpool, Wolverhampton, Southend-on-Sea, Brighton, Blackpool; (2) Stoke-on-Trent, Torbay, Hull, Grimsby, Hastings, Bournemouth, Plymouth, Eastbourne; (3) Nottingham, Derby, Bristol, Leicester, Oxford; (4) Southampton, Luton, Portsmouth, York, Bath, Exeter, Ipswich, Lincoln, Gloucester, Reading.

individuals.[10] This is obviously a difficult hypothesis to test directly when the relevant agent has not been identified. Increases in population density or conditions that in other ways greatly increase the level of social contact will also tend to promote unaccustomed contacts between susceptible and infected individuals, particularly when people come together from a variety of different origins as was the case in rural new towns during their period of rapid growth. In such conditions significant increases of leukaemia at ages 0–4 have been found.[12]

Population influxes are far from being the only causes of increased social contact. Wider car ownership, better roads, and faster trains now permit many people to live considerable distances from their work, for example in more desirable areas or where housing is less expensive or to avoid moving house. These travel patterns are one of the most striking of modern demographic changes. Information on these patterns is used by central government in defining travel-to-work (employment) areas, which form the basis for determining the allocation of financial aid for new businesses, besides other uses. They have also been the subject of much work by geographers.[6-8] Inevitably therefore much new contact, both direct and indirect, takes place between people from different communities in their areas of work or in the course of commuting. Thus in 1981 the number of people making daily journeys across Oxford's boundaries to reach their work was equivalent to half (50·5%) of that city's population—or alternatively the daily number of such boundary crossings was equivalent to its total population.

In accord with our hypothesis, the present study finds that in 28 county districts leukaemia incidence both at ages 0–14 and 0–4 shows a significant (positive) trend with increasing commuting change. The increase is not steady, however, and only with the most marked commuting increases is there a significant excess of leukaemia, either in individual (table II) or grouped county districts (table III). It may be noted that the absence of a steady trend is typical of many infectious diseases in which outbreaks or epidemics occur only when the density, or the numbers, of infected and susceptible individuals in a population reaches some critical point specific for the agent in question.

It was recognised at the outset of the study that if a high level of commuting *were* capable of increasing the incidence of childhood leukaemia, this might well be temporary as in epidemics of most infectious disorders, ending when the number of susceptible people declined below some critical level. Even in 1921 many areas of England and Wales had commuting levels of over 20%.[11] None of the districts with the highest commuting levels either in 1971 or 1981 had experienced any great commuting *increases*, and this may be the reason for their not showing any excesses of leukaemia (table IV, F and G).

When the effects of changes in the commuting-out level (table IV, D) of the county districts were examined separately from those of commuting-in, only the latter was associated with a significant excess of leukaemia (table IV, E). This difference is of uncertain significance, however, as three of the five districts in the highest tenth for "commuting-*in*" change also belonged to the highest tenth for total commuting increase.

It is noteworthy that the county district with the greatest increase in commuting is Reading. This is also the only district entirely contained within an area in which an excess of childhood leukaemia had already been observed, arousing concern that it might be related to the nearby nuclear establishments in west Berkshire at Aldermaston and Burghfield.[34] In fact, Reading children represented about half the child-population of that study area. This comprised those wards with half or more of their area within 10 km of these nuclear sites. This area showed a significant increase at ages 0–14 based on 41 cases, in the same period as our study (1972–85), due to an increase at ages 0–4 (29 observed, 14·42 expected). This excess is not appreciably different in magnitude from the excess found in the study in Reading itself or in group X of total commuting change, excluding Reading. Of the 29 cases aged 0–4, 12 were in Reading and were represented also in our study (O/E ratio 1·74).

It is likely that cases of leukaemia outside Reading but within the west Berkshire excess are also related to commuting increases, for these have occurred greatly throughout this area, much of it lying within so-called "Silicon Valley". Boundary changes in 1974 impede examination of such increases in the same way as Reading. Thus substantial amounts of

TABLE VI—*Commuting details for county districts (CDs) at least partly in Aldermaston-Burghfield (A–B) study area and nominal effects of 1974 boundary changes*

County districts (CD)	Number LADs in 1971	1971 Commuting and % nominal loss by 1974 boundaries		Commuting change (CD) 1971–81†	Rank*	% Children of A–B study area
Reading	1	40 000	0%	9·4%	27	49·6%
Wokingham	2	38 760	13·7%	10·4%	22	15·5%
Newbury	5	48 760	37·6%	9·1%	31	23·8%
Basingstoke	3	31 380	51·4%	7·6%	53	10·8%
S Oxfordshire	6	44 840	17·0%	3·9%	174	0·3%

LAD = Local authority district total (in + out). *Among 402 CDs (1 = highest). †As % of 1971 total population. The small part of Wantage rural district has been ignored.

commuting as recorded by the 1971 census would have been concealed had the 1974 boundaries existed, for many journeys would then have occurred within the new area without any boundary crossing. Workingham district was least affected in this respect as it is composed of only two complete pre-1974 areas, Wokingham metropolitan borough and rural district. The new area experienced a greater commuting increase (10·4%) even more than Reading; it also contributed seven cases of leukaemia at ages 0–4 (expected 3·0) to the excess in the Aldermaston study area. However, no less than 38% and 51%, respectively, of the total commuting in 1971 in what were later Newbury and Basingstoke districts would have been "lost" if the 1974 boundaries had been in force (table VI). Despite this, however, the increases from 1971 to 1981 in commuting level in those enlarged districts as defined in 1974, places them close (9·1 and 7·6%) to Reading, and within the range of group X in the present study (7·2–10·6%). It may be noted that none of the other county districts in group X are within 10 km (or even 25 km) of a nuclear installation.

The present hypothesis preceded the collection of both the childhood leukaemia and the commuting data, about which we previously knew nothing except for the recently reported excess of the disease in the Aldermaston-Reading area. The relation therefore seems unlikely to be due to chance or bias. Another possibility however is that the relation is indirect, reflecting some leukaemogenic factor that is related in some way to increases in commuting. If so, we have been unable to discover it in the census data for the 28 districts we have subsequently examined with respect to social class, changes in social class, and migration. Similarly, we have not found any distinctive changes in the organisation of schools in the group X districts of table III that might be relevant to the hypothesis about population mixing.

The recent findings imply that a commuting increase equivalent to, say, 10% of a large town's population may produce more effective contacts between infected and susceptible individuals for the postulated infection than a 10% (or even a 25%) increase in its residential population.[1 12] Large commuting increases with their many direct and indirect opportunities for new contacts and adding to the tides of almost daily ebb and flow may thereby exert more widespread effects than a similar-sized influx of new residents. These suggested effects on the immune response of large populations do not imply that the excess cases of leukaemia in the group X towns will necessarily be in the children of commuters themselves.

The towns in the highest tenth in table III had not only the greatest commuting *increase* through the 1970s but by 1981 had reached high absolute levels of commuting. The combination of marked increase with a reaching of a high absolute commuting level may therefore be important. The populations of many of the towns studied declined in the 1970s and none showed any marked increase (table I). Such population changes as there were showed no relationship with leukaemia (table V, H). However, when leukaemia incidence was analysed by change in commuting level simultaneously with population change, the only category that showed a significant increase was highest for each measure (table V). The possibility is therefore raised that populations changes, which alone may have little effect, may nevertheless compound the effects of commuting increases. If so, it may be relevant, for example, that several of the areas linked by commuting to the Aldermaston study area have themselves been subject to marked population increases during the study period, of up to 33%. These include the expanding town of Basingstoke, the new town of Bracknell and the large housing development in Earley on the east side of Reading that extends into Wokingham county district.

A significant excess of childhood malignancies other than leukaemia in the period 1971–80 was found in the districts of Reading, Newbury, and Basingstoke,[13 14] which include much of the Aldermaston study area. A study has therefore been initiated of the incidence of such malignancies (by subtype), as well as adult leukaemias, in relation to commuting change.

Investigations by the Committee on Medical Aspects of Radiation in the Environment indicate that the tiny amounts of radiation released into the environment from Aldermaston and Burghfield are too small to cause the increased incidence of leukaemia in their vicinity, which they were unable to explain. However, they regarded a hypothesis about disturbances of herd immunity by population mixes as irrelevant because there had been no sudden population influx into a somewhat isolated area as in the first reported test of the idea.[1] The present study offers an explanation that is consistent with that hypothesis and with the observations in new towns.[1 2] Moreover it is supported by the finding of similar excesses in areas without nuclear installations but which, like the area around Aldermaston and Burghfield, have recently experienced large increases in commuting levels.

A relevant question is whether the prevalence of any infectious disease has also increased in the districts that have experienced the greatest increases of commuting. Published data are limited to only a few infectious diseases, but none show any clear increase in the highest tenth group (data not shown). However, it may be noted that none of those diseases shows a close similarity to the type of disorder to which childhood leukaemia is postulated as belonging.

These findings are consistent with other evidence about the relevance of increases in social contact to the aetiology of childhood leukaemia. As such they represent further support for an infection-based hypothesis for the disease. More specifically they suggest that these contacts can occur (a) between adults, therefore affecting children only indirectly and (b) not only in the home community,[2] but also at work or in travelling to work between residents of different communities. These characteristics are far from unique. Meningococci and the polio viruses are examples of agents that can be transmitted not only among children but also among adults and from adults to children. The present study as well as other work[12] suggest that, because of their relevance to herd immunity, population dynamics in their *widest* sense should be considered in communities in which excesses of childhood leukaemia are recorded.[9] In the case of individual-based studies, such effects may not be reliably detected by comparison of cases with controls drawn from the same community.

We thank Helena Strange for clerical help, David Dipple, Janette Wallis and Fiona O'Brien for computing help, and Susan Hill for secretarial assistance. We are also grateful to Dr Paula Cook-Mozaffari and Dr Eve Roman for providing estimated proportions of the children in the Aldermaston and Burghfield study area by county district, and to Dr Robin Mole and Professor David Galton for helpful comments on an earlier draft. We thank the Office of Population Censuses and Surveys, the information and statistics division of the Common Services Agency of the Scottish Health Service, the registrar general for Scotland, regional cancer registries, clinical trial organisers and the UK Children's Cancer Study Group for providing notifications of childhood leukaemia cases. We are grateful to colleagues at the Childhood Cancer Research Group for their work on the national registry of childhood tumours, in particular Mr M Loach for computing and Mrs M Allen and Dr E L Lennox for their part in collecting medical data.

The CRC Cancer Epidemiology Research Group is entirely funded by the Cancer Research Campaign from which LJK holds a Gibb Fellowship. The Childhood Cancer Research Group is supported by the Department of Health and the Scottish Home and Health Department.

Addendum

A correction for multiple comparisons, omitted from table III, changes the significance levels, so that $p < 0.001$ becomes $p < 0.01$ and $p < 0.01$ becomes $p < 0.05$.

1 Kinlen L. Evidence for an infective cause of childhood leukaemia: comparison of a Scottish new town with nuclear reprocessing sites in Britain. *Lancet* 1988;**ii**:1323.

2 Kinlen LJ, Clarke K, Hudson C. Evidence from population mixing in British new towns 1946–85 of an infective basis for childhood leukaemia. *Lancet* 1990;**360**:577.

3 Barton CJ, Roman E, Ryder HM, Watson A. Childhood leukaemia in west Berkshire. *Lancet* 1985;**ii**,1248.

4 Roman E, Beral V, Carpenter L, *et al*. Childhood leukaemia in the West Berkshire and Basingstoke and North Hampshire District Health Authorities in relation to nuclear establishments in the vicinity. *BMJ* 1987;**294**,597.

5 Stiller CA. Descriptive epidemiology of childhood leukaemia and lymphoma in Great Britain. *Leuk Res* 1985;**6**:671.

6 Lawton R. The journey to work in Britain: some trends and problems. *Regional Studies* 1968;**2**:27.

7 Hall P, Thomas R, Gracey H, Drewett R. *The containment of urban England: 1. Urban and metropolitan growth processes or Megalopolis denied*. Allen & Unwin: London, 1973.

8 Champion AG, Green AE, Owen DW, Ellin DJ, Coombes MG. *Changing places*. Edward Arnold: London, 1987.

9 Kellett CE. Acute leukaemia in one of identical twins. *Arch Dis Child* 1937;**12**:239.

10 Smith PG. Spatial and temporal clustering. In: Schottenfeld D, Fraumeni JR, eds. *Cancer epidemiology and prevention*. Philadelphia: W B Saunders, 1982.

11 Census of England and Wales 1921. *General Report. Part XI. Workplaces*. HMSO: London, 1927.

12 Langford I, Bentham G. Infectious aetiology of childhood leukaemia (letter). *Lancet* 1990;**360**:945.

13 Committee on Medical Aspects of Radiation in the Environment (COMARE). *Third Report: Report on the incidence of childhood cancer in West Berkshire and North Hampshire area, in which are situated the Atomics Weapons Research Establishment, Aldermaston and the Royal Ordnance Factory, Burghfield*. Chairman: Professor M. Bobrow. HMSO: London, 1989.

14 Cook-Mozaffari PJ, Ashwood FL, Vincent T, Forman D, Alderson M. *Cancer incidence and mortality in the vicinity of nuclear installation. England and Wales, 1959–80*. London: HMSO, 1987. (Office of Population Censuses and Surveys. Studies on Medical and Population Subjects, No. 51.)

33: Leukaemia in children and paternal radiation exposure at the Sellafield nuclear site

MARTIN J GARDNER

Childhood cancer around nuclear installations has been studied in recent years, particularly in the United Kingdom but also in other countries. The early studies were prompted by the suggestion of a 10-fold raised level of childhood leukaemia around the Sellafield nuclear site in England, which was confirmed and followed by the identification of generally smaller excesses around some (but not all) other nuclear sites in the United Kingdom. Pronounced excesses have not been reported in other countries. The increased leukaemia rate around Sellafield has been further investigated by examining individual cases in detail in epidemiological cohort and case-control studies. The raised incidence seems to have been concentrated in children born in the local area, but not among children who moved in after birth, and was particularly associated with fathers who had experienced higher levels of occupational external ionising radiation exposure at Sellafield before their relevant child's conception. The underlying cause of this statistical association is not yet clear, but the findings have important potential implications for radiobiology and for protecting radiation workers and their children.

The Sellafield site is located in north west England on the coast of west Cumbria. The site was acquired in 1947 for the production of plutonium for defence purposes, two nuclear reactors and a spent fuel reprocessing plant were in operation by 1952. These reactors and the reprocessing plant were subsequently closed and replaced between 1956 and 1963 with five additional nuclear reactors (one of which was closed in 1981); in 1964, the reprocessing plant was replaced. The Sellafield plant reprocesses spent fuel from nuclear power stations in the United Kingdom and abroad and has both stored and discharged to the sea low-level radioactive waste—solid and liquid waste, respectively.

A 1983 television documentary suggested that the rate of childhood leukaemia was high in the locality of the Sellafield site and alleged that these high rates were linked to the environmental discharges of radiation from the plant. A committee of inquiry into the allegations reported in 1984,[1] and three features are relevant here. Firstly, geographical analyses of routinely collected cancer registration and mortality data on children enabled the committee to conclude that leukaemia rates in the vicinity of Sellafield were indeed high, if not totally extreme, in the regional and national picture. Secondly, analyses using models of the average radiation dose to the bone marrow received as a consequence of the radioactive discharges from Sellafield did not support the view that an environmental pathway was involved. Thirdly, the report recommended carrying out detailed epidemiological studies in an attempt to explore further the childhood leukaemia excess and any potential explanations.

Epidemiological studies

COHORT STUDIES

The village of Seascale, which is about 3 km south of Sellafield site, had been particularly implicated as having a raised level of childhood leukaemia. It was therefore decided to study all children who at some stage of their lives had resided in the village, particularly to overcome some of the disadvantages of geographical analyses and to include observations on children after they had moved away from Seascale. These cohort studies included, as far as possible, all children born since 1950 who at some age lived in Seascale.[23] Their names and other particulars were identified from birth and school registers, and the cohorts comprised 1068 children born in Seascale and a further 1546 children who attended schools in Seascale after having been born elsewhere. Records of mortality and cancer registration on these children were obtained, and the findings confirmed the geographical analyses of a raised level of leukaemia among Seascale children. However, the excess appeared to be concentrated among children born in Seascale in contrast to those moving in after birth to attend one of the local schools (table I). Thus there was a 10-fold excess of leukaemia and a twofold excess of other cancers among the births, with no increased rates

TABLE I—*Leukaemia and other cancer cases during 1950–86 in Seascale birth and school cohorts*

Diagnosis cohort	No of cases			95% Confidence interval for O/E
	Observed (O)	Expected (E)*	O/E	
Leukaemia				
Birth	6†	0·6	10·0	3·7 to 21·8
Schools	0	0·6	0	0 to 6·2
Other cancers				
Birth	6	2·2	2·7	1·0 to 5·9
Schools	4	3·4	1·2	0·3 to 3·0

*At rates specific for age, sex, and calendar period for England and Wales.

†Five children with leukaemia were diagnosed while resident in Seascale and are included in the case-control study (see fig).

among the schoolchildren who moved to Seascale after birth. The differential findings in the birth and school cohorts suggested that one or more factors might have acted on a locality-specific basis before birth or early in life to produce the increased childhood leukaemia rate.

CASE-CONTROL STUDY

A case-control study has been carried out including all cases of leukaemia and lymphoma diagnosed at less than 25 years of age in the west Cumbria area between 1950 and 1985.[45] This area was chosen to include coastal and inland areas where concern had been raised about potential risks from radiation contamination due to discharges to sea and air from the nuclear plant and to cover the places of residence of the Sellafield workforce.

The aim was to obtain information on individual cases and control subjects that might help to explain the excesses found in the geographical and cohort studies. Factors examined included prenatal *x* ray exposure as the only generally accepted cause for childhood leukaemia, various suspected risk factors (such as viral illnesses, social class, and maternal age), behavioural habits (for example, eating fresh seafood and playing on the beach, which might have enhanced exposure to radionuclides released from Sellafield), and parental occupation and radiation exposure at Sellafield. The control children for the study were taken from the same birth registers into which the case subjects' births were entered. For each case subject, two sets of eight control subjects were taken of the same sex and adjacent in date of birth, with one set covering the total birth registration area (area control subjects) and the other set confined to the same local village where the case subject was born (local control subjects).

The identifying details on the parents of the case and control subjects

TABLE II—*Relative risks for childhood leukaemia by father's external ionising radiation dose during employment at Sellafield before child's conception*

Radiation dose (mSv)	No of cases	Local control subjects	Odds ratio	95% Confidence interval
Total before conception				
0	38	236	1·0	
>0–49	3	26	0·8	0·2 to 3·0
50–99	1	11	0·8	0·1 to 7·7
⩾100	4	3	8·4	1·4 to 52·0
Six months before conception				
0	38	246	1·0	
>0–4	3	24	1·1	0·3 to 4·9
5–9	1	3	3·0	0·3 to 32·6
⩾10	4	3	8·2	1·6 to 41·7

were cross linked with the past and present Sellafield workforce file; when matches were found, individual records of external ionising radiation exposure were obtained from British Nuclear Fuels. It was in this respect that the most important result was identified, although the expected geographical distribution of leukaemia and association with prenatal *x* rays were also found.[4]

The relation between preconceptual radiation dose of the fathers during their employment and leukaemia in their children is shown in table II for local control subjects. High relative risks are found for paternal exposures over 100 millisieverts (mSv) accumulated during their total preconceptual employment period and over 10 mSv during the six months before their relevant child's conception, albeit based on small numbers. Three of the four cases in the upper ranges were born in Seascale. Of the remaining three Seascale case children with leukaemia shown in table I, the father of one had an accumulated preconceptual radiation dose of 96 mSv, and the father of another has not yet been linked to the Sellafield workforce file; the third case was diagnosed after leaving west Cumbria and was therefore excluded from this case-control study. The findings in relation to local control subjects for Seascale case children are shown in the figure, which shows that each of the four linked case fathers had higher radiation doses than all the matched control fathers. Comparable results were found for area control subjects. Data from questionnaires to parents did not suggest any relation of childhood leukaemia to potential sources of enhanced exposure to radionuclides discharged to sea from the nuclear site. Similar results in relation to father's employment at Sellafield were found for non-Hodgkin's lymphoma, although the number of cases was smaller, but not for Hodgkin's disease. The contrast is interesting because Hodgkin's disease is not thought of as a radiation-related condition.

297

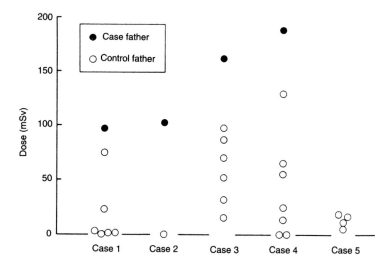

FIG 1—*Accumulated external ionising radiation dose during employment at Sellafield before children's conception in fathers of Seascale leukaemia case subjects and Seascale control subjects (the father of case 5 has not yet been linked to radiation dosimetry records).*

Discussion

The association of childhood leukaemia with the father's dose of radiation during employment at Sellafield is sufficiently strong to explain statistically the excess incidence rate in Seascale, but the interpretation in terms of a related causal mechanism, if there is one, is not known. Although there is one animal laboratory study that suggests a pathway involving radiation of the father,[6] the examination of radionuclides and other occupational exposures is under way. In the meantime, radiation exposure of workers at Sellafield has been declining from the peak levels of the 1950s, and no cases of children with leukaemia born since 1975 in Seascale are currently known. Further potential preventive measures, such as trials of personal dosimeters that emit an audible signal at a given raised dose rate, together with educational diagrams and leaflets, are being used.

In other countries, geographical analyses have not consistently found raised levels of childhood leukaemia near nuclear installations as in the United Kingdom. However, the geographical areas used have sometimes been too large for a localised effect to be shown. Consideration is now being given to case-control studies, such as described in this chapter, being carried out in the United States and France. Two other studies are currently under way in the United Kingdom.

1 Black D for the Independent Advisory Group. *Investigation of the possible increased incidence of cancer in west Cumbria.* London: HMSO, 1984. (Black report.)

2 Gardner MJ, Hall AJ, Downes S, *et al.* Follow up study of children born to mothers resident in Seascale, west Cumbria (birth cohort). *BMJ* 1987;**295**:822–7.

3 Gardner MJ, Hall AJ, Downes S, *et al.* Follow up study of children born elsewhere but attending schools in Seascale, west Cumbria (schools cohort). BMJ 1987; **295**:819–22.

4 Gardner MJ, Snee MP, Hall AJ, *et al.* Results of case-control study of leukaemia and lymphoma among young people near Sellafield nuclear plant in west Cumbria. *BMJ* 1990;**300**:423–9.

5 Gardner MJ, Hall AJ, Snee MP, *et al.* Methods and basic data of case-control study of leukaemia and lymphoma among young people near Sellafield nuclear plant in west Cumbria. *BMJ* 1990;**300**:429–34.

6 Nomura T. Parental exposure to X-rays and chemicals induces heritable tumours and anomalies in mice. *Nature* 1982;**296**:575–7.

34: Incidence of leukaemia and other cancers in birth and schools cohorts in the Dounreay area

ROGER J BLACK, JAMES D URQUHART,
STEPHEN W KENDRICK, KATHRYN J BUNCH,
JAN WARNER, DAVID ADAMS JONES

An excess of childhood leukaemia in the Dounreay area of Caithness, Scotland, has been observed. To examine whether the excess was in children born to local mothers or in those who moved to the area after birth (and also whether any cases of cancer have occurred in children born near Dounreay who may have moved elsewhere) a follow up study was undertaken of 4144 children born in the Dounreay area during 1969–88 (birth cohort) and 1641 who attended local schools during the same period but who had been born elsewhere (schools cohort). Main outcome measures were cancer registration records linked to birth and schools records by using computerised probability matching methods.

Five cancer registrations were traced from the birth cohort compared with 5·8 expected on the basis of national rates (observed to expected ratio 0·9; 95% confidence interval 0·3 to 2·0). All five cases were of leukaemia (2·3; 0·7 to 5·4). In the schools cohort three cases were found (2·1; 0·4 to 6·2), all of which were of leukaemia (6·7; 1·4 to 19·5). All eight children lived in the Dounreay area at the time of diagnosis; thus no cases were found in children who had been born in, or had attended school in, the study area but had subsequently moved away.

The raised incidence of childhood leukaemia in both the birth and schools cohorts suggests that place of birth was not a more important factor than place of residence in the series of cases of leukaemia observed near the Dounreay area.

Introduction

In 1986 a higher than expected incidence of leukaemia was observed in young people resident in the vicinity of the Dounreay nuclear reprocessing plant. This finding arose in a study carried out in anticipation of a local public inquiry into a proposed development of the plant.[1-3] Results of the study were referred to the Committee on Medical Aspects of Radiation in the Environment (COMARE) for further consideration. The committee accepted the evidence of a raised incidence of leukaemia in young people in the Dounreay area and made two recommendations for further epidemiological studies.[4] The first of these, a case-control study of young people registered as cases of leukaemia or non-Hodgkin's lymphoma, investigated a range of potential risk factors and has been presented elsewhere.[5] The committee also called for a study of birth and schools cohorts to assess, firstly, whether the excess of leukaemia cases occurred in children born to mothers resident in the Dounreay area or in children who moved to the area after birth and, secondly, whether any cases occurred in children born near Dounreay who may have moved elsewhere. This chapter reports the results of an investigation of cancer incidence in birth and schools cohorts in the Dounreay area, carried out in response to the second COMARE recommendation.

The sequence of investigation described above mirrors very closely that already undertaken in relation to the Sellafield nuclear fuel reprocessing plant in west Cumbria. Indeed, the rationale and aims of the present study are identical to those described by Gardner et al in two papers reporting studies of birth and schools cohorts in Seascale, a civil parish near the Sellafield plant.[6 7] Gardner et al pointed to two methodological weaknesses in earlier studies of cancer incidence and mortality in the Sellafield area[8 9] that also apply to the Dounreay incidence studies. Firstly, in conventional geographical analyses of disease incidence the person years for the risk of contracting the disease in the area of interest are estimated either from population estimates for large adminstrative areas or, if these are not available, by interpolation of census counts between census years. In the Dounreay studies the interpolation method was used. However, population estimates derived in this way cannot take account of variations in the local birth rate that might influence the person years at risk in young age groups. Furthermore, the Dounreay area has been shown to have experienced rapid demographic change in the 1960s.[10] Large numbers of young families

301

settling in an area in a relatively short period of time might result in an unusual or unstable pattern of births. The cohort (follow up) approach overcomes these potential problems by linking incident cases directly to population denominators. Secondly, the earlier Dounreay studies were based on children's places of residence at the time of diagnosis. This means that cases that might have been diagnosed in children who moved from the area were not included in calculating the local incidence of leukaemia. Conversely, cases in children moving to the Dounreay area before diagnosis would have been included.

The Seascale cohort studies showed that the excess leukaemia mortality in children resident in the parish had occurred mainly in those who were also born there.[67] More recent evidence from the case control study of leukaemia in west Cumbria suggests that the excess incidence of childhood leukaemia in Seascale might be explained by occupational exposures of fathers to radiation in the period immediately before conception.[11] Taken together, these observations suggest that place of birth might be more important than place of residence at the time of diagnosis in the aetiology of childhood leukaemia. The cohort approach used in this study addresses the question of place of birth by treating as two distinct groups those born in the Dounreay area and those who attended school there, having been born elsewhere.

The Sellafield and Dounreay sites differ from most other nuclear installations in that both are involved in reprocessing spent nuclear fuel. Although there are important differences in levels of discharges to the environment, the similarity of the plants' operations has been interpreted as potentially important in attempting to reach an explanation for the higher than expected incidence of leukaemia observed near both sites. This chapter aims to present an analysis of cancer incidence in birth and schools cohorts in the Dounreay area which, within the constraints of the availability of basic data, is comparable with the Seascale cohort studies.

Methods

SCHOOL RECORDS

The Dounreay site became operational in 1958. The original intention of the study was to seek school records of children born from 1958 who attended primary schools in the area. In defining schools to be included in the study, those in the parishes of Reay, Halkirk, Thurso, Olrig, and Bower were chosen because, firstly, the geography of these areas approximates to the 25 km zone around the Dounreay site analysed by COMARE;[4] secondly, birth records in Scotland are organised in registration districts which, in the Caithness area, are coterminous with parishes; and, thirdly, the parishes chosen form the western district as defined by Caithness County Council's education department in the period up to 1974. With the

TABLE I—*Schools in Dounreay area admitting children born since 1958*

Parish	School	Year opened	Year closed	Records available
Reay	Dounreay		1968	Yes
	Reay	1968		Yes
Halkirk	Scotscalder		1962	No
	Spittal		1970	No
	Halkirk			Yes
	Altnabreac		1978	No
	Lieurary	1978		Yes
Thurso	West Public		1967	No
	Janetstown		1970	No
	Weydale		1968	No
	Miller Academy			Yes
	Pennyland	1962		Yes
	Mount Pleasant			Yes
Olrig	Murkle		1970	No
	Castletown			Yes
Bower	Bower			No

assistance of Highland Regional Council's education department, 16 primary schools that could have admitted pupils born since 1958 were identified (table I).

In general the availabilty of admission records depended on whether or not schools had remained open after local government reorganisation in 1974. Inquiries were made at the Caithness district office of Highland Regional Council's education department in Wick, the regional council headquarters in Inverness, the regional archivist, local libraries, and public offices in an attempt to trace the admission records of schools closed before 1974. In addition, retired head teachers and county council officials were approached. These inquiries were unsuccessful and a reassessment of the feasibility of the study was made. It was decided to limit the study to children born since 1969 as, firstly, computer records of births in Scotland were available from 1969 and, secondly, complete coverage of school records for the study area was available only from 1971 (table I). It was thought to be important to achieve complete coverage of school records for a defined area so that children could be allocated to the appropriate cohorts. This reduced the number of potentially relevant schools to nine: Reay, Halkirk, Altnabreac, Lieurary, Miller Academy, Pennyland, Mount Pleasant, Castletown, and Bower. Of these, Bower and Altnabreac were excluded because they serve populations that are largely outside the 25 km zone around Dounreay. Admission records were available for the remaining seven schools.

Permission to extract identifying information from the records was sought from head teachers and this was granted in every case. The figure shows the boundaries of the areas chosen for analysis and the locations of

303

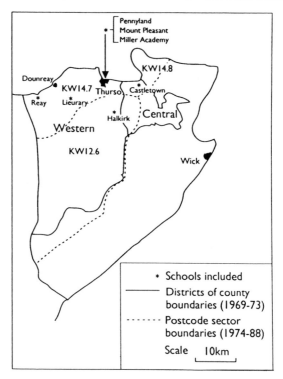

Study area of and location of schools in Caithness county from which records were obtained.

the schools included in the study. Children's full names (including second forenames and alternative surnames where recorded), sex, date of birth, and year of admission to school were keyed directly from photocopies of admission books for the period up to the end of 1988. These records were then verified and checked clerically in preparation for data analysis. Table II shows the numbers of admissions to each school.

BIRTH RECORDS

Registrations of births in Scotland are held by the General Register Office (Scotland) in the form of computer records from 1969. Before 1974 births were required to be registered in the registration district in which they occurred. Thereafter births could be registered at any office, often the nearest to a mother's usual place of residence. However, Scottish birth records contain allocation codes indicating mother's usual place of residence. These are based on districts of county and small burghs before 1974 and postcodes thereafter. Thus the general registrar office was able to supply a listing of births to mothers resident in the study area from which

TABLE II—*Numbers of children born in the period 1969–88 admitted to primary schools in the Dounreay area*

School	No of admissions
Reay	161
Halkirk	458
Lieurary*	260
Miller Academy	1355
Pennyland	1203
Mount Pleasant	936
Castletown	510
Total	4883

*Annual school rolls rather than admission books obtained.

the child's full name, sex, date of birth, registration district, and entry number were abstracted. Table III shows numbers of births ascertained in each of the study areas.

DATA LINKAGE

For allocating children to the birth or schools cohorts, the school admission records and the birth records were linked by using computerised probability matching techniques. The matching algorithms were based on techniques developed by the Oxford Record Linkage System[12] and Statistics Canada[13] and were part of an extensive programme of medical record linkage being carried out in the Common Services Agency of the Scottish Health Service. In addition, the results of the linkage were manually checked at each stage of the procedure. In a preliminary phase, the school records were linked internally to identify multiple entries for individual children which occurred, for example, where children had moved from one school to another. This linkage reduced the 4883 admission records to 3976

TABLE III—*Numbers of births to mothers resident in the Dounreay area, by area of residence and period of birth, 1969–88*

Area	Period of birth		Total
	1969–73	1974–88	
Thurso small burgh	756		756
Western district (of Caithness county)	247		247
Central district (of Caithness county)	147		147
KW14·7 postcode sector*		1568	1568
KW14·8 postcode sector		1144	1144
KW12·6 postcode sector		282	282
Total	1150	2994	4144

*Only the portion of KW14·7 within Caithness local government district was included.

TABLE IV—*Numbers of children allocated to birth and school cohorts by period of birth and school of first admission*

	Period of birth				
	1969–73	1974–78	1979–83	1984–88	Total
Birth cohort	1150	996	1077	951	4144
Schools cohort:	778	511	340	12	1641
Reay	36	13	12		61
Halkirk	51	45	43	1	140
Lieurary	2	2	2		6
Miller Academy	247	181	105	1	534
Mount Pleasant	77	58	48	9	192
Pennyland	272	166	95	1	534
Castletown	93	46	35		174

identifiable individuals. For 34 children either the date of birth or the sex was unknown and these records were excluded. The remaining 3942 records of identified school pupils were then linked with the birth records and 2301 were found to have been born in the study area, leaving a cohort of 1641 children who attended primary school in the study area, having been born elsewhere (the schools cohort). The birth cohort was made up of all children born in the study period from 1969 to 1988, including the 2301 who subsequently attended local schools. Table IV summarises the allocation of children to the two cohorts.

The Scottish national cancer registration scheme, administered by the Common Services Agency, holds records collected by five regional registries since 1959. Registrations of leukaemia in the 0–24 age group in the period 1968–81 have been reviewed and amended in a validation exercise[14] and the ascertainment rate and accuracy of data for this disease in more recent years is thought to be high.[1] For other childhood cancers, incidences calculated from Scottish cancer registration data are comparable with those of England and Wales and other northern European countries. The ascertainment rate is thought to be over 90%.[15] A file of registrations up to 31 December 1988 of cancers in those born since 1969 was extracted from the national data set. This was then linked with the birth and schools records by using the probability weighted matching procedures already described. All potential links were checked by tracing the manual records held at the regional registries and, if necessary, by referring to hospital notes. To verify the results of this linkage exercise and to attempt to ascertain cases that might have been registered outside Scotland, the birth and schools records were also linked with data held by the National Registry of Childhood Tumours.[16]

ANALYSIS

Expected numbers of cases were calculated by the allocation of person

TABLE V—*Numbers of children admitted to schools in the Dounreay area by cohort, period of admission, and age at admission*

	Birth cohort	Schools cohort
Period of admission:		
1969–73	1	
1974–78	819	563
1975–83	669	578
1984–88	812	500
Age at admission (years):		
3	268	48
4	1115	435
5	856	583
6	21	153
7	15	139
8	12	109
9	7	76
10	2	67
11	3	26
⩾12	2	5
No admission record	1843	
Total	4144	1641

years at risk based on Scottish national rates broken down by tumour site, sex, age, and calendar year of registration. For the birth cohort the person years at risk were allocated from the year of birth to the end of the study (31 December 1988) and for the schools cohort from the year of first admission to a local school to the end of the study. As no information on deaths or emigration was available no withdrawals were accounted for in calculating person years at risk. Results are expressed as ratios of observed to expected cases with Poisson based confidence intervals calculated by standard methods.[17]

Results

Table V shows a breakdown of year and age at first admission to schools in the study area for children allocated to the birth and schools cohorts. As might be expected from the pattern of births over time shown in table IV, the numbers of admissions to schools of children born in the study area fell from 819 in 1974–8 to 669 in 1979–83 and rose again to 812 in 1984–8. In the schools cohort the numbers of admissions over the period 1974–83 remained fairly constant at about 115 a year before falling to about 100 a year thereafter. A total of 1066 (65%) children in the schools cohort first attended a school in the study area at or before the age of 5.

Table VI shows the areas of residence at birth of the 2233 children who were born in the study area in the period 1969–83 and were admitted to local schools. The overall proportion (70%) seems to be consistent between

TABLE VI—*Numbers (and percentages of all births in area) of birth cohort children admitted to local schools by period of birth and area of residence at birth*

Period of birth and area of residence	No	Percentage of all births in area
No (%) born 1969–73:		
Thurso small burgh	514	68
Central district of county	104	71
Western district of county	172	70
No (%) born 1974–83:		
KW14·7 postcode sector	743	68
KW14·8 postcode sector	531	71
KW12·6 postcode sector	169	83
Total	2233	70

the areas and time periods considered. This implies a fairly constant outward movement before school age of about 30% of children born in the area. Children born in the last time period, 1984–8, have been excluded from this table as most would not have attained school age by the end of the study period.

In table VII the observed numbers of cancer registrations in the birth and schools cohorts are compared with expected numbers based on Scottish national rates. In the birth cohort five registrations were found compared with 5·8 expected (a ratio of 0·9; 95% confidence interval 0·3 to 2·0). All five cases were of leukaemia (2·3; 0·7 to 5·4). One case had originally been registered as non-Hodgkin's lymphoma and all were previously known to COMARE.[4] All were resident in the Dounreay area at the time of diagnosis; thus no cases were found in children who were born

TABLE VII—*Observed and expected registrations of malignant neoplasms (ICD 140–208) by tumour site and cohort*

Cohort and site	No observed (O)	No expected (E)	O·E ratio (95% confidence interval)
Birth cohort:	5	5·8	0·9 (0·3 to 2·0)
Leukaemia and non-Hodgkin's lymphoma	5	2·2	2·3 (0·7 to 5·4)
Hodgkin's disease		0·3	0 (0·0 to 13·8)
Other cancers		3·4	0 (0·0 to 1·1)
Schools cohort:	3	1·4	2·1 (0·4 to 6·2)
Leukaemia and non-Hodgkin's lymphoma	3	0·4	6·7 (1·4 to 19·5)
Hodgkin's disease		0·2	0 (0·0 to 24·2)
Other cancers		0·8	0 (0·0 to 4·5)

in the study area but who subsequently moved away. In the schools cohort, three registrations were found where 1·4 would be expected from national rates (2·1; 0·4 to 6·2). Again, all the cases were of leukaemia (6·7; 1·4–19·5). One case was included in the COMARE analysis.[4] COMARE was also aware of one other case, originally registered in 1986 as non-Hodgkin's lymphoma but considerd by COMARE to be leukaemia, although not included in the principal analysis. The third case, in a boy aged 16 at diagnosis in 1988, was previously unknown to COMARE. All three children were resident in the study area at the time of diagnosis. One child was born in Strathclyde region, the second in England, and the third in Highland region outside Caithness.

Table VIII shows that no particular pattern was evident in the years of birth or age at diagnosis of the cases found in the birth cohort, but all five cases in the birth cohort were registered in 1979–83. In the schools cohort, the existence of only three cases means that it is unlikely that there would be any discernible patterns, but, as with the cases in the birth cohort, all three occurred after 1979. School of first admission was not of interest even when the schools attended by children in the birth cohort were considered. One of the five birth cohort children died before school age, two attended Pennyland school, and the remaining two attended Lieurary and Castletown schools.

Discussion

The first aim of this study was to consider whether the excess of registrations of leukaemia and non-Hodgkin's lymphoma in children and young adults resident in the Dounreay area occurred in those born there or those who were born elsewhere. We have shown that the incidence of leukaemia and non-Hodgkin's lymphoma was raised in both the birth and schools cohorts (observed to expected ratios of 2·3 and 6·7 respectively). The second main aim of the study was to attempt to ascertain cases of leukaemia, non-Hodgkin's lymphoma, and other cancers in those born in the Dounreay area who might have moved elsewhere before being registered as cancer cases. No such cases were found.

A secondary intention in the study was to assess the incidence of leukaemia and non-Hodgkin's lymphoma in the Dounreay area on the basis of the exact allocation of person years at risk and the follow up method of ascertainment. Taken separately, the incidence of these diseases in the birth and schools cohorts studied is raised, but significantly so only in the schools cohort. Considered together, the observation of eight cases of leukaemia and non-Hodgkin's lymphoma compared with 2·6 expected on the basis of national rates (3·0; 1·5 to 5·5) is not inconsistent with the eight cases of leukaemia and non-Hodgkin's lymphoma observed in the 25 km zone in the period 1968–84 compared with 3·9 expected (2·1; 1·0 to 3·7)

TABLE VIII—*Observed and expected registrations of malignant neoplasms (ICD 140–208) by cohort, period of birth, age, sex, period of follow up, and school of first admission*

	No observed (O)	No expected (E)	O/E ratio (95% confidence interval)
	Birth cohort		
Period of birth:			
1969–73	1	2·5	0·4 (0·1 to 2·2)
1974–78	3	1·6	1·9 (0·4 to 5·6)
1979–83	1	1·2	0·8 (0·0 to 4·4)
1984–88		0·5	0 (0.0 to 7·1)
Age:			
0		0·7	0 (0·0 to 5·5)
1–4	3	2·5	1·2 (0·3 to 3·6)
5–9	2	1·4	1·4 (0·2 to 5·1)
10–14		0·7	0 (0·0 to 5·2)
15–19		0·6	0 (0·0 to 6·4)
Sex:			
Male	2	3·3	0·6 (0·1 to 2·2)
Female	3	2·5	1·2 (0·2 to 3·5)
Period of follow up:			
1969–73		0·5	0 (0·0 to 7·3)
1974–78		1·2	0 (0·0 to 2·9)
1979–83	5	1·7	3·0 (1·0 to 7·0)
1984–88		2·4	0 (0·0 to 1·5)
	Schools cohort		
Period of birth:			
1969–73	2	1·0	2·1 (0·3 to 7·5)
1974–78	1	0·3	2·9 (0·1 to 15·9)
1979–83		0·1	0 (0·0 to 39·1)
Age:			
5–9		0·5	0 (0·0 to 6·7)
10–14	2	0·5	4·4 (0·5 to 15·9)
15–19	1	0·4	2·6 (0·1 to 14·5)
Sex:			
Male	1	0·8	1·2 (0·4 to 6·9)
Female	2	0·6	3·3 (0·4 to 11·9)
Period of follow up:			
1974–78		0·2	0 (0·0 to 22·0)
1979–83	1	0·4	2·4 (0·1 to 13·5)
1984–88	2	0·8	2·4 (0·3 to 8·7)
School:			
Reay		0·1	0 (0·0 to 60·0)
Halkirk		0·1	0 (0·0 to 36·4)
Lieurary		0	0 (0·0 to >99·9)
Miller Academy	2	0·5	4·4 (0·5 to 15·9)
Mount Pleasant		0·2	0 (0·0 to 21·7)
Pennyland	1	0·5	2·1 (0·1 to 24·6)
Castletown		0·2	0 (0·0 to 23·5)

reported by COMARE.[4] Thus, even though the mobility of the population at risk has been shown to be high, the incidence rates of leukaemia and non-

Hodgkin's lymphoma reported in the earlier geographical studies did not overestimate risk in the local population.

CHOICE OF METHOD

The similarities of the operations carried out at Sellafield and Dounreay, even though levels of discharges to the environment were greater at Sellafield, and the findings of raised leukaemia incidence near both sites lead inevitably to the need to consider the results reported here for the Dounreay area in the light of those reported by Gardner *et al* for Seascale. Important differences in the methodologies used in the two studies must, however, be considered. Ascertainment in the Seascale studies was by manual searches of the NHS central register, principally for notifications of death. In contrast, the present study used computerised methods to link school and birth records to cancer registration records. There were three main reasons for this choice of method. Firstly, the present study included many more subjects: 5785 compared with 2614 in the Seascale studies. Secondly, computerised birth and cancer registration records were available for the period for which school admission records were also available. Thirdly, the improving prognosis for many childhood cancer patients, particularly those with leukaemia (the five year survival rate in the 0–4 age group in Scotland in 1978–82 was 53%), means that incidence data are now a more reliable basis than mortality data for estimating the risk of these diseases.

An advantage of using searches of the NHS central register is that emigrants and subjects dying from causes other than cancer can be withdrawn from the calculation of person years at risk of dying from cancer. No such adjustment was made in the present study. If the proportion of emigrants and deaths from other causes in the Seascale schools cohort study were to apply to the Dounreay area then the person years at risk would be overestimated by approximately 5%. Overestimation of this order would not affect the interpretation and overall conclusions drawn from this study. In the Seascale studies, the success of the searches of the register in tracing all cases of leukaemia expected from earlier studies led the authors to express confidence in the method of ascertainment. In the present study, all cases anticipated on the basis of the COMARE investigation of the Dounreay area were found.

CASE FINDING

Of the eight cases described in the COMARE report in the 25 km zone around Dounreay in the period 1968–84, five were found in the birth cohort and one in the schools cohort. The remaining two cases were subjects born before 1969, the earliest year for which births were included. One had been born in England and the other in Caithness, within the area covered in the present study. Thus all cases expected in this study were found by the computerised record linkage method used. The range of values of the linkage scores (which are proportional to the probability that two linked records relate to the same individual) for those cases expected was 24·6 to 36·6, but any potential matches with scores of 10·0 or more were checked manually. Thus it is unlikely that the absence of any cancer registrations in subjects who move away from the Dounreay area could be an artefact of the method of ascertainment used.

Although an investigation of the levels of population mobility was not one of the aims of this study, the basic results obtained are broadly comparable with those from Seascale. About 30% of children born in the Dounreay area did not attend schools there, compared with 43% in the Seascale studies. Of those assumed to have moved to the Dounreay area after birth, 65% did so before attaining school age compared with 60% in the Seascale studies.

CONCLUSIONS

The main finding of this study is the raised incidence of leukaemia and non-Hodgkin's lymphoma in both the birth and schools cohorts. Although the ratio of leukaemia mortality in the Seascale birth and schools cohorts was not significantly greater than unity, the finding that most cases occurred in the birth cohort and the more recent results of the west Cumbria case control study[11] focused attention on potential risk factors associated with place of birth rather than place of residence at the time of diagnosis of the cases of leukaemia found in the Seascale and Dounreay areas. The results of the present study and the previously reported case-control study[5] suggest that place of birth is not a more important factor than place of residence at diagnosis in the series of cases of leukaemia and non-Hodgkin's lymphoma observed in the Dounreay area. Furthermore, no important trends in the years of birth of the cases were found. In an analysis of periods of birth and diagnosis and of sex and age at diagnosis only the period of diagnosis seemed to be important. All eight cases of leukaemia were diagnosed after 1978, six of these in the period 1979–83. The most remarkable features of this series of cases in the Dounreay area remain their concentration in a relatively short period of time and the common diagnosis of leukaemia with a complete absence of all other types of childhood cancer.

We thank the General Register Office (Scotland) and in particular Miss Christine Rae and Mr Jack Arrundale for their valuable advice on birth records in Scotland; Highland Regional Council Education Department; and the head teachers of the schools in Caithness from which we sought admission records. We also thank the Office of Population Censuses and Surveys, the regional cancer registries, and the many organisations and individuals who contribute to the national cancer registers in Scotland and in England and Wales, and the National Registry of Childhood Tumours at the Childhood Cancer Research Group. We thank Mr Graeme Hunter,

Miss Jill Morrison, Miss Antonia Romero, and other staff of Common Services Agency Information and Statistics Division involved in the collection and preparation of data. We are grateful to Professor M Bobrow, Dr G J Draper, and Professor M J Gardner, who kindly commented on an earlier version of the chapter. The study was partially funded from a Scottish Home and Health Department grant. The Childhood Cancer Research Group is supported by the Department of Health and the Scottish Home and Health Department.

1 Heasman MA, Urquhart JD, Kemp IW, Black RJ. Childhood leukaemia in Northern Scotland. *Lancet* 1986;**i**:266,385.

2 Heasman MA, Urquhart JD, Black RJ, Kemp IW, Glass S, Gray M. Leukaemia in young persons in Scotland: a study of its geographical distribution and relationship to nuclear installations. *Health Bull (Edinb)* 1987;**45**:147.

3 Bell AG. *Report of the Dounreay EDRP public local injury relating to the planning application for the siting of the European Demonstration Reprocessing Plant (EDRP) for fast reactor fuel (Caithness, 7 April–25 November 1986)*. Edinburgh: Scottish Office, 1989.

4 Committee on Medical Aspects of Radiation in the Environment. *Investigation of the possible increased incidence of leukaemia in young people near the Dounreay nuclear establishment, Caithness, Scotland* London: HMSO, 1988. (COMARE 2nd report.)

5 Urquhart JD, Black RJ, Muirhead MJ, Sharp L, Maxwell M, Eden OB, *et al*. Case control study of leukaemia and non-Hodgkin's lymphoma in children in Caithness near the Dounreay nuclear installation. *BMJ* 1991;**302**:687–92.

6 Gardner MJ, Hall AJ, Downes S, Terrell JD. Follow up study of children born elsewhere but attending schools in Seascale, west Cumbria (schools cohort). *BMJ* 1987;**295**:819–22.

7 Gardner MJ, Hall AJ, Downes S, Terrell JD. Follow up study of children born to mothers resident in Seascale, west Cumbria (birth cohort). *BMJ* 1987;**295**:822–7.

8 Black D for the Independent Advisory Group. *Investigation of the possible increased incidence of cancer in west Cumbria*. London: HMSO, 1984. (Black report.)

9 Gardner MJ, Winter PD. Mortality in Cumberland during 1959–78 with reference to cancer in young people around Windscale. *Lancet* 1984;**i**:216–7.

10 Kinlen L. Evidence for an infective cause of childhood leukaemia: a comparison of a Scottish new town with nuclear reprocessing sites in Britain. *Lancet* 1988;**ii**:1323.

11 Gardner MJ, Snee MP, Hall A, Powell CA, Downes S, Terrell JD. Results of a case-control study of leukaemia and lymphoma among young people near the Sellafield nuclear plant in west Cumbria. *BMJ* 1990;**300**:423–9.

12 Baldwin JA, Acheson ED, Graham WJ, eds. *Textbook of medical record linkage*. Oxford: Oxford University Press, 1987.

13 Newcombe HM. *Handbook of record linkage*. Oxford: Oxford University Press, 1988.

14 Glass S, Gray M, Eden OB, Hann IM. Scottish validation study of cancer registration data for childhood leukaemia 1968–81. *Leuk Res* 1987;**2**:881.

15 Stiller CA, Kemp I, Draper GJ, Fearnly H, Lennox EL, Roberts EM, *et al*. United Kingdom—Scotland: National Registry of Childhood Tumours, 1971–80. In: Parkin DM, Stiller CA, Draper GJ, Bieber CA, Terracini B, Young JL, eds. *International incidence of childhood cancer*. Lyon: International Agency for Research on Cancer, 1988. Scientific publication, No 87.)

16 Draper GJ, Stiller CA, Fearnly H, Lennox EL, Roberts EM, Sanders BM. United Kindgom—England and Wales: National Registry of Childhood Tumours, 1971–80. In: Parkin DM, Stiller CA, Draper GJ, Bieber CA, Terracini B, Young JL, eds. *International incidence of childhood cancer*. Lyon: International Agency for Research on Cancer, 1988. (Scientific publication, No 87.)

17 Breslow NE, Day NE. *Statistical methods in cancer research*. Vol II. *The design and analysis of cohort studies*. Lyon: International Agency for Research on Cancer, 1987. (Scientific publication, No 82.)

35: Cancer in Cumbria and in the vicinity of the Sellafield nuclear installation, 1963–90

G J DRAPER, C A STILLER, R A CARTWRIGHT,
A W CRAFT, T J VINCENT

The Black advisory group reported a possible excess of malignant disease, particularly childhood acute lymphoid leukaemia and non-Hodgkin's lymphomas, near the Sellafield nuclear installation. To assess whether any excess of malignant disease had occurred among people in the area aged 0–24 during 1984–90—that is, since the Black report—incidences of cancer were calculated for all people aged up to 75 resident in: England and Wales, the county of Cumbria, the county districts Allerdale and Copeland within Cumbria, and Seascale ward within Copeland.

Data were obtained, from population based cancer registries and special surveys, of the number of cases and incidence of cancer (particularly of lymphoid leukaemia and non-Hodgkin's lymphomas) in all residents in the above areas aged 0–75, but with particular reference to those aged 0–24.

Previous reports of an increased incidence of cancer, especially leukaemia, among people aged 0–24 in Seascale up to and including 1983 are confirmed. During 1984–90 there was an excess of total cancer among those aged 0–24, based on four cases (including two of non-Hodgkin's lymphoma but none of leukaemia). In the same period there was an increased, but non-significant, incidence of other cancers among those aged

15–24, based on two cases (one pinealoma and one Hodgkin's disease), but not in those aged 0–15 and not before 1984. In the immediately surrounding area—that is, the county districts of Allerdale and Copeland excluding Seascale and in the remainder of Cumbria—there was no evidence of an increased incidence of cancer among those aged 0–24 in either period.

It is concluded that during 1963–83 and 1984–90 the incidence of malignant disease, particularly lymphoid leukaemia and non-Hodgkin's lymphomas, in people aged 0–24 was higher in Seascale than would be expected on the basis of either national rates or those for the surrounding areas. Although this increased risk is unlikely to be due to chance, the reasons for it are still unknown.

Introduction

In the past 10 years there have been many suggestions of an increased incidence of cancer, or of clusters of cases, near nuclear installations. The most detailed investigations have concerned the Sellafield nuclear reprocessing plant in west Cumbria. An advisory group chaired by Sir Douglas Black investigated the suggestion that there was an increased incidence of cancer near this installation. This group produced a report discussing the discharges around the site and the extent of radiation exposures and giving estimates of the likely risks.[1] The report included a series of epidemiological analyses and also contained lists of patients resident in Seascale and the surrounding area. The analyses covered a variety of diagnostic groups, age groups, and periods.

Few other areas have been the subject of systematic epidemiological studies: in the United Kingdom such studies include those of Dounreay,[2] of Aldermaston and Burghfield,[3] and of nuclear installations generally.[4]

Since the Black report further cohort and case-control studies of the area around Sellafield have been carried out,[5-7] but there has been no comprehensive analysis of cancer incidence.

The report includes analyses of the incidence of cancer among people aged 0–24 years during the period up to 1983. These analyses are based on more complete data than were available to the authors of the Black report. Although the data are not directly comparable with those in previously published analyses, they are nevertheless subject to the major criticism of the studies discussed in the Black report—namely, that the results were vitiated by biased selection of diagnostic groups, age groups, calendar

315

periods, and areas. Although the Black report does not contain any explicit statement about the period that it covers, none of the analyses on which it is based go beyond 1983. Our report is mainly concerned with 1984 onwards. In planning our analyses we were concerned to avoid the biases that affected the analyses of the period up to and including 1983; it was agreed in advance, at a meeting of a working group of the Committee on Medical Aspects of Radiation in the Environment, that the principal hypothesis to be tested should be that "no excess of leukaemia or other cancer in 0–24 year olds has occurred in the area of the Sellafield plant from 1984 to the present," and that the diagnostic groups, areas, and calendar periods to be analysed should be those set out below.

Methods

DIAGNOSTIC GROUPS

In planning this report it was agreed that the analyses would cover both total malignant disease around Sellafield and also several individual diagnostic groups. The diagnostic groups were defined as follows, the disease categories in brackets referring to the standard classification for childhood cancer:[8] (a) lymphoid leukaemia and non-Hodgkin's lymphomas, including Burkitt's lymphoma, unspecified lymphoma, and hairy cell leukaemia (I(a), I(b), II(b), II(c), II(d), plus ICD-O M code 9940/3; (b) all other and unspecified leukaemias (I(c), I(d), I(e) except ICD-O M code 9940/3; (c) Hodgkin's disease (II(a)); (d) brain and spinal tumours, including non-malignant tumours (III(a) to III(e)); and (e) all other malignant diseases (II(f), IV to XII).

Diagnostic group (a) was chosen in the light of discussions in the report on Dounreay (paras 2.27–2.30)[2] and of the conclusion of the working group that acute lymphoblastic leukaemia could be adequately distinguished from other leukaemia in our data. Chronic lymphocytic leukaemia never occurs in childhood, and so in children lymphoid leukaemia is equivalent to acute lymphoblastic leukaemia. Hairy cell leukaemia is now regarded as a variant of chronic lymphocytic leukaemia and has been grouped with it.[9]

Langerhans cell histiocytosis (histiocytosis X) was not included in the analyses as this group of diseases is not now regarded as neoplastic.

AREAS

The areas used throughout the study (figure) were (a) Seascale ward; (b) Allerdale and Copeland county districts (without Seascale), the two county districts nearest to Sellafield; (c) Cumbria county (without Allerdale and Copeland). All boundaries came into force with the local government reorganisation of 1974. Cases were assigned to areas according to their residence address at diagnosis as defined for the national cancer registration scheme.[10]

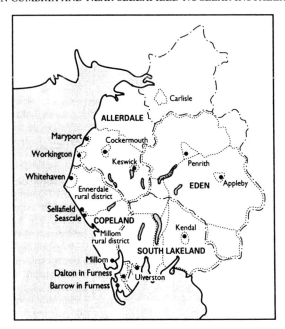

County of Cumbria showing districts before (----) and after (—·—·—·) its creation in 1974 (based on figure 2.3 of Black report[1])

CALENDAR PERIODS

Data are presented for 1963–83 and for 1984–90. The period 1984–90 does not overlap with any of the analyses covered in the Black report.

CASE ASCERTAINMENT

For the analyses of childhood cancers including leukaemias—that is, those diagnosed in children aged 0–14 years—data were obtained from the national registry of childhood tumours at the childhood cancer research group.[11] Cases are ascertained from cancer registries, the Northern region children's malignant disease registry (for 1968 onwards),[12] the Manchester children's tumour registry (for cases occurring before 1974 in the area now called south Cumbria),[13] death certificates, entries to the Medical Research Council leukaemia trials (1970 onwards), and the register of the United Kingdom Children's Cancer Study Group (1977 onwards). Details of the methods of ascertainment of cases and verification of diagnostic and other information have been published elsewhere.[11] For the areas in our study there was a high degree of completeness of ascertainment from 1968 onwards for children aged 0–14 because these areas are included in the data collected prospectively for the Northern region children's malignant dis-

317

ease registry and all these cases were included in the national registry of childhood tumours.

The analyses for people aged 15–24 were based mainly on data from the Northern region children's malignant disease registry, which originally covered only children aged 0–14 years but was extended, as a result of the recommendations of the Black advisory group, to people aged 15–24. For 1969–83 registrations at age 15–24 were obtained from the Northern region cancer registry and (for 1969–73 in what is now south Cumbria) the North Western regional cancer registry; in general, no further effort was made to ascertain cases.

Assertainment through regional cancer registries may not be complete,[13] and so a special search of hospital and pathology department records was made to ascertain any cases of leukaemia or lymphoma in Allerdale and Copeland for 1969–83 that might not previously have been registered. This resulted in the inclusion of a further four cases in addition to the 27 previously registered. From 1984 onwards cases have been ascertained direct from hospitals throughout the Northern region. Cumbria has been included in the Leukaemia Research Fund data collection study[9] since it began in 1984. The data collection study also ascertains cases of leukaemia and lymphoma direct from diagnostic sources within hospitals in its study areas, and these are cross checked with cancer registration records; ascertainment for these diagnositic groups is believed to be virtually complete. For 1984–90 a comparison between the Northern region's children's register and the data collection study found no additional cases for Allerdale and Copeland, but for the rest of Cumbria seven were added to the register.

Among people aged 25–74 the only analyses in this chapter are of leukaemia and lymphoma for 1984–90, using data derived from the data collection study.

POPULATION DATA

For the calculation of incidences we needed population estimates for five year groups for each of the years 1963–90. Census data and estimates from the Office of Population Censuses and Surveys were used wherever these were available. For Seascale in 1986 estimates from CACI Ltd were used. For other years estimates were made by linear interpolation, a proportionate adjustment being made if the total of the estimates so obtained for individual age groups did not agree with the independent estimate from the Office of Population Censuses and Surveys for all ages taken together.

INCIDENCE

Incidences were expressed as annual rates per million population. For ages 0–14 and 15–24 age standardised rates were calculated as simple averages of the age specific rates for the five year age groups they contained.

318

Standardised registration ratios were calculated by expressing the observed number of cases as a percentage of the expected number, the expected number being calculated by applying the national age specific rates calculated by applying the national age specific rates for each five year age group to the number of people in the population being considered.

COMPARISONS WITH NATIONAL DATA

On the one hand, the most obviously appropriate analyses of the incidences are comparisons of Seascale with the rest of Copeland plus Allerdale and of each of these areas with the rest of Cumbria, but such comparisons are based on comparatively small numbers. On the other hand, comparisons with national data may be less relevant in that there may be broad geographical variations either in incidence or in case ascertainment that would make it difficult to assess whether an increase in Seascale or Allerdale and Copeland was a local effect (and hence possibly related to Sellafield) or whether it affected the whole of Cumbria. By calculating rates for each of these areas it is possible to examine the geographical extent of any apparently local increase.

National data of the same quality used for the present analyses were not always available, though even 20% underregistration, which is unlikely, would not have affected the conclusions of this report. We compared the incidence in the study areas with national data using the following sources: for childhood cancer, data from the national registry of childhood tumours for 1969–87; for young people aged 15–24, cancer registration statistics for England and Wales for 1971–86, though these data were not subjected to the review processes carried out for the specialist registries; for leukaemias and lymphomas in those aged 25–74, data from the data collection study covering about one third of the population of England and Wales.[9]

Results

POPULATION ESTIMATES

Estimates for five year age groups and the calendar years 1963–90 are summarised in table I.

NATIONAL DATA ON CANCER REGISTRATIONS

Age standardised annual incidence of specific cancers for England and Wales is given in table II.

CASES OF CANCER IN YOUNG PEOPLE IN SEASCALE SINCE 1953

Table III lists all cases of cancer diagnosed during 1953–91 in people aged 0–24 in Seascale. We checked as far as possible the information for the cases listed in tables 2.1 to 2.4 of the Black report; in table III cross

TABLE I—*Summary of population estimates for areas within Cumbria*

Year	Age (years)		
	0–14	15–24	25–74
	Seascale		
1961*	606	176	—
1966†	604	218	—
1971*	602	259	—
1976†	506	299	—
1981*	411	339	—
1986‡	320	291	1126
1990†	302	234	1129
	Copeland and Allerdale minus Seascale		
1961*	41 990	21 852	—
1966†	41 718	23 215	—
1971‖	39 898	23 441	—
1976‖	37 694	24 101	—
1981‖	34 224	25 719	—
1986‖	30 885	25 514	98 988
1990‖	30 717	22 836	102 614
	Rest of Cumbria		
1961*	67 854	37 794	—
1966†	69 227	39 683	—
1971‖	70 400	42 200	—
1976‖	69 200	42 400	—
1981‖	61 049	46 624	—
1986‖	56 721	49 464	189 621
1990‖	55 926	44 855	196 978

*Census.
†Interpolated.
‡CACI Ltd.
‖Office of Population Censuses and Surveys.

references are given to the cases listed in these tables of the Black report and, when necessary, the information has been corrected. Ten cases diagnosed during 1963–90 (cases 4–13) were included in our analyses. One from the most recent period, 1984–90 (case 10 in table III), was included in the Black report but with the year of diagnosis given wrongly as 1983 instead of 1984. This case was notified to the Black advisory group during the course of its investigation and does not appear in any of the analyses in its report. We therefore included the case in our analysis for the post-Black period 1984–90 as this information should be regarded as testing rather than generating the Seascale hypothesis. One further patient (case 15 in table III) had a second address in another part of Britain, to which he should correctly be allocated under the rules followed by the national cancer registration scheme; he has therefore been excluded from the analyses. Four other cases in table III were excluded from our analyses

TABLE II—*Age standardised annual incidence* of specific cancers per million, England and Wales*

	Age 0–14 years†		Age 15–24 years‡	
	1969–83	1984–7	1971–83	1984–6
Lymphoid leukaemia and non-Hodgkin's lymphomas	35·5	39·6	18·8	19·8
Other leukaemias	8·5	7·6	11·1	9·0
Hodgkin's disease	4·5	5·5	33·5	31·1
Brain tumours (including benign)	25·5	27·6	27·7	24·4
Other malignant tumours	35·5	41·1	93·1	90·6
All registrations	109·4	121·3	183·8	174·9

*Calculated for populations with equal numbers in each five year age group for the age range shown.
†National registry of childhood tumours.
‡Cancer registration statistics for England and Wales.

TABLE III—*Details of cases of cancer occurring among people aged 0–24 years who were resident in Seascale at diagnosis, 1953 onwards*

Case No	Year of birth	Year of diagnosis	Age (years)	Sex	Diagnosis	Included in present analysis	Reference No in Black report
1	1948	1954	6	M	Neuroblastoma	No	22
2	1947	1955	7	F	Acute lymphoblastic leukaemia	No	1
3	1957	1960	2	M	Acute myeloid leukaemia	No	3
4	1957	1968	11	M	Acute lymphoblastic leukaemia	Yes	2
5	1964	1968	4	M	Acute lymphoblastic leukaemia	Yes	5
6	1968	1971	2	F	Acute lymphoblastic leukaemia	Yes	6
7	1960	1975	15	F	Rhabdomyosarcoma*	Yes	26
8	1974	1979	5	F	Acute lymphoblastic leukaemia	Yes	7
9	1974	1983	9	M	Non-Hodgkin's lymphoma	Yes	16
10	1982	1984	1	F	Non-Hodgkin's lymphoma	Yes	17
11	1966	1985	18	M	Pinealoma	Yes	—
12	1965	1988	23	F	Non-Hodgkin's lymphoma	Yes	—
13	1970	1988	17	F	Hodgkin's disease	Yes	—
14	1975	1991	16	M	Acute lymphoblastic leukaemia	No	—
15	1958	1978	20	M	Chronic myeloid leukaemia	No	4†

*Previously described as retroperitoneal sarcoma.
†This patient also had an address in another region of England where he was resident at the time of diagnosis, and he is therefore excluded from all the analyses.

TABLE IV—*Age standardised annual incidence of specific cancers per million children aged 0–14 years in specified areas of Cumbria*

Year	Seascale ward No	Seascale ward Age standardised rate	Allerdale and Copeland minus Seascale ward No	Allerdale and Copeland minus Seascale ward Age standardised rate	Rest of Cumbria No	Rest of Cumbria Age standardised rate
		Lymphoid leukaemia and non-Hodgkin's lymphomas				
1963–83	5	459·1	19	24·2	50	35·8
1984–90	1	511·2	7	32·5	26	66·4
1963–90	6	470·7	26	26·0	76	42·5
		Other leukaemias				
1963–83	0	0·0	7	8·7	11	7·8
1984–90	0	0·0	3	13·8	4	10·0
1963–90	0	0·0	10	9·9	15	8·3
		Hodgkin's disease				
1963–83	0	0·0	0	0·0	4	2·7
1984–90	0	0·0	1	4·5	4	9·7
1963–90	0	0·0	1	0·9	8	4·2
		Brain tumours (including benign)				
1963–83	0	0·0	21	26·2	44	31·1
1984–90	0	0·0	4	18·6	6	15·2
1963–90	0	0·0	25	24·5	50	27·6
		Other malignant tumours				
1963–83	0	0·0	31	39·3	43	30·8
1984–90	0	0·0	12	55·8	14	35·9
1963–90	0	0·0	43	42·8	57	32·0
		All registrations				
1963–83	5	459·1	78	98·4	152	108·2
1984–90	1	511·2	27	125·2	54	137·1
1963–90	6	470·7	105	104·1	206	114·7

because they fell outside the period covered: cases 1–3 occurred before complete registration data were available, and case 14 occurred in 1991 after the decision had been taken to make 1990 the final year of the analysis.

CANCER INCIDENCE AT AGES 0–14 YEARS, 1963–90

Table IV shows the numbers of cases of cancer together with the age standardised rates in children aged 0–14 years for each diagnostic group in the three study areas during 1963–83 and 1984–90. The rates of malignant disease and specifically of lymphoid leukaemia and non-Hodgkin's lymphomas for children in Seascale were substantially higher than those for the remainder of Copeland and Allerdale, Cumbria, and England and Wales. In Allerdale and Copeland (excluding Seascale) the rates for lymphoid leukaemia and non-Hodgkin's lymphomas were lower than those for other

TABLE V—*Age standardised annual incidence of specific cancers per million people aged 15–24 in specified areas of Cumbria*

Year	Seascale ward		Allerdale and Copeland minus Seascale ward		Rest of Cumbria	
	No	Age standardised rate	No	Age standardised rate	No	Age standardised rate
Lymphoid leukaemia and non-Hodgkin's lymphomas						
1969–83	0	0·0	12	32·4	9	14·4
1984–90	1	542·9	4	22·6	4	11·9
1969–90	1	192·8	16	29·6	13	13·5
Other leukaemias						
1969–83	0	0·0	4	11·2	5	7·6
1984–90	0	0·0	2	11·5	3	8·9
1969–90	0	0·0	6	11·2	8	8·1
Hodgkin's disease						
1969–83	0	0·0	15	41·3	19	31·1
1984–90	1	500·0	11	63·2	15	44·7
1969–90	1	133·0	26	48·3	34	35·2
Brain tumours (including benign)						
1969–83	0	0·0	8	21·7	12	18·4
1984–90	1	500·0	6	34·6	2	6·0
1969–90	1	133·0	14	25·9	14	14·2
Other malignant tumours						
1969–83	1	181·2	24	65·8	45	70·1
1984–90	0	0·0	8	46·2	18	53·4
1969–90	1	133·0	32	59·4	63	64·4
All registrations						
1969–83	1	181·2	63	172·3	90	141·5
1984–90	3	1542·9	31	178·2	42	124·8
1969–90	4	591·8	94	174·4	132	135·3

parts of Cumbria and for England and Wales. In the remainder of Cumbria the rates were higher than those for England and Wales.

Thus there is no evidence over the period from 1963 onwards that the excess found in Seascale extends to a wider area around Sellafield, though for the most recent period there was a slight increase in the incidence of lymphoid leukaemia and non-Hodgkin's lymphomas in the rest of Cumbria, particularly among children aged 0–4 years.

CANCER INCIDENCE AT AGES 15–24 YEARS, 1969–90

Results, mainly from data from the Northern region children's malignant disease registry, for those aged 15–24 for 1969–90 are given in table V. In Seascale there were four cases, of which three were diagnosed during 1984–90 (one non-Hodgkin's lymphoma, one Hodgkin's disease, and one pineal tumour). Again this represents a considerable increase over the national rates whether one considers lymphoid leukaemia and non-Hodgkin's lymphomas or all malignant disease and for both 1963–90 and 1984–90. In the remainder of Copeland and Allerdale and in the rest of Cumbria the rates were unremarkable.

LEUKAEMIA AND LYMPHOMAS AT AGES 25–74 YEARS, 1984–90

Table VI shows the numbers of cases of leukaemia and lymphomas for 10 year age groups in the age range 25–74, together with age specific and overall incidence rates, in the three study areas during 1984–90. In Seascale there were two cases of non-Hodgkin's lymphoma, both occurring at ages 55–64. On the basis of the national rates in the data collection study one case would be expected. Thus the excess found among young people does not extend to the older age groups.

RATES OF MALIGNANT DISEASE IN SEASCALE AT AGES 0–24 YEARS, 1963–83 AND 1984–90

The rates for Seascale were based on very small numbers. The method used to carry out a formal analysis of the hypothesis that there is no raised incidence of cancer among young persons aged 0–24 was the same as that in the Black report and was based on a comparison with the national rates for England and Wales summarised in table II. It is clear from a comparison of the rates in tables II, IV, and V that much the same results would be obtained if the rates for Cumbria or for Allerdale and Copeland were used. Expected numbers of cases are calculated on the assumption that the true rates are the same as those for England and Wales. In table VII we compared the observed numbers of cases with those expected for lymphoid leukaemia and non-Hodgkin's lymphomas, for all other cancers, and for all cancers combined separately for 1963–83 and 1984–90.

In 1963–83 a total of six cases, of which five were lymphoid leukaemia and non-Hodgkin's lymphomas, occurred. The expected number of cases of lymphoid leukaemia and non-Hodgkin's lymphomas on the basis of national rates is 0·49 (standardised registration ratio = 1015); the expected number for all malignant disease is 2·18 (standardised registration ratio = 275). The probabilities of such high values occurring by chance are respectively $p = 0·00016$ and $p = 0·024$. These probabilities are low and support the findings of the Black report, though they exaggerate the significance of the findings because there was no prior hypothesis, formulated independently of the observed data, in determining the diagnostic groups, age groups, periods, or area to be studied.

This criticism does not extend to analyses of subsequent periods. In table VII we analyse also the data for cancer occurring among young people in Seascale during 1984–90, when a total of four cases occurred in those aged 0–24 years. The expected number of cases of lymphoid leukaemia and

324

TABLE VI—*Age specific annual incidence of leukaemia and lymphomas per million people aged 25–74 in specified areas of Cumbria, 1984–90*

	Age (years)											
	25–34		35–44		45–54		55–64		65–74		Total 25–74	
	No	Rate	No	Rate	No	Rate	No	Rate	No	Rate	No	Rate
Seascale ward												
Lymphoid leukaemia and non-Hodgkin's lymphomas	0	0·0	0	0·0	0	0·0	2	1176·5	0	0·0	2	252·0
Other leukaemias	0	0·0	0	0·0	0	0·0	0	0·0	0	0·0	0	0·0
Hodgkin's disease	0	0·0	0	0·0	0	0·0	0	0·0	0	0·0	0	0·0
Allerdale and Copeland minus Seascale ward												
Lymphoid leukaemia and non-Hodgkin's lymphomas	4	23·5	4	24·9	17	126·9	23	175·7	46	442·8	94	134·3
Other leukaemias	1	5·9	2	12·4	6	44·8	16	122·2	18	173·3	43	61·4
Hodgkin's disease	2	11·7	4	24·9	1	7·5	2	15·3	4	38·5	13	18·6
Rest of Cumbria												
Lymphoid leukaemia and non-Hodgkin's lymphomas	5	16·0	21	69·8	28	111·0	62	241·5	105	482·5	221	165·0
Other leukaemias	6	19·2	8	26·6	6	23·8	13	50·6	31	142·4	64	47·8
Hodgkin's disease	4	12·8	10	33·2	6	23·8	11	42·8	6	27·6	37	27·6

TABLE VII—*Observed numbers of cases at ages 0–24 years in Seascale, 1963–90, and Poisson probability of observed or greater number of cases**

	Lymphoid leukaemia and non-Hodgkin's lymphomas	Other cancers	All malignant
1963–83:			
No of cases in Seascale	5	1	6
Probability of obtaining at least			
this No of cases	0·000161	0·816	0·0242
1984–90:			
No of cases in Seascale	2	2	4
Probability of obtaining at least			
this No of cases	0·00702	0·0831	0·00335

*Calculated from estimates of incidence in England and Wales as given in table II.

non-Hodgkin's lymphomas in this period and age group is 0·12 (standardised registration ratio = 1620). For all diagnostic categories taken together the expected number is 0·60 (standardised registration ratio = 667). Whether we consider just the two cases of lymphoid leukaemia and non-Hodgkin's lymphomas or the total of four cases there was a significant (p = 0·0070 and p = 0·0034, respectively) excess of cases in Seascale in this period.

Discussion

Two principal questions are considered in this chapter. Firstly, do the findings of the Black report relating to the period up to and including 1983 remain unchanged now that more comprehensive data sets and analyses are available? Secondly, did the excess incidence of childhood leukaemia in Seascale found in the various analyses summarised in the Black report persist in later years? The present report covers the periods 1963–90 for children aged 0–14 years, 1969–90 for people aged 15–24, and 1984–90 for leukaemia and lymphomas in adults. As explained in the introduction, the diagnostic groups, age groups, calendar periods, and areas to be analysed were agreed in advance of the analyses being carried out.

The conclusions of the Black report are confirmed in so far as they relate to malignant disease occurring in young people between 1963 and 1983; on the basis of the six cases included in table III we conclude that the excess in Seascale is unlikely to have arisen by chance (table VII). All of the six cases are included in the report by Craft *et al.*[14] We omitted from these analyses case 15 in table III because this person had an address in another part of Britain which was regarded as his area of residence for the purposes of the national cancer registration scheme.[10] Inclusion of this case would have strengthened our conclusion about the period 1963–83.

For the period before 1984 our analyses rely on much the same evidence as the Black report, though more complete registration data are now available. There is, however, no way of overcoming the objection that analyses of Seascale data for this period are not amenable to any rigorous statistical evaluation because the area, age group, and types of disease to be studied were selected as a result of the observed clustering of cases.

This criticism cannot be applied to the results for 1984–90. Even the case from this period that was included in the Black report (with the year of diagnosis wrongly given as 1983 rather than 1984) was diagnosed after concern had been raised about the high incidence in Seascale. For those aged 0–24 there is an excess of malignant disease that is highly unlikely to have arisen by chance (table VII). These more recent data therefore strengthen the suggestion that there is an increased incidence in Seascale among those aged 0–24 years, but whereas the original findings related mainly to lymphoid leukaemia in those aged 0–14 years, there were no leukaemias and only one case below age 15 during 1984–90. Of the four cases found in this period two had non-Hodgkin's lymphomas, one Hodgkin's disease, and one a pineal tumour; the excess is mainly attributable to non-Hodgkin's lymphomas. We have excluded from these analyses case 14 in table III because this case occurred beyond the period specified in planning the analysis (see introduction). The occurrence of this case does, however, strengthen the conclusion that there is an excess of lymphoid leukaemia and non-Hodgkin's lymphomas among those aged 0–24 years in Seascale. As regards other cancers in this age group, there is a small, non-significant excess during 1984–90 but no overall excess if the whole period 1963–90 is considered.

There is no evidence that the raised incidence in Seascale extends to the two county districts nearest to Sellafield or to Cumbria generally. There was an apparently raised incidence of lymphoid leukaemia and non-Hodgkin's lymphomas in the rest of Cumbria in 1984–90 among those aged 0–4 years, but this is based on only 13 cases and is difficult to interpret. Birth records have been obtained for the 42 children with cancer diagnosed up to the age of 4 years throughout Cumbria during 1984–90 in order to investigate the possibility that some of these children had been born in Seascale and then moved, but in fact only the child resident in Seascale at diagnosis was also domiciled there at birth.

EXPLANATIONS FOR OUR FINDINGS

We consider some of the main hypotheses that might account for our findings.

Firstly, the results may simply be due to chance because a search for clusters is likely to show some spatial aggregations of cases even if there is no causal explanation: this is particularly true if the age groups, areas, calendar periods, and diagnostic groups to be studied are not specified in advance. When claims were originally made concerning a cluster at Seascale it seemed quite possible that this was the explanation. The accumulation of further data since the original reports and the analysis in table VII suggest that this is not the correct explanation.

Secondly, the most obvious suggestion is that the cases are caused by the direct effects of environmental radiation on the child or fetus. The results of calculations based on estimates of environmental discharges and on modelling of risks attributable to such radiation suggest that the doses delivered to the child or fetus were far too low to explain the cluster unless either the discharges were considerably underestimated or the assumptions made in computing the risks were grossly incorrect.[15]

Thirdly, Gardner *et al*, in their case-control study of leukaemia and lymphoma diagnosed during 1950–85 among young people in west Cumbria, concluded that the excess occurred among children whose fathers had high levels of exposure to radiation before the child was conceived, and perhaps particularly in the preceding six months; they suggested that some cases were the result of paternal germ cell mutations, and that this could explain the excess in this geographical area.[7] Again, the level of risk implied by this explanation seems inconsistent with the dosimetry and previous estimates of genetic risk. The measured dose of external radiation might be a surrogate measure for internal exposure to radionuclides or to chemicals; such alternative explanations are still open to the objection that there are no generally accepted data on humans to support this. Our analysis includes the geographical area covered by Gardner *et al* but follows it too closely in time to provide data to test their findings; only cases 12–14 in table III (one non-Hodgkin's lymphoma, one leukaemia, one Hodgkin's disease) were diagnosed after the period covered by the Gardner study and moreover all three were conceived before the parents moved to Seascale.

The only published study that can be directly compared with the Gardner report is that by McLaughlin *et al* on workers at nuclear facilities in Ontario; they found no increased risk of leukaemia in the children of fathers working in these facilities.[16] In particular, although the numbers of cases and the prevalence of exposures in the highest dose categories considered by Gardner *et al* were similar for the control fathers in the two studies, the Ontario study found no evidence of a risk associated with such doses. Differences between the studies include the fact that Canadian workers "receive a substantial proportion (20–40%) of their total exposure as an internal dose (largely due to tritium)," that workers in Ontario did not have the types of chemical exposure received by the Sellafield workers, and that some of the control fathers with high doses were uranium miners.

Little is known about risk factors for childhood leukaemias and lymphomas. In a series of papers Stewart and colleagues have shown a significant association, now widely accepted as causal, between obstetric radiography and childhood leukaemia and other cancers.[17] For children born in the late 1950s and early 1960s this could have accounted for perhaps 5% of cases; as Gardner et al showed it does not explain the increased incidence in Seascale.[7] Kinlen et al have carried out a number of analyses relating to areas in which there has been increased population mixing and have found an increased incidence of childhood leukaemia in some of these areas.[18 19] They attribute this to an increased likelihood of exposure to a leukaemogenic virus or viruses. The high incidence in Seascale occurred over an extended period, and we are not sure whether this could be explained by Kinlen's hypothesis. A number of studies (see, for example, Draper et al[20]) have suggested that childhood leukaemia is more common among higher socioeconomic groups, and it has also been suggested that the risk of childhood acute lymphoblastic leukaemia is doubled in isolated towns and villages,[21] but the excess in Seascale is too large to be accounted for in these ways.

In conclusion, we confirm that there is good evidence of an increased incidence of lymphoid leukaemia and non-Hodgkin's lymphomas among young people in Seascale, though we are unable to identify the cause of this increase; nor can we say that our data and analyses either support or detract from the conclusions of Gardner et al.[7]

We thank the Office of Population Censuses and Surveys, regional cancer registries, specialised childhood tumour registries, and members of the UK Children's Cancer Study Group for providing copies of notifications of childhood cancer cases, and haematologists in Whitehaven and Carlisle hospitals for information on leukaemia and lymphoma cases. We thank many colleagues, particularly Jim Miller, Shirley Wilson, and Lorna More; and the registry and computing staff at the Childhood Cancer Research Group for help with data collection; and Sue Medhurst for secretarial help. Support for this work was received from the Department of Health, the Scottish Home and Health Department, the Leukaemia Research Fund, and the North of England Children's Cancer Research Fund.

1 Black D for the Independent Advisory Group. *Investigation of the possible increased incidence of cancer in west Cumbria.* London: HMSO, 1984. (Black report.)
2 Committee on the Medical Aspects of Radiation in the Environment. *Investigation of the possible increased incidence of leukaemia in young people near the Dounreay nuclear establishment, Caithness, Scotland.* London: HMSO, 1988. (COMARE 2nd report.)
3 Committee on the Medical Aspects of Radiation in the Environment. *Report of the incidence of childhood cancer in the west Berkshire and north Hampshire area, in which are situated the Atomic Weapons Research Establishment, Aldermaston and the Royal Ordnance Factory, Burghfield.* London: HMSO, 1989. (COMARE 3rd report.)
4 Cook-Mozaffari PJ, Darby SC, Doll R, Forman D, Hermon C, Pike MC, et al. Geographical variation in mortality from leukaemia and other cancers in England and Wales in relation to proximity to nuclear installations, 1969–78. *Br J Cancer* 1989;59:476–85.
5 Gardner MJ, Hall AJ, Downes S, Terrell JD. Follow up study of children born to mothers resident in Seascale, west Cumbria (birth cohort). *BMJ* 1987;295:822–7.

6 Gardner MJ, Hall AJ, Downes S, Terrell JD. Follow up study of children born elsewhere but attending schools in Seascale, west Cumbria (schools cohort). *BMJ* 1987;**295**:819–22.
7 Gardner MJ, Snee MP, Hall AJ, Powell CA, Downes S, Terrell JD. Results of case-control study of leukaemia and lymphoma among young people near Sellafield nuclear plant in west Cumbria. *BMJ* 1990;**300**:423–9.
8 Birch JM, Marsden HB. A classification scheme for childhood cancer. *Int J Cancer* 1987;**40**:620–4.
9 Cartwright RA, Alexander FE, McKinney PA, Ricketts TJ. *Leukaemia and lymphoma. An atlas of distribution within areas of England and Wales 1984–88.* London: Leukaemia Research Fund, 1990.
10 Swerdlow AJ. Cancer registration in England and Wales: some aspects relevant to interpretation of the data. *Journal of the Royal Statistical Society [Series A]* 1986;**149**:146–60.
11 Stiller CA, O'Connor CM, Vincent TJ, Draper GJ. The national registry of childhood tumours and the leukaemia/lymphoma data for 1966–83. In: Draper G, ed. *The geographical epidemiology of childhood leukaemia and non-Hodgkin lymphomas in Great Britain 1966–83.* London: HMSO, 1991;7–16. (OPCS Studies in Medical and Population Subjects, No 53.)
12 Craft AW, Amineddine HA, Scott JES, Wagget J. The Northern Region Children's Malignant Disease Registry 1968–82: incidence and survival. *Br J Cancer* 1987;**56**:853–8.
13 Birch JM. United Kingdom—Manchester Children's Tumour Registry 1954–1970 and 1971–1983. In: Parkin DM, Stiller CH, Draper GJ, Bieber CA, Terracini B, Young JL, eds. *International incidence of childhood cancer.* Lyons: International Agency for Research on Cancer, 1988:299–304. (IARC Scientific Publications, No 87.)
14 Craft AW, Parker L, Openshaw S, Charlton M, Newell J, Birch JM, Blair V. Cancer in young people in the north of England 1968–85. Analysis by census wards. *J Epidemiol Community Health* (in press).
15 Committee on Medical Aspects of Radiation in the Environment. *The implications of the new data on the releases from Sellafield in the 1950s for the conclusions of the report on the investigation of the possible increased incidence of cancer in west Cumbria.* London: HMSO, 1986. (COMARE, 1st report.)
16 McLaughlin JR, Anderson TW, Clarke EA, King W. *Occupational exposure of fathers to ionising radiation and the risk of leukaemia in offspring—a case-control study.* Ottawa: Atomic Energy Control Board, 1992.
17 Bithell JF, Stewart AM. Pre-natal irradiation and childhood malignancy: a review of British data from the Oxford survey. *Br J Cancer* 1975;**31**:271–87.
18 Kinlen LJ, Clark K, Hudson C. Evidence from population mixing in British new towns 1946–85 of an infective basis of childhood leukaemia. *Lancet* 1990;**336**:577–82.
19 Kinlen LJ, Hudson C. Childhood leukaemia and poliomyelitis in relation to military encampments in England and Wales in the period of national military service, 1950–63. *BMJ* 1991;**303**:1357–62.
20 Draper GJ, Vincent TJ, O'Connor CM, Stiller CA. Socio-economic factors and variations in incidence rates between country districts. In: Draper G, ed. *The geographical epidemiology of childhood leukaemia and non-Hodgkin lymphomas in Great Britain 1966–83.* London: HMSO, 1991;37–45. (OPCS Studies in Medical and Population Subjects, No 53.)
21 Alexander FE, McKinney PA, Ricketts TJ, Cartwright RA. Community lifestyle characteristics and risk of acute lymphoblastic leukaemia in children. *Lancet* 1990;**336**:1461–5.

36: Case-control study of leukaemia and non-Hodgkin's lymphoma among children aged 0–4 years living in west Berkshire and north Hampshire health districts

EVE ROMAN, ANN WATSON, VALERIE BERAL, SANDRA BUCKLE, DIANA BULL, KRYS BAKER, HILARY RYDER, CAROL BARTON

To investigate the relation between parental employment in the nuclear industry and childhood leukaemia and non-Hodgkin's lymphoma in the West Berkshire and the Basingstoke and North Hampshire District Health Authorities, a case-control study of 54 children aged 0–4 years (who were diagnosed during 1972–89, had been born in the study area, and lived there when cancer was diagnosed) was undertaken. Six controls were selected for each case: four from hospital delivery registers and two from live birth registers maintained by the NHS central register. Controls were matched for sex, date of birth (within six months), and area of residence at birth and at time of diagnosis. The outcome measures were parents' employment by the nuclear industry and exposure to ionising radiation at work.

Five (9%) of the 54 patients and 14 (4%) of the 324 controls had one or both parents who had been employed by the nuclear industry (relative risk 2·2; 95% confidence interval 0·6 to 6·9). Nuclear industry employees who work in areas where exposure to radiation is possible are given film badges to monitor their exposure to external penetrating ionising radiation. Three fathers of patients and two fathers of controls (and no mothers of either) had been monitored in this way before the conception of their children (relative risk 9·0; 95% confidence interval 1·0 to 107·8). No father (of a patient or a control) had accumulated a recorded dose of more than 5 millisieverts (mSv) during the time he was monitored before his child was conceived, and no father had been monitored at any time in the four years before his child was conceived. A dose-response relation was not evident among fathers who had been monitored.

These results suggest that the children of fathers who had been monitored for exposure to external penetrating ionising radiation in the nuclear industry may be at increased risk of developing leukaemia before their fifth birthday. This finding is based on small numbers and could be due to chance. If the relation is real the mechanisms are far from clear, except that the effect is unlikely to be due to external radiation; it is possibly caused by internal contamination by radioactive substances or some other exposure at work. The above average rates of leukaemia in the study area cannot be accounted for by these findings.

Introduction

We previously found an increased incidence of childhood leukaemia in the West Berkshire and the Basingstoke and North Hampshire District Health Authorities during 1972–85.[1] The excess was concentrated in children under 5 years who were living within 10 km of the atomic weapons establishments at Aldermaston and Burghfield. We report here the results of a case-control study set up to investigate whether the excess was related to parents' employment in the nuclear industry.

Subjects and methods

The study was carried out in the West Berkshire and the Basingstoke and

North Hampshire District Health Authorities. Information about children under 5 years old living in the study area who had leukaemia or non-Hodgkin's lymphoma diagnosed between 1972 and 1989 was ascertained from multiple sources. Children with non-Hodgkin's lymphoma were included because of the current understanding, based on immunological studies, that acute lymphoblastic leukaemia and non-Hodgkin's lymphoma represent opposite ends of the same range of disease.[23] Most cases were notified by consultants at the Royal Berkshire District Hospital, the Basingstoke District Hospital, and hospitals in the surrounding districts. General practitioners within the study area also provided details of children with cancer. In addition, listings of children with leukaemia or non-Hodgkin's lymphoma were obtained from the Childhood Cancer Research Group's national registry of childhood tumours.[4] All diagnoses were histologically confirmed.

We studied only children who were born and had cancer diagnosed in the study area. The mothers of 56 of the 71 children diagnosed during 1972–89 were living in the study area at the time of their child's birth. Two of these 56 children are not included in the analyses; both died in the early 1970s shortly after having non-Hodgkin's lymphoma diagnosed, and we were unable to verify their parents' names or dates of birth.

Six control children were selected for each case: two from birth registers maintained by the NHS central register in Southport and four from delivery registers in the two district hospitals in the study area.

The two birth registry controls were chosen by staff employed at the central register. The entry for the case was located in the birth register and the first preceding and the first succeeding entries were selected who matched the case with respect to sex, date of birth (plus or minus six months), district of birth registration, and family health services authority of the child's first general practitioner. Controls were further matched with cases for residence in the study area at time of diagnosis. Control children who were found to have died or to have moved out of the study area before their matched case had cancer diagnosed were replaced.

Mother's address is not recorded in the birth registers maintained by the central register. To allow matching for proximity of mother's residence to a nuclear establishment at the time of her child's birth a further series of controls was selected from locally held hospital delivery registers. Mother's address as recorded in the delivery register was used to assign births to 5 km bands round the nuclear establishments in the study area, and controls were chosen from the same 5 km band as their associated case. These 5 km bands correspond to the boundaries used in our previous analyses.[1] Selecting controls from delivery registers also enabled matching for mother's age (plus or minus five years), child's sex and date of birth (plus or minus six months), district health authority of birth, and residence in the study area at the time of diagnosis. Controls selected from the delivery register were chosen by locating the birth entry of the case and selecting the two closest preceding and the two closest succeeding entries fulfilling the matching criteria. For the 10 case children who were not born in maternity units within the study area (eight were born at home and two in hospitals in adjacent health authorities) the place in the register where the birth would have been entered was located and controls were chosen as above.

Children were considered ineligible to be controls if they were a twin, were adopted, or had a serious congenital defect. Controls whose mother had died (two) or was unavailable because of ill health (one) and controls whose father could not be identified (eight) were also considered ineligible. As control families were traced through their general practitioner with the facilities offered by the central register, families who emigrated before the study began (five) and those whose current family health services authority was not recorded (five) or incorrectly recorded (11) were replaced by the next eligible control in the series. One control was selected from both the delivery register and birth register. This child was assigned to the delivery register series and another control was chosen from the birth register.

DATA COLLECTION

Information about case and control children and their parents was obtained from four sources: the child's birth certificate, personal interview of parents, mother's obstetric notes, and employment and health physics records held by the nuclear industry (table I).

Birth certificates of cases and controls were obtained from the Office of Population Censuses and Surveys. Mother's and father's names, mother's address, and father's occupation are routinely recorded on the birth certificate. This information was used to confirm residential details and parental names. Father's occupation and social class were coded by the Office of Population Censuses and Surveys 1980 classification scheme.[5] Father's occupation was assigned to one of eight groups on the basis of knowledge of the industries in the area and of previous reports of association between parental occupation and childhood cancer.[6-8]

Parents of cases and controls were interviewed by a trained nurse interviewer using a structured questionnaire. Separate questionnaires were used for mothers and fathers. A full residential and occupational history, including specific questions about employment at nuclear establishments, was recorded for each parent. To improve the quality of information obtained at interview, a form asking parents to list the places in which they had lived and the jobs they had had was sent out in advance of the interview. Parent's social class and occupation was coded in the same way as the information on birth certificates. During the interview, mothers and fathers were also asked to confirm their own names and dates of birth and about their own health and habits. Additional questions about pregnancies,

334

TABLE I—*Information obtained about parents of cases and controls*

Information	No (%) of cases (n = 54)	No (%) of controls* (n = 324)
Name:		
Mother	54 (100)	324 (100)
Father	53 (98)	324 (100)
Date of birth:		
Mother	54 (100)	312 (96)
Father	52 (96)	290 (90)
Father's occupation recorded on birth certificate	52 (96)	323 (99)
Completed questionnaire:		
Mother	51 (94)	223 (73)†
Father	49 (91)	219 (72)†
Obstetric notes abstracted‡	37 (88)	196 (88)

*Six controls were sought for each case.
†Mothers and fathers of three case children were not interviewed and interviews were not sought for their 18 corresponding controls.
‡Obstetric notes were sought for only the 42 cases born at Royal Berkshire District Hospital or Basingstoke District Hospital and their 222 corresponding controls.

the index child, and other children in the family were incorporated in the mother's questionnaire. Because of the seriousness of the disease, interviewers knew whether they were approaching the parents of a case or control child.

The parents of three case children did not wish to be interviewed, and interviews with the corresponding controls of these children were not arranged. All mothers of the remaining 51 case children were interviewed but two fathers were not (table I). Of the parents of the 306 matched controls for these 51 cases, 223 (73%) mothers and 219 (72%) fathers were interviewed. Among the 83 controls for whom neither parent was interviewed, 58 sets of parents declined an interview, 14 were not approached on the advice of their general practitioner, and the current addresses of the remaining 11 were not traced. For each of the 51 case children whose mother was interviewed at least one mother of a corresponding control was also interviewed: the numbers of case children for whom 1, 2, 3, 4, 5, and 6 corresponding control mothers were interviewed were 1, 3, 3, 21, 15, and 8 respectively. For the 49 case children whose father was interviewed the numbers for whom 1, 2, 3, 4, 5, and 6 corresponding control fathers were interviewed were 1, 3, 5, 18, 15, and 7 respectively.

We located the obstetric notes of 37 of the 42 (88%) mothers of case children born at the Royal Berkshire District Hospital or the Basingstoke District Hospital. The obstetric notes of 196 of the 222 (88%) controls associated with these 37 cases were also obtained (table I). Information about the pregnancy and delivery and about the name and date of birth of the father (where recorded) were abstracted from the obstetric notes. Obstetric data were abstracted for at least one control for the 37 cases. The numbers of cases for which 1, 2, 3, 4, 5, and 6 controls gave obstetric data were 1, 0, 2, 2, 11, and 21 respectively.

Parents' names, including mothers' maiden names, and dates of birth were checked against the employment and health physics records of past and present employees held by the Atomic Weapons Establishment, the Atomic Energy Authority, and the National Registry of Radiation Workers. These records were primarily compiled for epidemiological studies of the health of nuclear industry workers.[9-11] Parents' surname, forename(s), sex, and date of birth were linked to these databases by industry staff. Different spellings of names were also checked. Eight potentially matching people with the same or similar names but missing or incomplete dates of birth were eliminated as true matches after thorough cross checking. Details about dates of employment and health physics records were obtained for all parents confirmed as having been employed at a nuclear establishment before their child's cancer was diagnosed (or, for controls, before the date of diagnosis of the corresponding case).

ANALYSIS OF DATA

Data were entered on to a microcomputer with the database management system FOXPRO,[12] and tabulations were produced with the statistical program SPSS.[13] Relative risks were estimated as matched odds ratios by conditional maximum likelihood methods.[14] Information on exposure was considered up until the time of diagnosis for cases and until the date of diagnosis of the corresponding case for controls. Confidence intervals and p values for relative risks were calculated by conditional exact methods based on the binomial distribution with the computer package EGRET.[15] Two sided p values (given to two significant figures) and 95% confidence intervals are presented throughout.

Results

Table II gives the characteristics of children who had leukaemia or non-Hodgkin's lymphoma diagnosed during 1972–89 and who were born in the study area and resident there when their cancer was diagnosed. Fifty children had leukaemia diagnosed (39 had acute lymphoblastic leukaemia and 11 other forms of leukaemia) and six had non-Hodgkin's lymphoma. Of the 11 children with other forms of leukaemia, seven had acute myeloid leukaemia, two chronic granulocytic leukaemia, and two undifferentiated leukaemia. Two of the children with acute myeloid leukaemia, and both of the children with undifferentiated leukaemia, had Down's syndrome. The

TABLE II—*Characteristics of children who had leukaemia or non-Hodgkin's lymphoma diagnosed before their fifth birthday in the West Berkshire and the Basingstoke and North Hampshire District Health Authorities during 1972–89 and were born to mothers resident in the area*

	Acute lymphoblastic leukaemia	Other leukaemias*	Non-Hodgkin's lymphoma	Total
No of children diagnosed	39	11	6	56
No included in the analysis	39	11	4†	54
Sex:				
Male	21	4	2	27
Female	18	7	2	27
Age at diagnosis (years):				
⩽1	4	3	1	8
2	11	4	1	16
3	13	2	1	16
4	11	2	1	14
Year of diagnosis:				
1972–4	8	4	1	13
1975–7	9		1	10
1978–80	9	3		12
1981–3	6	1		7
1984–6	1	2	1	4
1987–9	6	1	1	8
Year of birth:				
⩽1970	6	3	1	10
1971–3	10		1	11
1974–6	8	3		11
1977–9	3	2		5
1980–2	5	2	1	8
⩾1983	7	1	1	9

*Includes seven children with acute myeloid leukaemia, two with chronic granulocytic leukaemia, and two with undifferentiated leukaemia. Two of the children with acute myeloid leukaemia and both of the children with undifferentiated leukaemia had Down's syndrome.

†Two children are not included in the analyses. Both died in the early 1970s, shortly after diagnosis. Only the child's name and diagnosis was known; parents' names and dates of birth were not verified and neither parent was traced.

numbers of children diagnosed and born each year fluctuated, but the numbers were small and there was no noticeable trend with time.

At the time of their child's birth, the parents of case and control children were similar with respect to their age, distance of residence from a nuclear establishment, and social class (table III). As expected, the matching to cases was best for controls selected from delivery registers. In the analyses that follow relative risks were estimated by using data from all available controls. Analyses were also performed with birth register and delivery register controls separately. The findings were similar, although the number of controls per case was small.

TABLE III—*Characteristics of the parents of cases and matched controls obtained from hospital delivery register and NHS birth register*

Parental characteristic at time of child's birth	No (%) of cases	No (%) of controls		
		Delivery register	Birth register	Total
All children	54	216	108	324
Mother's age (years)*:				
≤24	20 (37)	93	32	125 (39)
25–29	24 (44)	84	44	128 (40)
≥30	10 (19)	39	28	67 (21)
Not known			4	4 (1)
Father's age (years):				
≤24	10 (19)	44	17	61 (19)
25–29	26 (48)	73	36	109 (34)
≥30	16 (30)	77	45	122 (38)
Not known	2 (4)	22	10	32 (10)
Distance of mother's residence from a nuclear establishment (km)*:				
≤5	11 (20)	44	18	62 (19)
6–10	24 (44)	96	36	132 (41)
11–15	11 (20)	44	29	73 (23)
≥15	8 (15)	32	25	57 (18)
Social class†:				
I	4 (7)	18	10	28 (9)
II	11 (20)	43	16	59 (18)
III Non-manual	9 (17)	33	18	51 (16)
III Manual	20 (37)	79	43	122 (38)
IV	5 (9)	25	13	38 (12)
V	1 (2)	8	6	14 (4)
Armed forces	1 (2)	3		3 (1)
In adequately described	3 (6)	7	2	9 (3)

*Delivery register controls and cases were matched for these variables.
†Social class was assigned on the basis of father's occupation as stated on the birth certificate.

EMPLOYMENT BY NUCLEAR INDUSTRY

Fathers of children with leukaemia or non-Hodgkins lymphoma were more likely than fathers of control children to have been employed by the nuclear industry, but the excess was not significant. Linkage to nuclear industry databases identified four (out of 54) case fathers and 10 (out of 324) control fathers who were employed at some time before their child had cancer diagnosed (relative risk 2·5, p = 0·25, p = 0·25; table IV). All four fathers of case children and nine of the 10 fathers of control children were employed by the industry before their child was conceived (relative risk 2·8, p = 0·20).

Employees who work in areas where exposure to ionising radiation is possible are issued with personal film badges or other dosimeters to monitor their exposure. The risk of leukaemia or non-Hodgkin's lym-

TABLE IV—*Numbers of cases and controls and relative risks (95% confidence intervals) for childhood leukaemia and non-Hodgkin's lymphoma by father's employment and monitoring for exposure to ionising radiation at nuclear establishment*

| Father's employment at a nuclear establishment before child's diagnosis* | Cases (n=54) | Controls | | | Relative risk† (95% confidence interval) |
		Delivery register (n=216)	Birth register (n=108)	Total (n=324)	
Ever employed	4	5	5	10	2·5 (0·6 to 9·0)
Before conception	4	4	5	9	2·8 (0·6 to 10·5)
Conception to diagnosis	1	2	3	5	1·2 (0·1 to 10·7)
Ever monitored for ionising radiation	4	1	2	3	8·0 (1·4 to 54·6)
Before conception	3	1	1	2	9·0 (1·0 to 108·8)
Conception to diagnosis	1		1	1	6·0 (0·1 to 471·0)

*Based on search of nuclear industry databases.
†Estimated by using information matched sets.

phoma was significantly increased in children whose fathers had been thus monitored: four fathers of cases and three fathers of controls had been issued with monitoring devices before their child's illness was diagnosed (relative risk 8·0, p=0·02), and of these, three fathers of cases and two fathers of controls were monitored before their child's conception (relative risk 9·0, p=0·047).

The figure summarises information on timing of father's employment in the nuclear industry and radiation exposure, in relation to the birth of his child, for the seven fathers (four cases and three controls, of whom three and two respectively had been employed at the atomic weapons establish-

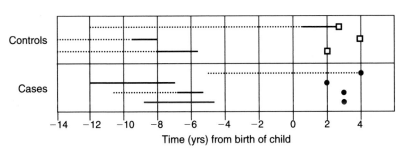

Time (yrs) from birth of child

Employment details of the seven fathers identified from nuclear industry databases as having been monitored for exposure to ionising radiation.—Employed and monitored for external radiation, ····· employed and not monitored for external radiation, ● indicates the age of child when leukaemia was diagnosed, □ indicates the age of child when leukaemia was diagnosed in the matched case

TABLE V—*Number of cases and controls and relative risks (95% confidence intervals) for leukaemia and non-Hodgkin's lymphoma in children by mother's employment at a nuclear establishment‡*

Mother's employment at a nuclear establishment before child's diagnosis	Cases (n = 54)	Controls			Relative risk† (95% confidence interval)
		Delivery register (n = 216)	Birth register (n = 108)	Total (n = 324)	
Ever employed	1	4	3	7	0·9 (0·2 to 7·2)
Before conception	0	4	2	6	0·0 (0·0 to 5·1)
Conception to birth*	1	1	1	2	3·0 (0·1 to 57·6)
Birth to diagnosis	0	0	0	0	0·0

*Based on search of nuclear industry.
†Estimated by using informative matched sets.
‡No mother had a record of monitoring for exposure to ionising radiation.

ments in the area) who were issued with dosimeters. No fathers were monitored for exposure at around the time of their child's conception, or in the four years preceding their child's conception. The recorded doses of external radiation received by the seven fathers were low. Of the five fathers issued with badges before their child was conceived, two (of three) fathers of cases and one (of two) father of a control accumulated a whole body dose of less than 1 mSv. The remaining two fathers (one case and one control) accumulated a whole body dose of 1–5 mSv. Data on dose for individual fathers are not presented because this information might enable them to be identified. As well as wearing film badges, some employees are investigated for internal contamination by radioactive substances if this is believed to have occurred, and one father of a case was tested for internal contamination by uranium in the year before his child had leukaemia diagnosed.

The malignancies in children whose fathers were monitored for exposure to ionising radiation were not unusual. All four children had acute lymphoblastic leukaemia diagnosed between the ages of 2 and 4 years, the year of diagnosis ranging from 1972 to 1988. None of the 11 children who had other forms of leukaemia and none of the four who had non-Hodgkin's lymphoma had fathers with a record of employment at a nuclear establishment.

We found no association with mother's employment in the nuclear industry. One mother of a case and seven mothers of controls were employed by the nuclear industry before their child's diagnosis (relative risk 0·9, p = 1·0). No mother of a case had worked at a nuclear establishment before her child's conception, and no mother had a record of being monitored for exposure to ionising radiation at any time before diagnosis (table V).

In our study of the incidence of childhood leukaemia during 1972–85 the excess was concentrated in the 50 electoral wards in which half or more of the area was within 10 km of the atomic weapons establishments at Aldermaston and Burghfield.[1] All four case children whose fathers were monitored for exposure to ionising radiation were born within this 10 km circle. When the analysis was restricted to only controls from the delivery register (who were matched to cases by distance of residence from a nuclear establishment) the risks associated with paternal monitoring before the child's diagnosis and before conception were 16·0 (95% confidence interval 1·6 to 788·0; p = 0·013) and 12·0 (1·0 to 630·0; p = 0·054) respectively.

The questionnaire administered to parents included specific questions about work at nuclear establishments and monitoring for exposure to ionising radiation. All employees identified by linkage to industrial records also reported that they had worked in the nuclear industry and no additional parents reported having been an employee. Employees' reports of monitoring for exposure to ionising radiation agreed with the industrial records, except for one mother of a case who reported being monitored, but there was no record of this in the industry databases. Employees of outside contractors sometimes work on nuclear sites, and information about them is not held on nuclear industry's employee databases. Three additional parents reported that they worked on contract at nuclear sites and had been monitored for exposure to radiation before their child was diagnosed (one father of a case, after conception; one father of a control, before conception). The risks estimated on the basis of information recorded at interview were consistent with those estimated on the basis of information obtained from the nuclear industry.

OTHER RISK FACTORS

Table VI compares the occupations of fathers of cases and controls who were assigned to one of seven occupational groups where potentially hazardous exposures might have occurred. The information recorded on the birth certificate refers to one point in time—when the child's birth was registered—whereas the information reported at interview refers to a period of employment of three months or longer, at any time from three years before the child's birth up until diagnosis. Hence, fathers are counted once only in the birth certificate analysis, but may appear more than once in the interview analysis. For the two sets of analyses the findings are similar, but the data overlap. None of the father's job descriptions given on the birth certificate referred to work at a nuclear establishment. Mother's occupation is not routinely recorded on the birth certificate. No notable associations between paternal or maternal occupation and leukaemia or non-Hodgkin's lymphoma in their children were evident from the birth certificate data or those collected at interview.

Information on possible risk factors for leukaemia and non-Hodgkin's

TABLE VI—*Number of cases and controls and relative risks (95% confidence intervals) for leukaemia and non-Hodgkin's lymphoma in children by father's occupation as recorded on the birth certificate and reported at interview*

Exposure group†	Recorded on child's birth certificate					Reported at interview*				
		Controls			Relative risk‡ (95% confidence interval)		Controls			Relative risk‡ (95% confidence interval)
	Cases	Delivery register	Birth register	Total		Cases	Delivery register	Birth register	Total	
Agriculture	2	9	2	11	1·1 (0·1 to 5·9)	3	10	5	15	0·8 (0·1 to 3·3)
Building and construction	5	25	14	39	0·8 (0·2 to 2·0)	11	20	9	29	1·8 (0·8 to 4·2)
Drivers and related	3	24	6	30	0·6 (0·1 to 2·0)	7	20	4	24	1·3 (0·4 to 3·2)
Electrical and electronic	8	14	8	22	2·5 (0·9 to 6·8)	9	13	8	21	2·2 (0·8 to 5·9)
Engineering and metal	8	25	20	45	1·1 (0·4 to 2·5)	12	22	15	37	1·5 (0·6 to 3·2)
Medical and laboratory	0	7	2	9	0·0 (0·0 to 3·0)	2	8	3	11	0·9 (0·1 to 4·0)
Wood	1	8	2	10	0·6 (0·0 to 4·2)	3	7	3	10	1·4 (0·2 to 5·5)
Other occupations	25	95	50	145	1·1 (0·6 to 2·0)	13	60	29	89	0·5 (0·2 to 1·0)
Total	52§	207	104	311		49	143	68	211‖	

*Father's occupation in the three years before birth up until diagnosis. Only periods of employment of at least three months are included.
†Codes from the Office of Population Censuses and Surveys classification of occupations§: agriculture 107, 166–70, 172; building and construction 18, 68, 82–4, 88–9, 92–4, 300–16, 330; drivers and related 52, 95, 100, 124, 127–8, 141, 161, 317–29, 331–2, 336, 338; electrical and electronic 12, 62, 71–2, 86–7, 121–2, 252–9, 273–4, 276, 283, 286; engineering and metal 69–70, 74–7, 81, 91, 231–51, 260–72, 275, 277, 285, 343–4; medical and laboratory 41–51, 61, 65–6, 73, 80, 153, 155–6, 220, 288; wood 203, 213–9, 224, 293.
‡Estimated using informative matched sets.
§The occupation of two case fathers was not stated and they and their corresponding controls are excluded.
‖Eight interviewed control fathers are excluded because their corresponding case fathers were not interviewed.

lymphoma reported at interview and recorded in the obstetric notes are summarised in table VII. Of the 37 cases and 196 controls for whom obstetric notes were retrieved, 34 (92%) cases and 140 (71%) controls were interviewed and are included in both analyses. The relative risks estimated on the basis of data collected at interview and on the basis of data from obstetric notes are generally similar. The only significant association was an increased risk of leukaemia and non-Hodgkin's lymphoma associated with first pregnancy. No differences were detected between case and control parents with respect to their own health or the numbers of diagnostic radiographs they reported before their child was conceived, or habits such as swimming in local rivers or canals, or in the children's histories of being breast fed, their preschool activities, allergies, or viral infections.

Discussion

This study was set up to investigate whether the raised incidence of leukaemia in children aged 0–4 years in the west Berkshire and north Hampshire health districts, which was 60% above the national average in 1972–85, was related to paternal employment in the nuclear industry.[12] The fathers of four and the mother of one of the 54 children who were born in and had leukaemia or non-Hodgkin's lymphoma diagnosed in the study area had been employed in the nuclear industry before their child was diagnosed (relative risk 2·2, 95% confidence interval 0·6 to 6·9). This excess was not significant and was insufficient to account for the increased rates of leukaemia in the area.

After this study began, Gardner and colleagues reported the results of their case-control study of childhood leukaemia and non-Hodgkin's lymphoma around the Sellafield reprocessing plant.[16 17] They found that children of men who had been exposed to external penetrating ionising radiation before their child was conceived were at an increased risk of leukaemia. Our results can be interpreted as supporting Gardner and colleagues' finding in that the fathers of three (out of 54) cases and two (out of 324) controls had been monitored for exposure to ionising radiation before their child was conceived (relative risk 9·0, 1·0 to 107·8).

VALIDITY OF DATA BIAS AND CHANCE

Although our result for paternal preconceptual exposure could be affected substantially by the play of chance because of small numbers, it is unlikely to be biased. Cases were ascertained from multiple sources, and it is doubtful that any were missed, although we cannot be certain. The exclusion of two children with non-Hodgkin's lymphoma (whose parents could not be traced) probably did not affect the results.

Information about parental employment and monitoring for exposure to

TABLE VII—Number of cases and controls and relative risks (95% confidence intervals) for leukaemia and non-Hodgkin's lymphoma in children by exposure to suspected risk factors as recorded in obstetric notes and reported at interview

Suspected risk factor in index child/pregnancy	Obstetric records					Reported at interview				
		Controls			Relative risk* (95% confidence interval)		Controls			Relative risk* (95% confidence interval)
	Cases	Delivery register	Birth register	Total		Cases	Delivery register	Birth register	Total	
Total	37	139	57	196		51	150	73	223	
Abdominal x rays	5	19	5	24	1·1 (0·3 to 3·7)	10	22	1	23	2·2 (0·8 to 5·6)
Ultrasound scans	13	44	25	69	1·1 (0·4 to 3·1)	22	68	30	98	1·2 (0·5 to 3·0)
Smoking	8	28	12	40	0·9 (0·3 to 2·5)	9	42	18	60	0·5 (0·2 to 1·2)
Drinking alcohol	3	8	2	10	1·8 (0·3 to 8·8)	29	96	30	126	1·1 (0·6 to 2·2)
Birthweight ⩾3500 g	9	47	20	67	0·6 (0·2 to 1·4)	16	41	28	69	1·0 (0·5 to 2·1)
Gestational age ⩾41 weeks	9	36	13	49	0·9 (0·3 to 2·3)	13	45	16	61	0·9 (0·4 to 1·9)
Caesarian delivery	4	12	5	17	1·3 (0·3 to 4·2)	5	14	5	19	1·2 (0·3 to 3·4)
First pregnancy	20	55	14	69	2·3 (1·0 to 5·3)	28	64	16	80	2·3 (1·2 to 4·9)
First livebirth	22	71	17	88	1·8 (0·8 to 4·2)	30	75	21	96	2·0 (1·0 to 4·1)

*Estimated by using informative matched sets.

ionising radiation was obtained from nuclear industry files and is likely to be complete and unbiased. The names and dates of birth of all parents of case and control children (regardless of whether or not they were interviewed) were cross checked against three databases of employees held by the nuclear industry, the completeness and accuracy of which are known to be high.[9-11] Employment and exposure records date from before the occurrence of leukaemia in the children, and the link to industry files was done by industry staff who did not know who were the parents of cases and who were the parents of controls. Not all parents were interviewed and self reported details on radiation exposure could be biased, so emphasis is given here to results obtained from industrial records.

The apparent excess of fathers monitored for radiation among children with leukaemia does not seem to be because the number of such fathers in the control group was unusually low by chance. On the basis of estimates of the size and composition of the nuclear workforces in the study area, national fertility rates, and local migration rates, we estimate that the expected numbers of control fathers who were employed and monitored for exposure to ionising radiation are in broad agreement with the numbers observed. Nevertheless, our results should be interpreted cautiously as they are based on only three monitored fathers and it is not possible to assess reliably how many of the three leukaemias, if any, were caused by paternal preconceptual exposure to some occupational factor.

CAUSE OF THE EFFECT

If the association between paternal preconceptual exposure to radiation and childhood leukaemia we found is not a chance finding, the effect is unlikely to be due to paternal exposure to the forms of external penetrating ionising radiation measured by monitoring devices. A more plausible explanation is that exposure to external radiation is a marker of exposure to some other hazard, such as internal contamination by a radioactive substance or a chemical.[16 18 19] The external doses recorded for the fathers in our study are orders of magnitude lower than the external doses received by survivors of the atomic bombs at Hiroshima and Nagasaki, whose children are not at an increased risk of childhood leukaemia.[20] No father (of a case or a control child) in this study had a recorded cumulative external exposure to penetrating radiation above 5 mSv before his child was conceived, and such low doses could accumulate from background radiation in about five years. Important differences between the exposures of atomic bomb survivors and nuclear industry workers are that nuclear industry workers are more likely to be contaminated internally by the ingestion, inhalation, or other intake of radioactive substances; to be exposed to other types of external radiation such as neutrons; and to be exposed to chemicals at work. Film badges monitor exposure to external penetrating and sparsely ionising radiation but not internal or other forms of radiation, and the fact of being issued with a film badge to monitor external penetrating radiation could, for certain workers, be a marker of exposure to other forms of radiation.

Insufficient is known about the radiobiological effects of many types of radiation and radioactive substances to which workers may be exposed, other than external penetrating radiation. Certain workers have been monitored for internal contamination by radionuclides and exposure to other forms of radiation such as neutrons since the 1950s, but this is not done routinely and monitoring methods can be unreliable.

COMPARISON WITH OTHER STUDIES

If being monitored for exposure to external penetrating radiation can be a marker of other exposures in the workplace, some of which might be hazardous, studies of the relation between men's exposure to external radiation and leukaemia in their children could yield apparently inconsistent results. Two other case-control studies have not found evidence of an increased risk of leukaemia in association with fathers' preconceptual exposure to external ionising radiation. This could be because exposure to the hazardous substance or substances did not occur in those populations or that being monitored for exposure to external radiation was not a marker of the relevant exposure.[19 21] The fact that Gardner *et al* found a dose-response relation between fathers' preconceptual external exposure to penetrating ionising radiation and childhood leukaemia and we did not could be because the cumulative dose was a marker of exposure to some hazardous substance or substances at Sellafield but not elsewhere.

Apart from the apparent relation with fathers' preconceptual exposure to ionising radiation, we found no other notable associations. The age and sex distribution of children who had acute lymphoblastic leukaemia diagnosed in the study area conformed to expected patterns, with slightly more boys and a peak age at diagnosis of 3 years; the excess of Down's syndrome in young children with non-lymphocytic forms of leukaemia is as would be expected.[22 23] The relation with pregnancy order is also compatible with the results of other studies, although its meaning is not clear.[24-26] Among the 50 children diagnosed as having leukaemia, no suggestion of an unusual distribution of leukaemic subtypes was found, although diagnostic information in the form of chromosome studies and cell markers became available only in recent years. The malignancies of children whose fathers were monitored for exposure to ionising radiation did not seem to be atypical: all had acute lymphoblastic leukaemia, their ages at diagnosis were not unusual, and the time of their diagnosis was not concentrated in any particular period.

CONCLUSIONS

The findings from this study, taken together with those of Gardner *et al*, suggest that the children of certain men who are monitored for exposure to external ionising radiation in the nuclear industry might be at an increased risk of leukaemia. Because the numbers are small and the results could be due to chance, studies of larger numbers of children are needed. A study investigating the occurrence of all cancers, not only leukaemia, and the incidence of other illnesses and conditions that could have a genetic cause among children of workers in the nuclear industry is under way.

If the effects seen in our study are real, the underlying mechanisms are far from clear. Nevertheless, the hazardous exposure is unlikely to be monitored external penetrating ionising radiation. The possibility that the effects could be due to internal contamination by radioactive substances, a chemical, or some other exposure at work should be explored.

The Department of Health funded AW and SB and the data collection phase of this study. We thank the parents who participated in the study, the general practitioners and hospital staff who helped us, and Lynn Aston, Jim Donovan, Gerald Draper, and Charles Stiller who advised and supported us throughout. We also thank the health physicists who supplied data, particularly Jane Jeffries, Gerry Kendall, Dallas Law, and Len Salmon. Pat Ansell and Margo Pelerin helped with data collection; Eva Alberman, Martin Bobrow, Pat Doyle, Dudley Goodhead, Hazel Inskip, Richard Peto, and Peter Smith commented on earlier drafts; and Sarah Jones and Juliet Jain produced the manuscript. We would especially like to acknowledge Martin Gardner, who died on 22 January 1993, who had advised us on the conduct of the study and commented on the final report.

1 Roman E, Beral V, Carpenter L, Watson A, Barton C, Ryder H, et al. Childhood leukaemia in the West Berkshire and Basingstoke and North Hampshire District Health Authorities in relation to nuclear establishments in the vicinity. BMJ 1987;294:597–602.

2 Committee on Medical Aspects of Radiation in the Environment. Report on the incidence of childhood cancer in the west Berkshire and north Hampshire area, in which are situated the Atomic Weapons Research Establishment, Aldermaston and the Royal Ordance Factory, Burghfield. London: HMSO, 1989. (COMARE 3rd report.)

3 Committee on Medical Aspects of Radiation in the Environment. Investigation of the possible increased incidence of leukaemia in young people near the Dounreay nuclear establishment, Caithness, Scotland. London: HMSO, 1988. (COMARE 2nd report.)

4 Stiller CA, O'Connor CM, Vincent TJ, Draper GJ. The national registry of childhood tumours and the leukaemia/lymphoma data for 1966–83. London: HMSO, 1991:7–16. (Studies on medical and population subjects, No 53.)

5 Office of Population Censuses and Surveys. Classification of occupations and coding index. London: HMSO, 1980.

6 Sanders BM, White GC, Draper GJ. Occupations of fathers of children dying from neoplasms. J Epidemiol Community Health 1981;35:245–50.

7 O'Leary LM, Hicks AM, Peters JM, London S. Parental occupational exposures and risk of childhood cancer: a review. Am J Ind Med 1991;20:17–35.

8 McKinney PA, Alexander FE, Cartwright RA, Parker L. Parental occupations of children with leukaemia in west Cumbria, north Humberside, and Gateshead. BMJ 1991;302:681–7.

9 Beral V, Fraser P, Carpenter L, Booth M, Brown A, Rose G. Mortality of employees of the Atomic Weapons Establishment, 1951–82. BMJ 1988;297:757–70.

10 Fraser P, Booth M, Beral V, Inskip H, Firsht S, Speak S. Collection and validation of data in the United Kingdom Atomic Energy Authority mortality study. BMJ 1985;291:435–9.

11 Kendall GM, Muirhead CR, MacGibbon BH, O'Hagan JA, Conquest AJ, Goodhill AA, *et al*. Mortality and occupational exposure to radiation: first analysis of the National Registry for Radiation Workers. *BMJ* 1992;**304**:220–5.

12 *FOXPRO: user's guide*. Perrysburg, Ohio: Fox Holdings, 1991.

13 SPSS. *Statistical package for the social sciences—X: user's guide*. New York: McGraw Hill, 1989.

14 Breslow NE, Day NE. *Statistical methods in cancer research*. Vol 1. *The analysis of case-control studies*. Lyon: International Agency for Research on Cancer, 1980.

15 *EGRET: user's guide*. Seattle: Statistics and Epidemiology Research Corporation, 1989.

16 Gardner MJ, Snee MP, Hall AJ, Powell CA, Downes S, Terrell JD. Results of case-control study of leukaemia and lymphoma among young people near Sellafield nuclear plant in west Cumbria. *BMJ* 1990;**300**:423–9.

17 Gardner MJ. Paternal occupations of children with leukaemia. *BMJ* 1992;**305**:715.

18 Beral V. Leukaemia and nuclear installations. *BMJ* 1990;**300**:411–2.

19 McLaughlin JR, Anderson TW, Clark EA, King W. *Occupational exposure of fathers to ionizing radiation and the risk of leukaemia in offspring—a case-control study*. Ottawa, Canada: Atomic Energy Control Board, 1992. (AECB project No 7.157.1.)

20 Yoshimoto Y, Mabuchi K. Mortality and cancer risk among the offspring (F_1) of atomic bomb survivors. *J Radiat Res (Tokyo)* 1991; suppl:294–300.

21 Urquhart JD, Black RJ, Muirhead MJ, Sharp L, Maxwell M, Eden OB, *et al*. Case-control study of leukaemia and non-Hodgkin's lymphoma in children in Caithness near the Dounreay nuclear installation. *BMJ* 1991;**302**:687–92.

22 Doll R. The epidemiology of childhood leukaemia. *Journal of the Royal Statistical Society* 1989;**152**:1–11.

23 Narod SA, Stiller C, Lenoir GM. An estimate of the heritable fraction of childhood cancer. *Br J Cancer* 1991;**63**:993–9.

24 Van Steensel-Mol HA, Valkenburg HA, Vandenbroucke JP, Van Zanen GE. Are maternal fertility problems related to childhood leukaemia? *Int J Epidemiol* 1985;**14**:555–9.

25 Kaye SA, Robison LL, Smithson WA, Gunderson P, King FL, Neglia JP. Maternal reproductive history and birth characteristics in childhood acute leukaemia. *Cancer* 1991;**68**:1351–5.

26 Greaves MF. Speculations on the cause of childhood acute lymphoblastic leukaemia. *Leukaemia* 1988;**2**:120–5.

37: Retinoblastoma in children of former residents of Seascale

Letter to the *British Medical Journal*

J A MORRIS, R BUTLER, R FLOWERDEW,
A C GATRELL

In 1990 three cases of retinoblastoma were reported in children whose mothers had spent part of their childhood in Seascale and whose maternal grandfathers had worked at Sellafield nuclear plant.[1] Subsequently a further two cases of retinoblastoma linked to Seascale came to light.[2] The common feature in these five cases is that the mother had been resident in Seascale at some time since the early 1950s, when the Sellafield nuclear plant came into operation.

We have estimated the size of the denominator population as an average of 31·4 births a year which, projected to a 41 year period (1950–90), gives 1287 births. Of the children born in Seascale 57% entered the village school; the others were assumed to have left the village. If the average age at school entry is 4·5 years this gives an outward migration rate of 12·5% a year (95% confidence interval 10·8% to 14·4%).

If it is assumed that the age structure of the inward flow and the outward flow is similar and that those who leave continue to reproduce at the same rate as those of a similar age who stay then an estimate of the number of births to women who leave can be made (table). Two methods of calculation are possible.

Method A assumes that women who leave in any one year will produce a × b children a year thereafter, where a = average number of children born in Seascale per year and b = the migration rate. The number born from 1950 to 1990 is obtained by summing over all years—that is, a × b (sum of 0·5 to 40·5). This will be an overestimate, however, as some of the births will be grandchildren, not children, of Seascale residents.

Method B corrects for this overestimate by using the average age at

Estimate of number of children born 1950–90 whose mothers had lived in Seascale at some time since 1950

Method and migration rate (%)	No of births		
	Outside Seascale	In Seascale	Total
Method A			
10·8	2850	1287	4137
12·5	3299	1287	4586
14·4	3800	1287	5087
Method B			
10·8	2518	1287	3805
12·5	2914	1287	4201
14·4	3357	1287	4644

which women give birth, which in England and Wales between 1950 and 1990 was 27·1 years.[5] The women who leave Seascale in 1950 will produce approximately $a \times b \times 27$ children, as will those who leave in 1951, and so on for 14 years. But then the number will reduce. An extimate is given by:

$$(a \times b \times 27 \times 14) + (a \times b \text{ (sum of } 0·5 \text{ to } 26·5))$$

The total number of births (table) is in the region of 4000–5000. Retinoblastoma occurs in 1 in 20 000 live births, and the expectation in 5000 children is 0·25 case. Five cases is a 20-fold increase (6·4 to 46·4; $p = 0·0001$).

There is a considerable increase in retinoblastoma in children whose mothers have lived in Seascale during the period of operation of the Sellafield nuclear plant. A longitudinal health study of this population is required to see if the incidence of other childhood cancers is increased.

1 Morris JA, Edwards JM, Buckler J. Retinoblastoma in grandchildren of workers at Sellafield nuclear plant. *BMJ* 1990;**301**:1257.
2 Morris JA, Buckler J. Retinoblastoma linked to Seascale. *BMJ* 1991;**302**:112–3.
3 Gardner MJ, Hall AJ, Downes S, Terrell JD. Follow up study of children born elsewhere but attending schools in Seascale, west Cumbria (schools cohort). *BMJ* 1987;**295**:819–22.
4 Gardner MJ, Hall AJ, Downes S, Terrell JD. Follow up study of children born to mothers resident in Seascale, west Cumbria (birth cohort). *BMJ* 1987;**295**:822–7.
5 Office of Population Censuses and Surveys. *Birth statistics.* London: HMSO, 1989.

38: Rural population mixing and childhood leukaemia: effects of the North Sea oil industry in Scotland, including the area near Dounreay nuclear site

LJ KINLEN, F O'BRIEN, K CLARKE, A BALKWILL, F MATTHEWS

To assess whether any excess of childhood leukaemia and non-Hodgkin's lymphoma was associated with certain striking examples of population mixing in rural Scotland produced by the North Sea oil industry, we studied the incidence of these cancers in young people aged under 25 in Scotland. Details were traced for over 30 000 workers involved in the construction of the large oil terminals in the Shetland and Orkney islands in northern Scotland or employed offshore. Home addresses of the 17 160 Scottish residents were postcoded, integrated with census data, and then classified as urban or rural. Rural postcode sectors, ranked by proportion of oil workers, were grouped into three categories with similar numbers of children but contrasting densities of oil workers. The incidence of leukaemia and non-Hodgkin's lymphoma was examined in these rural (and also in urban) categories in the periods 1974–8, 1979–83, and 1984–8.

A significant excess of leukaemia and non-Hodgkin's lymphoma was found in 1979–83 in the group of rural home areas with the largest proportion of oil workers, following closely on large increases in the workforce. The area near the Dounreay nuclear installation, where an excess of leukaemia is already well known, was within the rural high oil category.

The findings support the infection hypothesis that population mixing can increase the incidence of childhood leukaemia in rural areas. They also suggest that the recent excess in the Dounreay–Thurso area is due to population mixing linked to the oil industry, promoted by certain unusual local demographic factors.

Introduction

Evidence has mounted that the incidence of childhood leukaemia can be increased by population mixing, particularly in a rural area.[1-4] This implies an increase in contacts between susceptible and infected individuals for some unidentified transmissible agent whose transmission is more likely in areas of low population density where the prevalence of susceptible people tends to be higher than average. A striking example of rural population mixing has been produced in northern Scotland by the North Sea oil industry. The Sullom Voe oil terminal in Shetland, which can handle 70% of the United Kingdom's crude oil production, was Europe's largest construction site—moreover it is sited in Britain's remotest region.[5] Many thousands of men were transported and housed in specially built camps, drawn from places as diverse as the sparsely populated Scottish highlands and the densely populated conurbations of Britain. Similar arrangements applied to the smaller terminal at Flotta in Orkney. In addition, offshore work involves many thousands of men travelling to Aberdeen from all over Britain, to be ferried to installations by helicopter. Few children live close to these work sites (and, obviously, none offshore), but the regular home visits of these workers might occasion indirect exposure of their home communities to any effects of the mixing in those unusual worksites. We therefore studied leukaemia and non-Hodgkin's lymphoma in young people in the rural home areas of workers at Scottish oil terminal and offshore sites.

Methods

OIL INDUSTRY WORKERS

We concentrated on the three largest groups of workers in the oil industry ("oil workers") in northern Scotland in the late 1970s: construction workers of the oil terminal at Sullom Voe (Shetland); construction workers of the Flotta oil terminal (Orkney); and offshore workers on rigs and platforms. We could not identify all such workers as complete records have not survived and instead used the closest approximations possible—namely, records incorporating home address of all those (more than 17 000) attending the medical centre at the Sullom Voe oil terminal in Shetland during its construction phase (believed to represent a high proportion of all but short stay workers); 3500 construction workers at the Flotta oil terminal in Orkney (incomplete data); and more than 10 000 offshore workers, being all those who obtained an offshore survival certificate (required for such work) in Scotland in the period from June 1976 (the earliest date for which records have not been destroyed) to 1980. Substantial sections of the three workforces were covered in this way. For the purposes of this study, the three groups of oil workers have been combined. Many of these workers lived outside Scotland, particularly in the Tyneside and Teesside areas of England. After eliminating duplication due to men working at more than one site, the postcodes of all Scottish addresses were obtained.

LEUKAEMIA AND NON-HODGKIN'S LYMPHOMA

Details of leukaemia and non-Hodgkin's lymphoma in patients aged under 25 were provided by postcode sector by the Scottish cancer registration scheme for the 1970s and 1980s (from the start of the North Sea oil industry). Expected numbers for each sector were calculated by multiplying the five year age specific population of each sector in different calendar periods (see below) by the corresponding Scottish incidence rates for these diseases.

STUDY CATEGORIES: AREAS AND PERIODS

By integrating the postcoded details of oil workers with census small area statistics by postcode sector we calculated the proportions of oil workers among economically active men (those in work at the time of the census) in each postcode sector of Scotland. "Urban" areas were arbitrarily defined as those postcode districts that embrace Dundee, Aberdeen, and Scotland's central industrial belt stretching from Edinburgh to the Firth of Clyde west of Glasgow. The remainder of Scotland was regarded as "rural". To estimate the proportion of oil workers needed to influence the incidence of childhood leukaemia in a rural population, we created three categories containing different proportions of oil workers but with similar populations of children. We ranked rural postcode sectors in ascending order of proportions of oil workers among economically active men. By accumulating the calculated expected numbers of cases of leukaemia and non-Hodgkin's lymphoma below age 15 we then created three categories with (as far as possible) similar expected numbers. The ranges of density of oil workers in these categories were ≤ 4·81 oil workers per 1000 economically active men (low), 4·82–10·56 (medium), and ≥ 10·57 (high). These ranges were also used to examine urban areas. Aberdeen was examined separately because of its special place in the North Sea oil industry.

The three periods mainly considered were 1974–8, 1979–83, and 1984–8. The period 1979–83 centres on a census year, and 1974–8 and 1984–8 are of similar length (1988 is the latest year for which cancer registration data were available). For the period 1974–8, populations for 1976 were used, estimated as the mean of the relevant age specific numbers from the 1971 and 1981 censuses. For 1984–8, postcode sector populations by age group in 1986 were estimated by adjusting the 1981 figures by the proportionate regional changes in the 1986 age specific estimates of the registrar general's data. (When all sector populations estimated by this method were summed across ages 0–24, the total was 0·56% below the published Scottish figure for 1986.) There was a substantial increase in terminal and offshore activity in 1977–8,[6 7] reaching unprecedented levels shortly afterwards. In terms of their potential effects, the three periods may therefore be seen as pre-mixing, early post-mixing, and later post-mixing.

SPECIFIC INVESTIGATIONS

The incidence of leukaemia and non-Hodgkin's lymphoma was also investigated with respect to factors that may influence the prevalence of individuals susceptible to infective agents or the intensity of exposure. These include relative isolation, taken as more than 20 km from urban areas[8]; social class, defined as the proportion of the population in the registrar general's classes I and II; density of children, taken crudely as the number of enumeration districts in a given sector having 100 or more children (postcode sectors are fairly large, and acreages of enumeration districts are not available); and *increases* from 1971 to 1981 in the numbers of men working away from home in the construction and energy industries ("recent oil *impact* measure"). This measure of increases in men working away from home is unduly conservative but is the closest possible from census data, being the numbers of men in these industries who were working *outside* their local government district of residence in 1981 minus all men in the construction industry in 1971, expressed as a percentage of economically active men in 1981. (Details of men working outside their local government district in 1971 are not available.) It is relevant that these districts are large, in some cases similar to old counties, and that rural areas contained negligible numbers of oil workers in 1971 when the energy industry was not a census category.

STATISTICS

Significance levels (two sided) for the relative risks were calculated,

TABLE I—*Details of study categories*

| Type of area | Category | Oil workers | | | No of economically active men (1981) |
		Density (per 1000) economically active men)	No	No in Sullom Voe	
Rural	Low	0–4·81	555	291	208 570
	Medium	4·82–10·56	1470	794	196 650
	High	10·57–330·4*	5677	2935	182 070
			7702	4020	587 290
Urban (excluding Aberdeen city)	Low	0–4·81	390	235	129 210
	Medium	4·82–10·56	2832	1862	377 190
	High	10·57–40·83	4274	3113	285 290
			7496	5210	791 690
Aberdeen city	High	15·55–75·24	1962	156	61 760

*330·4 in Shetland; with the exception of certain tiny sectors, the highest mainland value was 56.

based on an assumed Poisson distribution. Point estimates for the relative risks were computed by using the observed to expected ratios in the individual exposure groups. Confidence intervals for these were calculated on the basis of the associated binomial probability.[9]

Results

Table 1 shows details of the 17 160 oil workers resident in Scotland, by category, together with the corresponding numbers of economically active men. Observed and expected numbers for leukaemia and non-Hodgkin's lymphoma were combined and are shown in table II for ages 0–4, 5–14, 15–24, and 0–24 by oil worker category in urban and rural Scotland and in the three periods. Of 18 categories only the rural high oil group in 1979–83, the early post-mixing period, showed a significant excess. This reflects an excess at ages 0–4 (31 observed, 16·60 expected) and is associated with a significant trend ($p < 0.01$) across the three rural categories, assuming a log linear model (table III). It is largely due to leukaemia (27 observed, 15·16 expected), mainly acute lymphatic leukaemia. The rural high oil category showed no significant excess in the other two periods in any age group, nor was there any (significant) excess in *any* period in the rural low or medium groups or any urban group. Incidence was also examined in 1969–73 (data not shown), but as in 1974–8 there was no excess in the rural high oil group. An excess at 0–4 years was present in the high category when the rural oil categories were reconstituted on the basis of ranked prevalence of workers

TABLE II—Observed (expected) numbers of cases of leukaemia and non-Hodgkin's lymphoma in young people by density of oil workers in urban and rural Scotland

Oil workers category	Urban areas				Rural areas			
	0–4 years	5–14 years	15–24 years	0–24 years	0–4 years	5–14 years	15–24 years	0–24 years
1974–78 (pre-mixing period)								
Low	8 (10·44)	12 (13·36)	7 (9·38)	27 (33·18)	19 (17·50)	19 (21·91)	14 (14·86)	52 (54·27)
Medium	43 (35·06)	43 (42·37)	27 (30·50)	113 (107·93)	19 (17·23)	25 (20·83)	9 (14·18)	53 (52·23)
High	24 (33·58)	37 (41·36)	38 (29·66)	99 (104·60)	17 (16·19)	23 (19·19)	16 (12·42)	56 (47·79)
Total	75 (79·08)	92 (97·09)	72 (69·54)	239 (245·71)	55 (50·92)	67 (61·93)	39 (41·40)	161 (154·29)
1979–83 (early post-mixing period):								
Low	9 (9·02)	7 (9·08)	9 (10·19)	25 (28·29)	11 (15·69)	15 (15·50)	20 (15·87)	46 (47·05)
Medium	23 (29·23)	25 (27·60)	32 (32·22)	80 (89·05)	15 (16·11)	18 (14·95)	14 (15·45)	47 (46·52)
High	26 (28·33)	27 (27·05)	28 (31·36)	81 (86·74)	31 (16·60)**	17 (14·83)	16 (13·93)	64 (45·37)**
Total	58 (66·38)	59 (63·73)	69 (73·77)	186 (204·08)	57 (48·40)	50 (45·28)	50 (54·25)	157 (138·94)
1984–88 (later post-mixing period):								
Low	12 (9·42)	9 (9·07)	9 (12·76)	30 (31·25)	15 (16·33)	17 (15·84)	16 (19·39)	48 (51·56)
Medium	30 (30·33)	29 (27·40)	35 (39·48)	94 (97·20)	17 (16·55)	15 (15·59)	22 (19·21)	54 (51·35)
High	27 (29·45)	22 (27·41)	48 (38·72)	97 (95·58)	18 (16·91)	19 (15·74)	17 (17·42)	54 (50·06)
Total	69 (69·20)	60 (63·88)	92 (90·96)	221 (224·03)	50 (49·79)	51 (47·17)	55 (56·02)	156 (152·97)

** $p < 0.01$.

TABLE III—*Regulations for leukaemia and non-Hodgkin's lymphoma in 1979–83 in children aged 0–4 years*

Oil worker category	No of cases			Relative risk (95% confidence interval)
	Observed	Expected	O/E	
Low	11	15·69	0·70	1·00
Medium	15	16·11	0·93	1·33 (0·55 to 3·22)
High	31	16·60	1·87	2·67 (1·30 to 5·88)*
Excluding area within 25 km of Dounreay	28	16·26	1·72	2·46 (1·20 to 5·44)*

* $p < 0.01$ for trend.

at Sullom Voe only (28 observed, 16·45 expected; $p < 0.01$), at Flotta only (24 observed, expected 16·27; $p < 0.08$), and offshore (29 observed, expected 16·55; $p < 0.01$).

When examined by single years of age from 0 to 4 (table IV), the rural high oil category showed excesses below age 1, at age 1, and particularly at

TABLE IV—*Annual incidence per 100 000 of leukaemia and non-Hodgkin's lymphoma by age in certain rural and urban categories by calendar period. Observed numbers are given in parentheses*

Age (years)	1974–8	1979–83	1984–8
	Rural high oil worker category		
0	(0)	13 (6)	2 (1)
1	6 (3)	9 (4)	2 (2)
2	9 (4)	38 (17)	15 (7)
3	14 (6)	5 (2)	12 (5)
4	5 (2)	5 (2)	9 (4)
	Rural low and medium oil worker categories		
0	3 (3)	(0)	6 (6)
1	10 (10)	5 (4)	7 (6)
2	9 (9)	9 (8)	6 (5)
3	12 (11)	13 (10)	13 (11)
4	6 (6)	5 (4)	5 (4)
	All urban categories		
0	3 (7)	1 (2)	3 (6)
1	6 (15)	3 (5)	6 (11)
2	10 (23)	13 (22)	11 (20)
3	6 (12)	10 (16)	6 (11)
4	8 (18)	8 (13)	12 (21)

age 2, when annual incidence peaked at 38/100 000/year. This peak at age 2 contrasts with that at age 3 (in all three periods) in the rural low and medium areas, as was found in the rural high oil group in the earlier period, 1974–8. In 1984–8, when incidence at ages 0–4 had declined, the rural high oil group continued to show a peak at age 2 as in urban areas in all three periods. Details of father's occupation in cancer registration and mortality records did not suggest any excess of oil related jobs among the fathers of cases living in rural high oil areas. Moreover, a comparison of the names of all rural oil workers with those of fathers of children with leukaemia or non-Hodgkin's lymphoma in 1979–83 (ascertained for another study) produced only a single match.

Incidence in the rural high oil category was examined in more isolated (> 20 km from urban areas) and less isolated sectors, and at higher and lower levels of certain factors, for which the division was made after ranking the sectors on the factor (disregarding isolation) at the point that as closely as possible halved the cumulative expected values at ages 0–14. The increased incidence at ages 0–4 was restricted to postcode sectors more than 20 km from urban areas, where it was greater in sectors of high social class (table V). There was also some indication of a higher incidence in sectors with a higher child density measure both at ages 0–4 and 5–24, and at both greater and lower degrees of isolation. In more isolated areas, where increases of construction workers working away from home in the 1970s (the recent oil impact measure) were greater, there was a higher incidence of leukaemia and non-Hodgkin's lymphoma at ages 5–24 (but not at 0–4) than in remaining areas. When these differences were investigated by this approach using *three* sub-groups of similar size, the recent oil impact measure in more isolated areas showed a significant trend at ages 5–24 ($p < 0.01$; table VI). Social class in more isolated areas showed a slight (but non-significant) trend in both age groups (table VI).

Discussion

The hypothesis underlying this study was confirmed by finding a signficant increase of childhood leukaemia in those *rural* areas of Scotland that were most affected by population "mixing" associated with the North Sea oil industry. Moreover, the effect occurred in the *early* post-mixing period and mainly in the 0–4 age group, in keeping with findings in rural new towns in their early growth period.[2] There can be concern in a study of this type that multiple testing may have resulted in certain conclusions being due to chance findings. However, the prior hypothesis led us to the findings in the rural high oil worker category (table II, both for all ages and the 0–4 age group. The only multiple testing therefore is within the time periods after population mixing (a total of two cells). However, the unusual

TABLE V—*Observed and expected numbers of cases of leukaemia and non-Hodgkin's lymphoma in rural high oil sectors*

Age (years)	Half*	<20 km from urban area				>20 km from urban area			
		Observed	Expected	O/E	Relative risk (95% confidence interval)	Observed	Expected	O/E	Relative risk (95% confidence interval)
Social class:									
0–4	Lower	9	4·204	2·14	1·00	6	4·056	1·48	1·00
	Higher	2	3·869	0·52	0·24(0·03 to 1·17)	14	4·473	3·13	2·12 (0·78 to 6·71)
5–24	Lower	9	7·436	1·12	1·00	8	7·226	1·11	1·00
	Higher	6	6·295	0·95	0·79 (0·22 to 2·45)	10	7·810	1·28	1·10 (0·42 to 3·41)
Density of children									
0–4	Lower	4	3·824	1·05	1·00	11	5·123	2·15	1·00
	Higher	7	4·249	1·65	1·57 (0·40 to 7·37)	9	3·406	2·64	1·23 (0·45 to 3·27)
5–24	Lower	6	6·967	0·86	1·00	8	9·133	0·88	1·00
	Higher	9	6·764	1·33	1·55 (0·50 to 5·27)	10	5·903	1·69	1·93 (0·70 to 5·70)
Recent oil impact measure:									
0–4	Lower	5	3·145	1·59	1·00	13	5·113	2·54	1·00
	Higher	6	4·928	1·22	0·77 (0·19 to 3·15)	7	3·416	2·05	0·81 (0·27 to 2·20)
5–24	Lower	7	6·059	1·16	1·00	7	9·184	0·76	1·00
	Higher	8	7·672	1·04	0·90 (0·28 to 2·88)	11	5·852	1·88	2·47 (0·86 to 7·51)

* The division into lower and higher was at the closest point possible to halving the total cumulative expected values (for ages 0–14, for the two distance categories combined) ranked on the relevant measure.

TABLE VI—*Effect of recent oil impact measure and social class on leukaemia and non-Hodgkin's lymphoma in rural high oil sectors > 20 km from urban areas*

	Age 0–4 years				Age 5–24 years			
	Observed	Expected	O/E	Relative risk (95% confidence interval)	Observed	Expected	O/E	Relative risk (95% confidence interval)
Recent oil impact measure:								
Low	10	3·74	2·67	1·00	3	6·85	0·44	1·00
Medium	5	2·98	1·68	0·63 (0·17 to 2·02)	7	5·17	1·35	3·09 (0·70 to 18·61)
High	5	1·81	2·76	1·03 (0·27 to 3·33)	8	3·02	2·64	6·04 (1·45 to 35·12)*
Excluding area within 25 km of Dounreay	2	1·47	1·36	0·51 (0·05 to 2·39)	5	2·00	2·50	5·70 (1·11 to 36·70)*
Social class:								
Low	4	2·92	1·37	1·00	5	5·17	0·97	1·00
Medium	8	3·45	2·32	1·69 (0·45 to 7·62)	7	6·00	1·17	1·20 (0·33 to 4·85)
High	8	2·16	3·71	2·71 (0·72 to 12·18)	6	3·86	1·55	1·61 (0·41 to 6·60)

* p<0·01 for trend.

nature of the mixing itself, as well as the areas it affected, warrants further discussion.

Much has been written about the technological challenge of North Sea oil, said to be second only to the American space programme in scale. The development of this industry by 1981 (costing £25 000m at 1980 prices) made a great impact on northern Scotland, a region of longstanding unemployment and depopulation. The building of oil terminals and platforms in the area, together with work offshore, provided unprecedented opportunities for employment. The most extensive operation was the construction in Britain's remotest region, Shetland, of the Sullom Voe oil terminal, the largest such site in Europe. The workforce (well over 20 000 men) contained many from the Highlands and Islands, though the largest numbers were drawn from industrial parts of Scotland (Clydeside) and England (Tyneside and Teesside) that were severely affected by unemployment.

For all this to take place in so remote an area required not only payment of high wages but elaborate logistic arrangements on a massive scale, particularly with the strict conditions laid down by the Shetlands Islands Council to protect both the environment and the local way of life. These conditions severely limited off site recreation. Non-local workers were transported by plane and housed in large, specially built camps or in adjacent accommodation ships. Work hours were long, 10–12 hours per day, $6\frac{1}{2}$ days a week, with a one week break taken away from the islands every four weeks.[5] Weather was often poor, and recreation centred around the bars provided. The high effective population density was further increased, as on any construction site, by the frequent arrival of new workers as others left. Conditions were often crowded. The bringing together of workers was therefore not only on a larger scale but also more continuous than at other oil industry sites, including the isolated platform construction yards at Kishorn, Nigg, and Ardeseir in Highland Region, where many workers travelled from home daily or at least went home at weekends. These differences may be significant given the potency of large and relatively prolonged aggregations for producing epidemics in experiments.[10]

The workforce at Sullom Voe increased from around 1500 early in 1977 to over 6500 in 1979 and over 7200 in 1980; in 1981 the number fell to over 3000 with further declines thereafter.[6] These numbers are exceptional for a construction site. Indeed a survey found that few such sites in rural Britain over the past 45 years reached even 3000. (Sellafield is the most striking exception in the numbers of nuclear and construction workers working together on the same site over most of a 40 year period.) Oil related activity in the North Sea also increased at this time, and helicopter flights to offshore sites reached record numbers in 1978.[7] Such activity would further promote contacts between individuals either susceptible to or infected with micro-organisms.

LEUKAEMIA

Ages 0–4—Leukaemia in Scottish rural areas showed a peak slightly later than in urban areas, at age 3 instead of age 2. This may be due to the very low population density—below 0·03 per acre; similar (slight) differences between rural and urban areas are well known in certain childhood infectious diseases.[11] In the rural high oil category, where incidence increased significantly in 1979–83 (table II), the peak moved during that period to age 2 as in urban areas, remaining there in 1984–8; in other rural areas it continued to be at age 3. The recent peak at age 2 in the rural high oil category might therefore be seen as an "urbanising" effect. Within this category, incidence at ages 0–4 was greatest in areas of relative isolation and higher social class (table VI) as in another recent study.[8] Here the prevalence of people susceptible to infectious agents would tend to be higher than in urban areas or in adjacent rural areas, which show no excess (tables II and VI).

Ages 5–24—There was no excess of leukaemia and non-Hodgkin's lymphoma at ages 5–24 in the rural high oil category. However, their incidence did show a highly significant trend with increasing oil impact measure among rural high oil sectors (p < 0·01; table V). All this is consistent with the absence of any effect of oil work in urban areas (table II): rural postcode sectors already supporting many construction workers (and Highlands Region has one of the highest levels of such workers in Britain) would be expected to be less affected by oil work than similar areas without such earlier "exposure" (that is, those in which the recent impact score was high). Areas with a relatively high density of children also seemed to have a higher incidence (table V), but a combined analysis was dominated by the recent oil impact measure. The absence of an increase [in cases of leukaemia] in the rural high oil category overall in 1979–83 is due to a deficiency that is almost significant in areas with a lower child density or a lower oil impact score—and which was not present in the previous period, 1974–8. Deficiencies at ages 5–24 were noted in new towns and the possibility was considered that they were due to immunising effects of a milder epidemic of the underlying infection.[2] If they were not due to chance, however, this may apply here. The subgroup analyses are, to a certain extent, exploratory.

COMMUNICABLE DISEASES

A severe epidemic of measles among local people in Shetland occurred in 1977–8 with more than 30% of people affected aged over 14 and 10% aged over 24.[12] Conditions at Sullom Voe were considered to have contributed to this epidemic as well as to unusual outbreaks of whooping cough, scarlet fever, and influenza (J D MacGregor, International Epidemiological Association, Edinburgh, 1981).[13] The role of large aggregations of individuals for appreciable periods is probably of central importance here. Such aggregations not only promote transmission of micro-organisms but through repeated exposure allow large doses of these. Large doses may be particularly important in relation to diseases that are uncommon responses to infection, such as feline leukaemia.

ASCERTAINMENT OF OIL WORKERS

Construction workers at the Sullom Voe oil terminal formed the largest group in this study. The proportion of the workforce covered by medical records (the source of our data) is probably greater than on most sites because a visit to the medical centre was one of the few legitimate reasons for breaking off work, so often made irksome by harsh weather. The other two groups were also not fully ascertained (in particular offshore workers who obtained their survival certificate before mid-1976). It is relevant, however, that their proportions in the populations were used only to *rank* the sectors (that is, for internal comparison). When we grouped the sectors approximately into local government districts and then ranked them on density of oil workers, this ranking coincided with that based on data for offshore workers in the 1981 census,[14] suggesting that our data were not affected by geographical bias.

The rural high oil category showed broadly similar excesses whether defined on the basis of all oil workers or of those only at Sullom Voe, at Flotta, or offshore. This probably reflects the fact that all such work tended to attract men from similar areas—those that were conveniently situated or with low levels of local employment. The excesses in the analyses of Flotta or offshore may therefore be indirectly due to the effects of Sullom Voe.

The above fundings on childhood leukaemia provide further evidence for horizontal transmission of some underlying infection of which leukaemia is a rare response[1-4 15] but made more likely in conditions of heavy exposure to the relevant agent, as in feline leukaemia.[2] They also suggest that the relevant agent (or agents) can be transmitted among adults, and thence to children, as suggested by other recent work involving occupational settings.[34] The excess of leukaemia and non-Hodgkin's lymphoma was not concentrated in the children of oil workers themselves, consistent with this being a community (or "herd") effect. The effects of the oil industry observed in this study are also consistent with long established observations on both experimental and human epidemics which Topley summarised 50 years ago as indicating that outbreaks of many infective diseases can be produced simply by "movements of susceptible and infected hosts in relation to one another, and aggregations or dispersals of human or animal herds."[10]

DOUNREAY–THURSO AREA

Among the rural areas with a high proportion of oil workers is the Dounreay–Thurso area, where a recent excess of childhood leukaemia is well known.[16-18] The relation of this excess to the present study has a rather complicated history—with the excess near Sellafield, it originally suggested the population mixing hypothesis, but what was then in mind was the mixing connected with the nuclear industry; an analogy with a new town was drawn.[1] Subsequent studies have supported the hypothesis that population mixing can influence the incidence of childhood leukaemia.[2-4] At the start of the present study and, indeed, until its analysis stage we did not associate the Dounreay–Thurso area with the oil industry, and finding that it contained a high proportion of oil workers was unexpected.

The 20 year interval between the first influx of nuclear workers in the late 1950s and the cluster of cases near Dounreay beginning in 1979 could not readily be explained as the excesses usually followed fairly quickly on other types of population mixing.[1-4] On the other hand, it would be incorrect to suppose that the first influx of nuclear workers in Thurso did not produce the twofold or greater increase noted in rural new towns: the only two cases at ages 0–14 in the period 1951–67 occurred in the five years after the influx in 1958 (expected 0·41; not significant). The well known excess of leukaemia began around 1979, at the same time as the increases found by this study in rural areas far removed from any nuclear installation—but all affected by population mixing associated with the oil industry. The (second) Dounreay–Thurso excess therefore followed closely on a striking example of population mixing.

Leukaemia

The excess of leukaemia and non-Hodgkin's lymphoma at ages 0–4 in 1979–83 in the area within 25 km of Dounreay was appreciable (8·8-fold), only six sectors in the rural high oil category having higher values (from 10·4-fold to 500-fold). The excess at ages 5–24 in this area is particularly noticeable and persistent, continuing up to 1988. The relation with the recent oil impact measure (table VI) has obvious relevance here and also to why all the Thurso cases are in the west of the town, with none in the east: west Thurso is largely composed of nuclear workers not native to the area (locally known as "atomics"), making it until about 10 years ago rather separate from the rest of the town. Compared with sector KW14·8 covering the east part of the town, a smaller proportion of residents in sector KW14·7, which covers the west part, worked in the construction industry in the pre-oil era (table VII). Indeed, the east part of Thurso has a tradition of "travelling workers"—men regularly working away from home on construction. The availability of work at terminals just to the north led to a much greater increase in construction workers (82% compared with 18%) in the western sector (KW14·7) than in the eastern sector (KW14·8), so

TABLE VII—*Leukaemia and non-Hodgkin's lymphoma 1979–88 in Thurso and certain demographic factors in Thurso area*

	West Thurso (post code sector KW14·7)	East Thurso (post code sector KW14·8)
Observed to expected ratios (observed/expected number of cases) of leukaemia and non-Hodgkin's lymphoma*		
Ages 0–4	3·1 (1/0·32)	0 (0/0·16)
Ages 5–24	8·7 (5/0·58)	0 (0/0·34)
Demographic factors in Thurso area†		
% Social classes I and II	44	28
Rank‡	106	57
Rank of recent oil impact measure	99	48
% Increase in construction workers 1971–81§	80	18
% Born outside Scotland (1971)	23	< 10
Rank‡	122	56

* Data for part of postcode sector in parish of Thurso.
† Data for whole of sector.
‡ Among 126 rural high oil sectors (lowest 1, highest 126).
§ Among economically active men relative to 1981.

that by 1981 their levels had become similar. The recent oil impact was therefore greater in the west, which had twice as high a rank as the east (table VII). Also relevant may be the greater density of children in west Thurso, given the evidence suggesting such an effect (table V) and its importance in epidemics.[10][11][19][20] Within the rural high oil category only three (small) sectors more than 20 km from urban areas had a higher rank than west Thurso when the recent oil impact and child density scores were combined.

In contrast, east Thurso (with no cases) may be seen as resembling the urban areas in our study in which the incidence of leukaemia was unaffected by the oil industry. The fewer susceptible people in urban areas would reflect the prior *sporadic* exposure to the widespread relevant agent, which would make them less vulnerable to an *epidemic* caused by new and sudden population mixing.

Intensity of exposure: incomes

The factor that may be decisive in explaining why the oil industry produced in west Thurso so great and prolonged an excess at ages 5–24 is the large number of incomers already associated with the nuclear industry. (An appreciable increase had also occurred in the late 1970s in the numbers of US servicemen and their families in the area). The 1971 census showed that the relevant postcode sector held almost the highest proportion (23%) of residents not born in Scotland of any sector in the rural high oil worker category, and indeed one of the highest in Scotland. Children who moved into west Thurso from other (and often distant) places would have been exposed quite suddenly (at school and elsewhere) to an unusual infective burden. Any such move makes probable the sudden exposure to new agents (or at least new strains) to which children born in the area, even if their parents had moved in, would already have developed some immunity. In the case of west Thurso such effects were likely to be compounded by the scale of exposure to infections among other incoming children, including possibly the infection of which childhood leukaemia is postulated to be a rare consequence. In a recent study of schools within 25 km of Dounreay, the proportion of incomers (born outside the county) among children was highest (namely, 50%) for the birth cohort 1969–74 (R Black, personal communication).[21] The proportion would have been even higher in the Pennyland Estate in west Thurso, for it was built by the nuclear authority specifically for incomers. All the cases of leukaemia in Thurso were centred on this estate, which lies just within 12·5 km of Dounreay, so that the excess there was much higher than in the next cumulative zone, which included the eastern half of the town (within 16·6 km), a difference that has been the subject of much comment.[18] It may not be a coincidence, therefore, that four of the five individuals who developed leukaemia at ages 5–24 in Thurso in the years 1979–88 were incomers—and also that four were born in the years 1969–74, the birth cohort with the greatest proportion of incomers. All three children with leukaemia at ages 0–4 within 25 km of Dounreay were born in the area. The absence of cases in west Thurso above age 4 among children born locally may at least partly reflect the immunity conferred by their recent exposure at earlier ages.

As mentioned previously, in its unusual level of incomers west Thurso resembles a new town, albeit on a smaller scale. Here, this earlier population mixing would have represented a leukaemogenic influence—and in a part of the town in which shortly afterwards a second and different type of mixing was occasioned by the oil industry. Other evidence has suggested that a double influence operates in the development of leukaemia at age 5–24, part early, the other late[15] (possibly analogous to the way that early and persisting pestivirus infection in cattle alters the response to later infection by a different strain).[22] The probable importance of large doses of the relevant agent (from either repeated exposures or particularly heavy exposures) has been emphasised previously in relation to childhood leukaemia.[2] This is established in feline leukaemia, of which the greatly increased incidence in households with many cats is due mainly to exposure of kittens to large doses of a virus that usually causes merely an immunising infection.[23] However, older cats are also at risk if introduced into those special households, but the exposure has usually to be longer.[24] The cases of leukaemia in Thurso at ages 5–24 seem to be analogous, for these occurred later (in 1983–8) than those at ages 0–4 (1980–1).

We cannot test independently the relevance of the high proportion of children not born locally in the isolated area that is west Thurso because no area within the rural high oil category is known to approach its high level. However, the only area (comprising three adjacent sectors) in this category with a comparable proportion not born in Scotland (though it is much less isolated) also showed an excess in the period 1979–83 at ages 5–24 (2 cases observed, 0·54 expected).

Previous studies have not investigated the role of population mixing in the Dounreay–Thurso area, though they have shown that the excess of leukaemia and non-Hodgkin's lymphoma there cannot be attributed to paternal nuclear employment or irradiation before the child's conception.[25] Furthermore, other evidence weighs strongly against radioactive discharges as the cause.[26] The present findings suggest that the excess is due to the population mixing associated with the oil industry causing an epidemic of the infection, to which childhood leukaemia is an uncommon response. Certain factors specific to the Dounreay–Thurso area would have tended to promote transmission and heavy exposure.

We thank Dr Iain Macaulay of British Petroleum, Dyce, Aberdeen, for providing access to records of the Sullom Voe medical centre; Sister Carol Fitzgerald, Sister M Drosso, Helen Wilkes, Wendy Metcalfe, and Marjorie Macleod for help in data extraction; Fiona Smith, Davina Patrizio, Susan Hill, and Janette Wallis for secretarial help; and Jan Warner and Dr Roger Black of the Scottish Cancer Registration Scheme for cancer registration details. We also thank Dr W Pyle and Mr David Sinclair of Flotta, Professor J N Norman and John Brebner of the Robert Gordon Institute in Aberdeen, the managers of the Sullom Voe and Flotta oil terminals, and Mr Falconer Waters of Thurso for their help. We are also grateful to Dr Freda Alexander, Dr Paula Cook-Mozaffari, and Helen Wilkes for their comments on the chapter.

1 Kinlen L. Evidence for an infective cause of childhood leukaemia: comparison of a Scottish new town with nuclear reprocessing sites in Britain. *Lancet* 1988;**ii**:1323–7.
2 Kinlen LJ. Evidence from population mixing in British new towns 1946–85 of an infective basis for childhood leukaemia. *Lancet* 1990;**336**:577–82.
3 Kinlen LJ, Hudson C, Stiller C. Contacts between adults as evidence for an infective origin of childhood leukaemia: an explanation for the excess near nuclear establishments in west Berkshire? *Br J Cancer* 1991;**64**:549–54.
4 Kinlen LJ, Hudson C. Childhood leukaemia and polyomyelitis in relation to military encampments in England and Wales in the period of national military service 1950–63. *BMJ* 1991;**303**:1357–62.
5 Carr BJ, Williamson JL. The Sullom Voe success story. *Proceedings of the Institution of Mechanical Engineers* 1982;**196**:239–58.
6 Project payroll by areas of work. *Sullom Voe Scene.* 1981;No 47 (December):11:(Aberdeen: British Petroleum.)
7 Alvares A. *Offshore: a North Sea journey.* London: Hodder and Stoughton, 1986.
8 Alexander FE, Ricketts TJ, McKinney PA, Cartwright RA. Community lifestyle characteristics and risk of acute lymphoblastic leukaemia in children. *Lancet* 1990;**336**:1461–5.
9 Breslow NE, Day NE. *Statistical methods in cancer research.* Vol 2. *The design and analysis of cohort studies.* Lyons: International Agency for Research on Cancer, 1987:95. (IARC scientific publications No 82.)

10 Topley WWC. The biology of epidemics. *Proc R Soc London* 1942;**130**:337–59.
11 Anderson RM, May RM. Directly transmitted infectious diseases: control by vaccination. *Science* 1982;**215**:1053–60.
12 MacGregorJD, MacDonald J, Ingram EA, McDonnell M, Marshall B. Epidemic measles in Shetland during 1977 and 1978. *BMJ* 1981;**282**:434–6.
13 MacGregor JD. Scarlet fever in Shetland: December 1979 to April 1980. *Communicable Diseases in Scotland Weekly Report* 1980;No 80/21.
14 Office of Population Censuses and Surveys. *Census 1981. Workplace and transport to work. England and Wales.* London: HMSO, 1984:147.
15 Alexander FE. Space-time clustering of childhood acute lymphoblastic leukaemia: indirect evidence for a transmissible agent. *Br J Cancer* 1992;**65**:589–92.
16 Heasman MA, Urquhart JD, Kemp IW, Black RJ. Childhood leukaemia in northern Scotland. *Lancet* 1986;**i**:266.
17 Heasman MA, Kemp IW, Urquhart JD, Black RJ. Leukaemia and lymphatic cancer in young people near nuclear installations. *Lancet* 1986;**i**:385.
18 Committee on the Medical Aspects of Radiation in the Environment. *Investigation of the possible increased incidence of leukaemia in young people near the Dounreay Nuclear Establishment, Caithness, Scotland.* London: HMSO, 1988. (COMARE 2nd report.)
19 Miles A. Herd infection and herd immunity. In: Wilson G, Miles A, Parker MT, eds. *Topley and Wilson's principles of bacteriology, virology and immunity.* Vol 1, 7th ed. London: Edward Arnold, 1983: 413–28.
20 Anderson RM, May RM. Population biology of infectious diseases: part 1. *Nature* 1979;**280**:361–7.
21 Black RJ, Urquhart JD, Kendrick SW, Bunch KJ, Warner J, Adams Jones D. Incidence of leukaemia and other cancers in birth and schools cohorts in the Dounreay area. *BMJ* 1992;**304**:1401–5.
22 Bolin SR, McClurkin AW, Cutlip RC, Coria MF. Severe clinical disease induced in cattle persistently infected with noncytopathic bovine viral diarrhea virus. *Am J Vet Res* 1985;**46**:573–5.
23 Onions DE, Jarrett O. Viral oncogenesis: lessons from naturally occurring animal viruses. *Cancer Surv* 1987;**6**:161–80.
24 Grant CK, Essex M, Gardner MB, Hardy WD Jr. Natural feline leukaemia virus infection and the immune response of cats of different ages. *Cancer Research* 1980;**40**:823–9.
25 Urquhart JD, Black RJ, Muirhead MJ, Sharp L, Maxwell M, Eden OB, *et al.* Case-control study of leukaemia and non-Hodgkin's lymphoma in children in Caithness near the Dounreay nuclear installation. *BMJ* 1991;**302**:687–92.
26 Darby SC, Dall R. Fallout, radiation dose near Dounreay, and childhood leukaemia. *BMJ* 1987;**294**:603–7.

39: Paternal preconceptual radiation exposure in the nuclear industry and leukaemia and non-Hodgkin's lymphoma in young people in Scotland

L J KINLEN, K CLARKE, A BALKWILL

To assess whether a relation exists between paternal exposure to relatively high levels of radiation in the Scottish nuclear industry and the risk of leukaemia and non-Hodgkin's lymphoma in subsequently conceived children, a matched case-control study with three controls for each case was undertaken throughout Scotland.

The fathers of 1024 children with leukaemia and 237 children with non-Hodgkin's lymphoma diagnosed at age 0–25 among those born in Scotland since nuclear operations began (in 1958) were compared with the fathers of 3783 randomly chosen control children. As some workers at one Scottish nuclear site live in north Cumbria, fathers of 80 children with leukaemia and 16 with non-Hodgkin's lymphoma in that area were also studied. Details of all fathers were then matched against records of the nuclear industry. Factors studied included paternal preconceptual exposure to radiation, particularly relatively high levels, during both lifetime and in the six and three months before conception.

No significant excess was observed in any subgroup and

there was no significant trend: fathers of three controls but no cases were exposed to lifetime preconceptual levels of 100 millisieverts (mSv) or more (Fisher's exact p value 0·84). In the six months before conception fathers of two cases and three controls received 10 mSv or more, odds ratio 2·3 (95% confidence interval 0·31 to 17·24). In the three months before conception the fathers of one case and two controls received 5 mSv or more, odds ratio 1·7 (95% confidence interval 0·10 to 30·24). The results for leukaemia and non-Hodgkin's lymphoma combined were similar.

No significant excess of leukaemia or of leukaemia and non-Hodgkin's lymphoma was found at any radiation level in any preconceptual period in any subgroup, and there was no significant trend.

Introduction

An unexpected association has been reported recently between high paternal radiation doses in the nuclear industry (at Sellafield) before conception and subsequent leukaemia and non-Hodgkin's lymphoma in young people.[1] Any test of this hypothesis requires the identification, among the records of men employed in the nuclear industry, of the fathers of affected (and control) children. In practice this involves tracing the dates of birth of many fathers of these children, many of whom died some years ago. In most of Britain this is far from straightforward, but in Scotland it is facilitated by the inclusion of additional details in birth and marriage registration records. We therefore investigated, by a case-control study covering the whole of Scotland, the possible relation between paternal preconceptual radiation in the Scottish nuclear industry and subsequent leukaemia and non-Hodgkin's lymphoma in young people.

Methods

CASES OF LEUKAEMIA AND NON-HODGKIN'S LYMPHOMA

Details were provided by the Scottish cancer registration scheme of cases of leukaemia and non-Hodgkin's lymphoma in the period 1958–90 among people aged under 25 who were born in or after 1958, the year in which nuclear operations began in Scotland. In addition, details of deaths from these causes were obtained from the registrar general and the names of the individuals concerned were then established in register house, Edinburgh.

In this way, individuals who were not represented in the incomplete early years of the cancer registration scheme could be covered. These formed the principal study group, and in addition an attempt was made to cover two much smaller groups: children born in Scotland but whose disease was diagnosed outside, and cases in north Cumbria.

Complete ascertainment of cases of these malignancies diagnosed in England and Wales in the relevant calendar period and age group among individuals who were born in Scotland was not possible, but we included cases known from the nationwide datasets held by the Oxford Survey of Childhood Cancer and the Childhood Cancer Reseach Group. Some additional cases were found by searching records of deaths from childhood cancer in England and Wales which, since 1968, have indicated country of birth.

Inclusion of cases of leukaemia and non-Hodgkin's lymphoma among individuals who were born in or after 1958 in England in the Carlisle, Eden, and Allerdale districts of north Cumbria was prompted by the fact that part of the workforce of the Chapelcross nuclear power station lives over the Scottish border in north Cumbria. Cases in this area were ascertained through the Childhood Cancer Research Group, from death registrations, and through the Northern young persons' malignant disease register.

SELECTION OF CONTROLS

Birth registration details were sought for the patients who were born in Scotland. For each birth certificate traced for a case child and which was associated with a paternal name, three control births of the same sex in the same county were chosen as follows. All the birth registers in the relevant county were examined (in a fixed order) to calculate the numbers of births registered in the county and year in question (cities being treated as counties). In this way each birth in the county could be identified by a unique number. Three random numbers were then generated, not exceeding the total number of births in the county concerned, each leading to a specific birth entry which identified a potential control for a given case. (In north Cumbria, controls were chosen using random numbers from within the Carlisle and Penrith birth registers.) If the entry selected concerned a child of inappropriate sex or without a named father, the first suitable control was chosen from the following entries. Similarly, if a control was found to be already in the study as a case or as a control, that selection was replaced by another. As a result no child with leukaemia or non-Hodgkin's lymphoma diagnosed in Scotland could be selected as a control. At a later stage, an opportunity was provided for all control children to be checked against the Scottish NHS central register. This enabled any control child diagnosed as having leukaemia or non-Hodgkin's lymphoma since 1970 after moving to England or Wales to be identified (and excluded). This exercise also allowed control children who died before the age at diagnosis of their matched case to be identified; these were replaced by the next eligible entry in the birth register.

TRACING PATERNAL DETAILS

We attempted to trace the paternal dates of birth of all case and control children, utilising the fact that in Scotland (uniquely in Britain) the birth certificate includes a reference to details of marriage (if any). In this way, paternal age at marriage could be obtained from the registration details of the marriage (if this took place in Scotland), and in turn, the father's date of birth by tracing his birth registration details (if he had been born in Scotland). In Scotland, the marriage certificate shows the names of the parents (including the maiden name of the mother) of the marrying couple, just as the birth certificate does for the parents of the child. Acceptance of a birth certificate as relating to the man mentioned on a marriage certificate required that not only his name but also the names of both parents and the maiden name of his mother agreed.

The fathers of children aged 0–14 at diagnosis were investigated first and then matched against the records of nuclear workers (see below). The relevant children of almost all successfully matched men were born in, or adjacent to, counties containing nuclear sites. In view of this, and the laborious nature of the method (at most three cases and their controls could be dealt with in an hour), paternal details of young people aged 15–24 at diagnosis, and of their controls, were sought only for those who were born in the "nuclear" counties of Caithness, Sutherland, Ayrshire, Dumfries-shire, Fife, Dumbartonshire, West Lothian, and Edinburgh.

DETAILS OF NUCLEAR WORKERS

Details of nuclear workers in Scotland were available from three sources.

(1) The four sections of the Scottish nuclear industry cooperated in the study by giving us access to details of all past and present male employees, hereafter referred to as nuclear workers. The industry comprises the Dounreay installation in Caithness (Atomic Energy Authority); the Hunterston and Torness power stations in Ayrshire and East Lothian respectively (Scottish Nuclear); the Chapelcross power station in Dumfriesshire (British Nuclear Fuels); and the Ministry of Defence, which includes naval and civilian employees at the Rosyth naval dockyard in Fife and the Faslane, Coleport, and Vulcan bases.

(2) The records of certain civilian workers in the Rosyth naval dockyard who receive only small radiation doses (less than 15 mSv in a year, though in practice usually much less) are governed by special provisions under which their radiation records are not classified with the permanent records of other workers, and need not be retained for more than three years. In the event, however, it was possible to cover such records as far back as 1980.

(3) In addition, the National Radiological Protection Board holds information about nuclear workers from the whole of the United Kingdom in the national register of radiation workers.[2] This will be used in a larger study of parental exposure to radiation and childhood cancer of which the present study will be a part. This register served as an independent check on the previous matching and also allowed some coverage of industrial radiographers and the employees of contractors working on nuclear sites as, except on Ministry of Defence sites, these are not represented in the records of the nuclear industry described above.

MATCHING

The above file of names and dates of fathers of cases and controls was matched against similar details of nuclear workers. We were provided with details of present and past employees at Hunterston, Torness, and Chapelcross. The Atomic Energy Authority and the Ministry of Defence, however, do not keep records of their Scottish employees separately. Partly for this reason, the matching exercise for employees at Dounreay and of the Ministry of Defence was carried out with our help in the central records section of those bodies. All matching was carried out in ignorance of the case or control status of each individual; paternal occupational details shown on birth or death certificates of the children; employment periods of the nuclear workers; the dates of birth of the relevant children; and the radiation exposures of the nuclear workers. Fathers whose date of birth was unknown were included in the matching exercise. Generous allowance was made for possible misspelling of surnames, incomplete forenames, and errors in parts of the birth dates. By this approach we aimed, besides identifying more obvious matches, to produce a series of possible matches which might then be the subject of detailed attention.

Possible matches were investigated, particularly through the national insurance section of the Department of Social Security, but also through the NHS central register and the primary health boards. All available identifying details were used, including NHS number, addresses, and occupation of our study subjects, and national insurance number and addresses held by the nuclear industry. The aim was to obtain positive grounds not only for regarding a match as definite but also for rejecting all others; rejection usually meant establishing that the records referred to separate identified individuals. Similar names were regarded as successfully matched if the dates of birth were identical, provided that the address and occupation as given on the child's birth certificate were (at least) not inconsistent with the nuclear industry records. If the nuclear employment had ceased before the child's birth, a place of birth on the child's birth certificate distant from the nuclear site was allowed if the NHS central register indicated a previous address close to the nuclear site, consistent with the employment records. For fathers of unknown date of birth, a match was accepted if the precise address agreed in the two sets of records and national insurance records had excluded confusion with any other individual. Also accepted were fathers stated on their child's birth certificate to have an occupation compatible with those in the Ministry of Defence when their names and postings agreed with Ministry of Defence records.

The above procedure was followed in the case of all Scottish fathers, irrespective of the period of "nuclear" employment. However, because of the greater difficulty already described of tracing paternal dates of birth in England, possible matches involving north Cumbrian fathers were pursued only if the possible "nuclear" employment preceded the relevant birth. For the same reason, the fathers of case children diagnosed in north Cumbria were matched against nuclear industry records irrespective of the child's place of birth. Only when a match remained possible was the birth certificate of the child checked to investigate whether he or she had been born in north Cumbria.

CHECKS ON THE MATCHING PROCEDURE

Details of paternal occupation on all birth and death certificates were carefully examined for any suggested employment at a nuclear power station, naval dockyard, or in the navy in case exposed individuals had been overlooked. Another check was provided by matching the file of study subjects against the national register of radiation workers.[2] This register does not claim to be complete—radiation workers who withheld their permission are not represented—and, in any case, any individual matched in this way who had been employed in the Scottish nuclear industry should have been identified by our previous matching exercise.

RADIATION DETAILS

For all men for whom a satisfactory match was made, radiation details were sought. These mainly referred to exposures in Scotland, though any exposures incurred during previous employment in the nuclear industry in England and Wales would also have been covered as details are routinely transferred to the new employer. Radiation details were obtained in the form of external total annual doses in millisieverts (mSv) for each year from first employment up to the time of the study. Detailed monthly doses were then requested for the three consecutive calendar years that included the six month period before conception of the relevant child, though this period was not specified in the request. Any records of neutron exposures were also obtained. Radiation doses were calculated for the critical periods proposed by Gardner et al—namely, the lifetime preconceptual exposure and the six months before conception.[1] In addition, we calculated doses in the three months before conception, in which it is biologically plausible that any effect on germ cells would be greatest. The date of conception was

TABLE I—*Leukaemia and non-Hodgkin's lymphoma in Scotland: number of cases by age group and calendar period of birth*

Age (years)	Leukaemia				Non-Hodgkin's lymphoma			
	1958–70	1971–80	1981–90	Total	1958–70	1971–80	1981–90	Total
0–4	302	219	164	685	64	26	10	100
5–14	279	145	35	459	84	56	6	146
15–24*	47	6	0	53	31	4	0	35
Total	628†	370	199	1197	179‡	86	16	281

* Nuclear counties only: Caithness, Sutherland, Ayrshire, Dumfriesshire, Fife, Dumbartonshire, West Lothian, Edinburgh.
† Forty cases identified only from death certificates.
‡ Twenty three cases identified only from death certificates.

taken to be 38 weeks (266 days) before the date of birth; six months was taken as 182 days, and three months as 91 days.

ANALYSIS

Radiation exposures were analysed by using dose categories that included those of Gardner and his colleagues.[1] The results were calculated by using conditional logistic regression analysis with the computer program EGRET,[3] which produces estimates of odds ratios approximating closely to relative risks, together with confidence intervals. When there were no cases in a particular category, Fisher's exact test was used on unmatched cases and controls to test a null hypothesis of homogeneity with the result shown as a p value. Evidence of a dose-response effect (linear trend) was examined using a likelihood ratio test.[4]

Results

A total of 1197 Scottish cases of leukaemia and 281 of non-Hodgkin's lymphoma were investigated, all diagnosed below age 25 in individuals born after 1957. Table I shows details of these 1478 cases by age group and calendar period of birth. In 1293 cases a Scottish birth certificate was traced so that (when 32 without a paternal name were excluded) the names of 1261 fathers were available, forming the principal subjects in this study (table II). Birth certificates could not be traced for the remaining 185; these would include name changes on account of adoption as well as births outside Scotland. For each of the 1261 (case) births associated with a paternal name, three control births were chosen at random from the births registered in the same year and county. When the controls were checked in the NHS central register no instance was found of leukaemia or non-

TABLE II—*Scottish cases of leukaemia and non-Hodgkin's lymphoma and their controls: numbers by availability of birth and paternal details*

	Cases			
	Leukaemia	Non-Hodgkin's lymphoma	Controls	Total
Diagnosed in Scotland	1197	281	NA	1478
Birth certificate traced in Scotland	1050	243	NA	1293
Known paternal name	1024	237	3783	5044
Paternal date of birth traced	875	202	3220	4297

NA = Not applicable.

Hodgkin's lymphoma in a control diagnosed after the person had moved to England or Wales, but this procedure resulted in replacement controls being chosen for 86 controls who died before the age at diagnosis of the relevant case. In this way, a total of 5044 names of fathers of cases and controls who were resident in Scotland at the birth of the children in question were assembled, 4297 with a date of birth. Added to these were 12 fathers of children with these malignancies who, though born in Scotland, had been diagnosed after moving to England and Wales, together with the fathers of 80 children with leukaemia and 16 with non-Hodgkin's lymphoma from north Cumbria, and their controls: this gave a grand total of 5476 fathers who were investigated in the personnel records of the nuclear industry.

Among these 5476 men, 60 were matched definitely in the records of the Scottish nuclear industry and 12 in those for non-classified workers at Rosyth. Many of these 72 fathers were exposed to radiation only after the relevant conception, and only 38 had some preconceptual exposure. Only one match was obtained which involved a child born in north Cumbria. Another 23 possible additional matches were found in the national register of radiation workers. None of these men belonged to the Scottish nuclear industry as defined above; all had been involved in industrial radiography. None therefore represented men who had been overlooked in the previous matching process. Again, most of the radiation exposure of these 23 men occurred after conception of the child, and only three definite matches were found involving preconceptual exposure. This gave a total of 41 case or control fathers who were found to have had some exposure to radiation before the conception of the relevant children (table III). Examination of paternal occupation as given on the birth certificate (together with associated checks) produced no instance of a match being overlooked. Each of the four sections of the Scottish nuclear industry was represented among the matched fathers and also among both the cases and controls with radiation

TABLE III—*Details of fathers identified in records of Scottish nuclear industry and the national register of radiation workers (NRRW)*

	No of definite matches	No with preconceptional radiation exposure		
		Cases	Controls	Total
Nuclear industry (excluding non-classified records)	60	11	27	38
Rosyth (non-classified records)	12	0	0	0
NRRW but not included above	(4–20)†	0	3	3
Total	≥76	11	30	41

* Including 1 from north Cumbria.
† Range given because attempt was made to establish definite matches only for individuals with preconceptual radiation exposure.

exposures before the relevant conception. Among the 60 fathers matched with nuclear industry records, the numbers who had worked at each non-Ministry of Defence site were roughly in proportion to the size of the total (ever employed) workforce: 25 at Dounreay, 12 at Hunterston, and seven at Chapelcross. (The numbers of men ever employed in Ministry of Defence nuclear work in Scotland is uncertain, many naval postings there being short term.) Fifty two of the above matched exactly on date of birth; of the other eight, for whom a date of birth had not been traced, five were described as servicemen on the child's birth certificate, their details matching with Ministry of Defence records of postings. In the three others, there was confirmation from the addresses and other particulars; in two, all three forenames matched.

Exposure details for the preconceptual period were traced for all but one of the fathers who were successfully matched with the occupational records. The exception, the father of a control for non-Hodgkin's lymphoma, was found in the national register of radiation workers and had worked in industrial radiography outside the Scottish nuclear industry from 1956 until 1986, accumulating a lifetime dose of 233 mSv. However, no dosage details were available by calendar period and, in particular, not for the period before the relevant conception (in 1959). He was included in the lowest lifetime exposure category (above zero but less than 50 mSv) but he was excluded from all analyses relating to the three and six month periods before conception. In addition, the father of one of the leukaemia controls warrants mention as the occupation on his child's birth certificate indicated employment in American nuclear powered submarines. However, the US Navy has informed us that no record of occupational exposure to radiation could be traced for this subject.

Table IV shows estimates of relative risk of leukaemia associated with any radiation exposure (that is, >0·0 mSv) before conception. Also shown

377

TABLE IV—*Relative risks for leukaemia in young people by external ionising radiation dose to father*

Father's exposure	Cases (n = 1115)	Controls (n = 3345)	Odds ratio (95% confidence interval)	Likelihood ratio test (df)	p Value
		Leukaemia			
Before conception:					
0	1104	3318	1·00		
Any	11	27	1·26 (0·59 to 3·90)	0·35 (1)	p = 0·55
		By dose			
Before conception:					
0	1104	3318	1·00		
0·01–49·99 mSv	9	21	1·32 (0·58 to 3·02)		
⩾50 mSv	2	6	1·04 (0·21 to 5·17)	0·43 (2)	p = 0·81
In 6 months before conception:					
0	1107	3328	1·00		
0·01–4·99 mSv	6	12	1·64 (0·55 to 4·89)		
⩾5 mSv	2	5	1·26 (0·22 to 7·19)*	0·81 (2)	p = 0·67
In 3 months before conception:					
0	1107	3329	1·00		
0·01–2·49 mSv	6	11	1·84 (0·66 to 5·70)		
⩾2·5 mSv	2	5	1·27 (0·22 to 7·26)†	1·15 (2)	p = 0·56

* Includes father of a control with dose of 5·05 mSv, of which 3·17 mSv was notional.
† Includes father of a control with dose of 3·92 mSv, of which 3·17 mSv was notional.

are the corresponding values by level of paternal radiation exposure in three periods before conception—namely, lifetime and in the six month and three month periods. No significantly increased risk was associated with any preconceptual radiation exposure, nor with any level in any of the three periods considered. There was no significant dose-response gradient. Part of the dose in the three month period before conception in the record of the father of one control was notional. If this dose were omitted, the trend test for leukaemia would be affected only slightly (p = 0·60; for the six month period, p = 0·69). The corresponding data for leukaemia plus non-Hodgkin's lymphoma are presented in table V; again, no dose-response effect or significant excess was found at any level of paternal exposure to radiation.

Details for the preconceptual dose levels at which significant excesses of leukaemia have been reported are given in table VI, namely for lifetime doses of 100 mSv or more and doses of 10 mSv or more in the six months before conception. These could not be included in tables IV and V because in those matched analyses the lack of cases in certain cells precluded estimation of the odds ratios. The odds ratio for the lifetime high level risk (0·00, Fisher's exact p value 0·84) and for the six month high level risk (2·30; 95% confidence limits 0·31 to 17·24) did not significantly deviate from unity. Also shown are the results of a matched analysis of four

TABLE V—*Relative risks for leukaemia and non-Hodgkin's lymphoma in young people by external ionising radiation dose to father*

Father's exposure	Cases (n = 1369)	Controls (n = 4107)	Odds ratio (95% confidence interval)	Likelihood ratio test (df)	p Value
	Leukaemia and non-Hodgkin's lymphoma				
Before conception:					
0	1358	4077	1·00		
Any	11	30	1·11 (0·53 to 2·33)	0·08 (1)	p = 0·78
	By dose				
Before conception:					
0	1358	4077	1·00		
0·01–49·99 mSv	9	24	1·14 (0·51 to 2·54)		
≥50 mSv	2	6	1·02 (0·20 to 5·06)	0·10 (2)	p = 0·95
In 6 months before conception:*					
0	1361	4087	1·00		
0·01–4·99 mSv	6	14	1·35 (0·47 to 3·82)		
≥5 mSv	2	5	1·25 (0·22 to 7·08)†	0·36 (2)	p = 0·84
In 3 months before conception:*					
0	1361	4089	1·00		
0·01–2·49 mSv	6	12	1·64 (0·55 to 4·89)		
≥2·5 mSv	2	5	1·26 (0·22 to 7·19)‡	0·81 (2)	p = 0·67

* One father of above 4107 controls excluded (dosage details not available by calendar period).
† Includes father of a control with dose of 5·05 mSv, of which 3·17 mSv was notional.
‡ Includes father of a control with dose of 3·92 mSv, of which 3·17 mSv was notional.

exposure levels for the three month period before conception: for levels of 5 mSv or more the odds ratio for leukaemia was 1·73 (0·10 to 30·76).

Few subjects in the study were recorded as having any neutron exposures before the relevant child was conceived: 0·4 mSv in each of two cases and 6·4, 9·3, 0·8, 8·2, and 0·1 mSv in each of five controls. One of these men, the father of a leukaemia control, received 4·94 mSv in the three months before the child was conceived, of which 1·0 mSv was from neutrons. No other case or control with neutron exposure was near the upper limit of any dose category in any period. If, as has been proposed,[6] a higher quality factor (than the current 10) for neutron exposure had been used, the effective dose in this subject would have risen from 4·94 to over 5 mSv in this three month period, causing the odds ratio shown in table VI for this dose level to fall from 1·73 to 1·07 (95% confidence limits 0·09 to 13·14) and for leukaemia and non-Hodgkin's lymphoma to 1·06 (0·09 to 12·87).

Discussion

This study of leukaemia and non-Hodgkin's lymphoma, like the recent

TABLE VI—*Number of cases and controls and odds ratio or Fisher's exact p value for the highest categories of father's external radiation exposure (mSv) before conception of child*

Father's exposure	No of cases	No of controls	Odds ratio (95% confidence interval)	Likelihood ratio test (df)	p Value
			Leukaemia		
Lifetime up to conception:					
< 100 mSv	1115	3342			
≥ 100 mSv	0	3	0·00		p = 0·84*
In 6 months before conception:					
< 10 mSv	1113	3342	1·00		
≥ 10 mSv	2	3	2·30 (0·31 to 17·24)†		
In 3 months before conception:					
< 5 mSv	1114	3343	1·00		
≥ 5 mSv	1	2	1·73 (0·10 to 30·76)†		
0	1107	3329	1·00		
0·01–2·49 mSv	6	11	1·84 (0·59 to 5·67)		
2·50–4·99 mSv	1	3	1·06 (0·11 to 10·25)‡		
≥ 5 mSv	1	2	1·73 (0·10 to 30·76)	1·22 (3)	p = 0·75
			Leukaemia and non-Hodgkin's lymphoma		
In 3 months before conception:					
0	1361	4089	1·00		
0·01–2·49 mSv	6	12	1·47 (0·51 to 4·27)		
2·50–4·99 mSv	1	3	1·04 (0·11 to 10·00)‡		
≥ 5 mSv	1	2	1·73 (0·10 to 30·76)	0·63 (3)	p = 0·89

* Fisher's exact p value.
† Odds ratios and confidence limits for leukaemia and non-Hodgkin's lymphoma are the same.
‡ Includes father of a control with a dose of 3·92 mSv, of which 3·17 was notional.

Canadian study of leukaemia,[7] found no significant association with paternal preconceptual exposure to radiation as reported by Gardner and colleagues.[1] The latter study, covering the area near Sellafield, found an odds ratio (using parish controls) of 8·30 (95% confidence interval 1·36 to 50·56) for these malignancies in the children of men with a lifetime dose (up to the time the child was conceived) of 100 mSv or greater. We found three men in this category, all fathers of controls (odds ratio 0·00), an unlikely finding if the true odds were 8·3 (0·028 is the conditional probability under this assumption) let alone the higher values of the confidence interval (up to 50·5). Our findings would also make unlikely a true odds ratio of 5·2, at the upper 95% confidence limit of our odds ratio. However, if all available evidence were to be used and our data were combined with that from the Canadian study (which found five controls but no cases in this category),[7] an appreciably lower level of risk could be excluded. Gardner *et al* reported an odds ratio of 5·0[1] (later corrected to 4·5[5]; 1·08 to 18·78) for leukaemia and non-Hodgkin's lymphoma in relation to exposures of 10 mSv or more in the six months before conception. (The period specified suggests greater precision than was available as the figures were based on a halving of the estimated dose in the year before conception.) In our study an odds ratio of 2·30 (0·31 to 17·24) was found for this dose level as actually recorded in the six months before conception (table VI).

If paternal radiation had an effect in the six months before conception, as postulated, it is biologically plausible that this effect would be greatest in the three months before conception. For this period our odds ratio for 5 mSv or more was 1·73 (0·10 to 30·76), based on one case and two controls. The wide confidence interval of our odds ratio for the six month preconceptual period makes it consistent with that in the original study,[1] although there the halving of the estimated dose in the 12 month period introduces a level of uncertainty. The number of workers exposed to relatively high levels in our study was small. Indeed, the potential effects on the odds ratio of minor changes is indicated by its decline from 1·73 for the high exposure level in the three months before conception to 1·06 if, as has been proposed,[6] a higher quality factor for neutron exposure than the current 10 had been used.

The proportion of fathers of controls exposed to radiation before the child was conceived was much smaller (0·8%) in our study than in the original study (15·9%) or in the recent Canadian study (6·0%). This is to be expected as those two studies were conducted in the vicinity of nuclear facilities whereas we covered the whole of Scotland. However, the concordant sets, all unexposed subjects, make no contribution to the results of these matched analyses, and the differences are less with respect to the absolute numbers of exposed fathers of cases and controls. Exposed fathers of leukaemia cases and controls number, respectively, 11 and 27 in this study, 9 and 45 in the original,[1] and 6 and 53 in the Canadian study.[7] The first two of these studies primarily concerned nuclear plant workers whose radiation exposure was monitored by monthly badge readings. The Canadian study included uranium miners whose radiation exposure (mainly due to radon) was until recently monitored differently, so that their external whole body exposures had to be inferred. If only exposed non-miners in that study are considered, the numbers are two cases and 31 controls.

A larger study of this subject covering England and Wales has been started using the databases of the Childhood Cancer Research Group, the Oxford Survey of Childhood Cancer, and the national register of radiation workers.[8] Our use of the national register to check our main findings provides an indication of its completeness and effectiveness for the larger study. Of the 60 fathers whom we successfully identified in the records of the nuclear industry, 47 were also found in the register, and of the remaining 13, 11 had no radiation exposure before the conception of the relevant child. This augers well for the newly launched study; its value is underlined by the importance of the subject and the relatively small numbers of exposed workers in the present study.

Our study fails to confirm the hypothesis that high doses of paternal preconceptual radiation can significantly increase the subsequent risk of childhood leukaemia. The study's statistical power is limited and the findings cannot exclude some relation, though they make it unlikely that the eightfold risk reported to be associated with high lifetime levels is correct. A striking aspect of this association found in the study in west Cumbria is its concentration in Seascale,[1] though most men who work at Sellafield live outside this parish. Suggested alternative explanations for the excess of leukamia and non-Hodgkin's lymphoma in Seascale include an unidentified chemical leukaemogen[10] and an (infective) epidemic promoted by the unusual population mixing in an isolated area of high social class,[11] though support from other studies exists only for the latter hypothesis.[11-15] But if the present study and the Canadian work fail to confirm the claimed relation with paternal preconceptual radiation they equally raise questions about the nature of the unexpected association in the original study.[1] This might reflect the throw of chance or an indirect relation between paternal radiation exposures and the true cause.

Even if paternal radiation were a genuine cause of childhood leukaemia it could not explain the Seascale excess. Of the 11 cases of leukaemia and non-Hodgkin's lymphoma in Seascale the fathers of only two have so far been reported to be associated with the lifetime external levels (100 mSv or more) before conception of the relevant child that Gardner and his colleagues linked to an excess of childhood leukaemia (a third case had been included inappropriately among the Seascale cases[16]). An additional two cases would qualify for inclusion if the high level category were redefined after inspection of the data as > 90 mSv. Attention has been drawn to the lack of information about any paternal radiation on three Seascale cases outside the original case-control study,[17] and this also applies to the two subsequently recorded cases.[16] It has recently been shown that four of these five cases were, like one of the cases in the case-control study,[1] not associated with appreciable paternal radiation before conception.[18] The hypothesis therefore originated largely in a subgroup of the cases that aroused the concern which led to the study. It is well known that hypotheses based on subgroups are often unreliable.

The findings provide little support for a relation between paternal preconceptual radiation and subsequent leukaemia and non-Hodgkin's lymphoma in the offspring. Indeed, if considered with the findings of studies of radiation workers in Canada[7] and of atomic bomb survivors[9] they weigh against such a relation.

We are grateful to the Committee on Medical Aspects of Radiation in the

Environment (COMARE) and the Health and Safety Policy Exchange Meeting of the UK Nuclear Operators for facilitating this study. We also thank the Scottish Cancer Registration Scheme and Jan Warner for providing cancer regression details; the Northern young persons' malignant disease register (Professor Alan Craft); the Childhood Cancer Research Group (Charles Stiller); and the Office of Population Censuses and Surveys for corresponding details for north Cumbria; Dr Louise Parker for choosing control births in north Cumbria; the Atomic Energy Authority (and particularly Len Salmon and Dallas Law), British Nuclear Fuels (Dr Roger Berry, Keith Binks, W Davies, Sheila Roe), the Defence Radiological Protection Service (Surgeon Captain John Harrison, Philip Sinkinson, Graham Hughes), and Scottish Nuclear (Dr Graham Stewart, Dr J McKeown, Dr Christopher Kalman) and the health physics department of the Rosyth Royal Dockyard (Julie Tooley) for providing workforce and radiation details; the National Radiological Protection Board (Dr G M Kendall, Mark Webb), Jean Luthwaite, and the Department of Social Security for help with certain doubtful matches; the NHS central register for Scotland (William McMaster); Francesca Michalak, Majorie Macleod, Vicky Stephenson, and Maureen Lumsden for their work in register house in Edinburgh; Dr Gillian Mann for details of certain diagnoses revised by COMARE; Helena Strange, Susan Hill, and Janette Wallis for clerical help; Mark Dickson and Richard Hickling for computing assistance; Fiona Smith and Sally Price for secretarial help, and Dr Valerie Beral, Dr Paula Cook-Mozaffari, Sir Richard Doll, and Professor P G Smith for their comments.

1 Gardner MJ, Snee MP, Hall AJ, Powell CA, Downes S, Terrell JD. Results of case-control study of leukaemia and lymphoma among young people near Sellafield nuclear plant in west Cumbria. *BMJ* 1990;**300**:423–9.
2 Kendall GM, O'Hagan JA, Rees S, Walker SM, Muirhead CR. Summary of the data held by the National Registry for Radiation Workers. London: HMSO, 1988. (NRPB-R219.)
3 Statistics and Epidemiology Research Corporation. *EGRET*. Seattle: SERC, 1991.
4 Breslow NE, Day NE. *Statistical methods in cancer research.* Vol I. *The analysis of case-control studies.* Lyons: International Agency for Research on Cancer, 1980.
5 Gardner MJ. Paternal occupations of children with leukaemia. *BMJ* 1992;**305**:715.
6 International Commission on Radiological Protection. *1990 Recommendations of the International Commission on Radiological Protection.* Oxford: Pergamon Press, 1991. (ICRP 60.)
7 McLaughlin JR, Anderson TW, Clarke EA, King W. *Occupational exposure of fathers to ionizing radiation and the risk of leukaemia in offspring—a case-control study.* Ottawa: Atomic Energy Control Board, 1992. (Research Report INFO-0424.)
8 Draper GJ, Kendall GM, Muirhead CR, Sarahan T, Fox AJ, Kinlen LJ. Cancer in the children of radiation workers. *Radiological Protection Bulletin* 1992;**129**:10–4.
9 Yoshimoto Y, Neel JV, Schull WJ, Kato H, Soda M, Eto R, *et al.* Malignant tumors during the first two decades of life in the offspring of atomic bomb survivors. *Am J Hum Genet* 1990;**46**:1041–52.
10 Evans HJ. Leukaemia and radiation. *Nature* 1990;**345**:16–7.
11 Kinlen L. Evidence for an infective cause of childhood leukaemia: comparison of a Scottish new town with nuclear reprocessing sites in Britain. *Lancet* 1988;**ii**:1323–7.
12 Kinlen LJ, Clarke K, Hudson C. Evidence from population mixing in British new towns 1946–85 of an infective basis for childhoood leukaemia. *Lancet* 1990;**336**:577–82.
13 Kinlen LJ, Hudson C, Stiller C. Contacts between adults as evidence for an infective origin of childhood leukaemia: an explanation for the excess near nuclear establishments in west Berkshire? *Br J Cancer* 1991;**64**:549–54.
14 Kinlen LJ, Hudson C. Childhood leukaemia and poliomyelitis in relation to military encampments in England and Wales in the period of national military service 1950–63. *BMJ* 1991;**303**:1357–62.

15 Kinlen LJ, O'Brien F, Clarke K, Balkwill A, Matthews F. Rural population mixing and childhood leukaemia: effects of the North Sea oil industry in Scotland—including the area near the Dounreay nuclear site. *BMJ* 1993;**306**:743–8.
16 Draper GJ, Stiller CA, Cartwright RA, Craft AW, Vincent TJ. Cancer in Cumbria and in the vicinity of the Sellafield nuclear installation, 1963–90. *BMJ* 1993;**306**:89–94.
17 Kinlen LJ. Leukaemia and lymphoma among young people near Sellafield. *BMJ* 1990;**300**:677.
18 Kinlen LJ. Can paternal preconceptional radiation account for the increase of leukaemia and non-Hodgkin's lymphoma in Scotland? *BMJ* 1993;**306**:1718–21.

40: Can paternal preconceptual radiation account for the increase of leukaemia and non-Hodgkin's lymphoma in Seascale?

L J KINLEN

Residents of the parish of Seascale, west Cumbria, aged under 25 years during 1951–91 who had leukaemia or non-Hodgkin's lymphoma were studied to assess whether these malignancies could be explained by paternal preconceptual exposure to radiation. Numbers of cases in people born in the parish and in those born elsewhere were compared, separately, with numbers expected on the basis of reference rates for England and Wales. Details of paternal radiation levels in milliseiverts (mSv) were sought for each case.

Significant excesses of leukaemia and non-Hodgkin's lymphoma at ages 0–24 were found in Seascale in those who were born there (ratios of observed to expected cases of these two malignancies were 8·6 and 20·2 respectively; $p < 0.01$). This also applied to those not born there (7·2 and 16·5; $p < 0.01$), a group often regarded as not showing an excess. The estimates were then conservatively recalculated so as to overestimate the risks among those born in Seascale and underestimate them among those born elsewhere. On this basis the six cases in those born in Seascale compare with 0·38 expected (15·8;

$p < 0.001$), of which two were associated with paternal preconceptual lifetime levels of 100 mSv or more and three others with levels of 90–99 mSv. Among those born elsewhere, there were five cases (expected 0.74; ratio 6.7, $p < 0.01$), of which only one was associated with a high level of such radiation.

Paternal preconceptual radiation cannot be the sole cause of the excess in Seascale as it will not explain the excess among those born outside Seascale. It follows that, unless two causes are to be postulated, any single cause must be a factor other than paternal preconceptual radiation. On this basis, the association found among those born there, if not partly due to chance, may reflect an indirect relation with the true cause. The hypothesis about such paternal radiation originated from a subgroup of the excess cases that aroused concern.

Introduction

An increased incidence of leukaemia and non-Hodgkin's lymphoma among young people in Seascale near the nuclear site of Sellafield in west Cumbria has been the subject of much study. Recent work has further strengthened the evidence of an excess, indicating its magnitude as well as its persistence into a recent period.[1] The suggested explanation for this excess that attracts most attention is the one concerning paternal preconceptual exposure to relatively high levels of radiation.[2] This association with leukaemia, which emerged from a study restricted to young people born in west Cumbria, is postulated to be causal and also to explain the excess in Seascale.[2] In fact, the relevant paternal exposure details have been reported only for those children born in Seascale—because no excess cases were considered to be present in young residents who were born elsewhere.[3 4] However, this view has been questioned, and the need for paternal details in cases of these malignancies among those born outside Seascale has been emphasised.[5] These aspects are examined here.

Methods

LEUKAEMIA AND NON-HODGKIN'S LYMPHOMA

Cases of leukaemia and non-Hodgkin's lymphoma occurring below age 25 in Seascale from 1951 to 1991 were identified. The particulars of cases up to 1983 that are listed in the report of the Black Advisory Group[6] have been supplemented by details obtained from a national series of death certificates, from relevant birth certificates, and from local clinicians. Cases diagnosed since 1983[1] have also been included.

Population details by five year age group up to age 24 for Seascale parish were obtained from the Office of Population Censuses and Surveys in the form of unpublished tables for the census years 1961, 1971, 1981, and 1991. The only age group below age 25 for which a 1951 census count is available is 0–14 years (383). Records of the local authority school in Seascale showed 181 children aged 5–15 on the roll for that year and this has been taken as approximating to the number of residents aged 5–14 years, implying a population of about 202 for the 0–4 age group. The proportion of the 1951 population aged 5–14 that were aged 5–9 and also the populations aged 15–19 and 20–24 were derived using the levels recorded in these age groups in the three subsequent censuses. The age specific populations in intercensal years were derived by linear interpolation. In this way person years by age group could be assembled for 1951–5 and for subsequent quinquennia to 1981–5 and also for the final period 1986–91.

For children born in Seascale, populations by single years of age and single calendar years were estimated by using details of the numbers of births to residents in the years 1950–83 and of moves from the parish by members of this cohort by age and calendar period reported in a previous study.[7] For the years before 1949 and after 1983 the numbers of births were assumed to be low—three a year before 1950 (when the school roll showed an average of around 40 children aged 5–15) and 15 a year after 1983. The levels of outward movement from Seascale among those born there were taken to be slightly higher than those reported,[7] thereby reducing the estimated numbers of those still resident there. These were calculated by rounding the fractions of those remaining in Seascale in each quinquennial calendar period in each age group (derived from table IVb in [7]) downwards to the nearest 0·05 (for example, 0·79 became 0·75 and 0·74 became 0·70). More importantly, it was assumed that the percentage who left at, say, ages 0–4 all migrated at under age 1. To further underestimate the populations in each single year of age and single calendar year, only the integer part of each number was used (for example, 12·9 was treated as 12).

Population estimates for those born elsewhere were derived by subtracting the details of those born in Seascale from the estimates for all residents of the parish. Because the numbers of those born within Seascale had been underestimated, the estimate for those born elsewhere would tend to be inflated, as would the corresponding expected numbers. Erring on the side of exaggerating the expected numbers for the group of special interest, namely those born elsewhere,[5] would lead to a conservative estimate of any excess in this group. As a check on this method it was applied to the births in the years 1950–83 covered in the earlier study.[7] Following up this group until mid-1986 by this method yielded a value of 7548 person years during residence in Seascale—appropriately smaller numbers than those published (8711).[7]

EXPECTED NUMBERS

The numbers of cases of leukaemia and non-Hodgkin's lymphoma observed in Seascale from 1951 to 1991 were compared with the numbers that would be expected. Expected numbers were calculated by applying national reference rates by age group and quinquennium to the corresponding population estimates for Seascale residents who were born there. A similar procedure was carried out for Seascale residents who were born outside the parish. For the period 1962–91, incidence rates for England and Wales from the national register of childhood cancers for ages 0–4, 5–9, and 10–14 and from the national cancer registration scheme for ages 15–19 and 20–24 were used. (Because of concern about incomplete registration of cases in those national schemes in the recent period it was judged prudent to use the rates for 1981–5 also for the period 1986–91.) For the earlier years 1951–61, for which reliable incidence data are not available, the corresponding national death rates were used both because incidence rates are not available for that period and because these malignancies were nearly always fatal.

RADIATION DETAILS

For the fathers of all individuals with leukaemia or non-Hodgkin's lymphoma, details were sought from the relevant nuclear bodies of any radiation exposures at Sellafield or elsewhere before the relevant conception, taken as 266 days (38 weeks) before the date of birth.

Results

The observed and expected numbers of leukaemia and non-Hodgkin's lymphoma in Seascale by age group and calendar period are shown in tables I and II, separately for those born in the parish and for those born outside. The use of different methods for estimating the age specific population for 1951 (consistent with the published census figure for the age group 0–14) had little effect on the expected numbers. No non-fatal case of either malignancy occurred in the years 1951–61, when national mortality was used as the standard. There was a significant excess of leukaemia during the period 1951–91 both among those born in Seascale (4 v 0·31 expected; ratio 12·9, $p < 0·001$) and also in those born elsewhere (3 v 0·58; 5·2, $p < 0·05$) (table I). There was also a significant excess of non-Hodgkin's lymphoma both among those born in Seascale (2 v 0·07; 28·5, $p < 0·01$) and among those born elsewhere (2 v 0·16; 12·5, $p < 0·05$). If these expected

TABLE I—*Leukaemia in young people in Seascale: observed and expected numbers by age group and calendar period 1951-91*

Age group	1951–60	1961–70	1971–80	1981–91	Total	Ratio of observed to expected cases	p Value
Cases among those born in Seascale (expected values in parentheses are underestimates)							
0–4	1 (0·04)	1 (0·05)	1 (0·04)	0 (0·04)	3 (0·17)		
5–9	0 (0·01)	0 (0·02)	1 (0·02)	0 (0·02)	1 (0·07)		
10–14	0 (0·00)	0 (0·01)	0 (0·01)	0 (0·01)	0 (0·03)		
15–19	0 (0·00)	0 (0·00)	0 (0·01)	0 (0·01)	0 (0·02)		
20–24	0 (0·00)	0 (0·00)	0 (0·00)	0 (0·01)	0 (0·01)		
0–24	1 (0·05)	1 (0·09)	2 (0·09)	0 (0·09)	4 (0·31)	12·9	<0·001
Cases among those born outside Seascale (expected values in parentheses are overestimates)							
0–4	0 (0·06)	0 (0·05)	0 (0·04)	0 (0·02)	0 (0·18)		
5–9	1 (0·04)	0 (0·05)	0 (0·04)	0 (0·02)	1 (0·15)		
10–14	0 (0·02)	1 (0·03)	0 (0·03)	0 (0·02)	1 (0·11)		
15–19	0 (0·01)	0 (0·02)	0 (0·03)	1 (0·03)	1 (0·09)		
20–24	0 (0·01)	0 (0·01)	0 (0·02)	0 (0·01)	0 (0·05)		
0–24	1 (0·15)	1 (0·16)	0 (0·16)	1 (0·11)	3 (0·58)	5·2	<0·05

TABLE II—*Non-Hodgkin's lymphoma in young people in Seascale: observed and expected numbers by age group and calendar period 1951–91*

Age group	1951–60	1961–70	1971–80	1981–91	Total	Ratio of observed to expected cases	p Value
Cases among those born in Seascale (expected values in parentheses are underestimates)							
0–4	1 (0·005)	0 (0·01)	0 (0·00)	1 (0·00)	2 (0·02)		
5–9	0 (0·00)	0 (0·01)	0 (0·01)	0 (0·00)	0 (0·02)		
10–14	0 (0·00)	0 (0·00)	0 (0·00)	0 (0·00)	0 (0·01)		
15–19	0 (0·00)	0 (0·01)	0 (0·00)	0 (0·01)	0 (0·01)		
20–24	0 (0·00)	0 (0·00)	0 (0·00)	0 (0·01)	0 (0·01)		
0–24	1 (0·01)	0 (0·02)	0 (0·02)	1 (0·02)	2 (0·07)	28·5	<0·01
Cases among those born outside Seascale (expected values in parentheses are overestimates)							
0–4	0 (0·01)	0 (0·00)	0 (0·00)	0 (0·00)	0 (0·02)		
5–9	0 (0·01)	0 (0·01)	0 (0·01)	1 (0·00)	1 (0·03)		
10–14	0 (0·01)	0 (0·01)	0 (0·01)	0 (0·01)	0 (0·03)		
15–19	0 (0·00)	0 (0·01)	0 (0·01)	0 (0·01)	0 (0·04)		
20–24	0 (0·00)	0 (0·01)	0 (0·01)	1 (0·01)	1 (0·03)		
0–24	0 (0·03)	0 (0·05)	0 (0·05)	2 (0·03)	2 (0·16)	12·5	<0·05

TABLE III—*Details of birthplace and paternal radiation in people aged 0–24 with malignancy who were resident in Seascale at diagnosis*

Case No (Draper et al[1])	Year of diagnosis	Age	Born in Seascale	Diagnosis	Paternal radiation category* (mSv)	Reference No in Black report
1	1954	6	No	Neuroblastoma	0	22
2	1955	7	No	Acute lymphatic leukaemia	0	1
†	1955	2	Yes	Non-Hodgkin's lymphoma	0	14
3	1960	2	Yes	Acute myeloid leukaemia	50–99[a]	3
4	1968	11	No	Acute lymphatic leukaemia	0·1–49[b]	2
5	1968	4	Yes	Acute lymphatic leukaemia	⩾100	5
6	1971	2	Yes	Acute lymphatic leukaemia	⩾100	6
7	1975	15	Yes	Rhabdomyosarcoma	0	26
8	1979	5	Yes	Acute lymphatic leukaemia	50–99[a]	7
9	1983	9	No	Non-Hodgkin's lymphoma	0	16
10	1984	1	Yes	Non-Hodgkin's lymphoma	50–99[a]	17
11	1985	18	No	Pinealoma	0·1–49[c]	NA
12	1988	23	No	Non-Hodgkin's lymphoma (Burkitt-like lymphoma)	⩾100	NA
13	1988	17	Yes	Hodgkin's disease	0·1–49[d]	NA
14	1991	16	No	Acute lymphatic leukaemia	0	NA
15‡	1978	19	Yes	Chronic myeloid leukaemia	⩾100	4
§‡	1954	3	Yes	Subacute lymphatic leukaemia	0	NA

[a] = in range 90–99 mSv; [b] = 5·5 mSv; [c] = 5 mSv; [d] = 0·5 mSv.
NA = Not applicable (diagnosed subsequently, etc).
* Father's lifetime paternal preconceptual (external) radiation.
† Inadvertently omitted initially and reported subsequently.[18]
‡ Diagnosed a few months after leaving Seascale for another address.
§ This case given by Gardner et al.[7]

numbers were not deliberately underestimated in those born in Seascale nor overestimated in the others (see Methods) then the observed to expected ratios for leukaemia become respectively 8·6 (p < 0·01) and 7·2 (p < 0·01). For non-Hodgkin's lymphoma the corresponding ratios are 20·2 (p < 0·01) and 16·5 (p < 0·01). All but one of the five born outside Seascale were born outside west Cumbria.

Details of the radiation exposures of the fathers of these young people before their conception are shown in table III, which uses the categories used by Gardner and colleagues.[2] For completeness, corresponding details are shown for other malignancies as included in the recent study of Draper et al.[1] The cases of leukaemia and non-Hodgkin's lymphoma are far from confined to the subgroup associated with lifetime preconceptual radiation levels of 100 mSv or more—the dosage category found to be associated with an increased relative risk of 8·3 for leukaemia and non-Hodgkin's lymphoma.[2] Of a total of 11 cases diagnosed while resident in Seascale, only three were associated with such high levels (though a further three had levels in the range 90–99 mSv). It is only if attention is restricted to those

TABLE IV—*Leukaemia and non-Hodgkin's lymphoma (NHL) in Seascale residents aged 0–24 years: numbers observed by paternal preconceptual radiation levels in those born in Seascale and those born elsewhere*

Paternal preconceptual radiation (lifetime; mSv)	Leukaemia	NHL	Leukaemia and NHL	Expected No	p Value
Born in Seascale					
Unexposed	0*	1	1		
0·01–49·9	0	0	0		
50–99·9	2	1	3		
>100	2*	0	2		
Total	4	2	6	0·37	<0·001
Born elsewhere					
Unexposed	2	1	3		
0·01–49·9	1	0	1		
50–99·9	0	0	0		
>100	0	1	1		
Total	3	2	5	0·74	<0·01
All residents	7	4	11	1·11	<0·001

* In each of these categories there is an additional individual who developed leukaemia within a few months of leaving Seascale for another address.

born in Seascale that a definite association with high levels of preconceptual radiation appears—shown by five of the six cases (table III). In contrast, in only one of the five cases among those born elsewhere is such an association present. Among the other four, only one father (of case No 4,[1] shown in table III) was recorded as having any radiation exposure before the relevant conception—namely, a lifetime preconceptual dose of 5·5 mSv, none of which was in the six months before conception. All radiation details given in the tables refer to external doses, as in the original study.[2] Inclusion of internal doses made only small absolute differences, though it moved one individual from the range 90–99 mSv to over 100 mSv.

Table IV summarises these details of leukaemia and non-Hodgkin's lymphoma. It would have been inappropriate to include in tables I, II, and IV the two cases of leukaemia that were diagnosed a few months after leaving Seascale. One is the case discovered in the birth cohort study in a child born in 1950 who died in 1954 age 3.[5] The second was diagnosed at age 19 in 1978 but, as was recently pointed out.[1] was inaccurately included in the Black report and also in the case-control study[2] as a Seascale case. Details of these cases are shown in parentheses in table III. The first child died of leukaemia within five months of being registered in the NHS central register at an address away from Seascale, and the other within two months of such a change. Nevertheless these two cases associated with Seascale undoubtedly represent an excess and are therefore relevant to the overall picture of those malignancies in relation to this parish: even if all those who were born in Seascale in the years 1940–91 had left Seascale (after 1951) they would contribute, in the first six months after leaving, only about 600 person years. It can be deduced from the fact that the 8816 person years (among those born in Seascale) yielded an expected value of 0·31, that the expected numbers of cases of leukaemia based on 600 person years would be tiny. Of those two cases, one was associated with a paternal preconceptual radiation level above 100 mSv; the father of the other had not been exposed to radiation.

Discussion

The study shows that, despite the not infrequent assertions to the contrary, a significant excess of leukaemia and non-Hodgkin's lymphoma in Seascale is not restricted to young people who were born there. It was among these that the hypothesis largely originated about paternal preconceptual radiation and the subsequent risk of leukaemia and non-Hodgkin's lymphoma in their children.[2] The present findings also indicate that high levels of such radiation cannot explain the significant excess among young people who moved into the parish.

Our findings for Seascale residents who were born elsewhere may seem to conflict with the reported absence of any excess of these malignancies among children born elsewhere but attending schools in Seascale.[3] A discrepancy is apparent, however, only if certain facts are overlooked. The previous study was not restricted to Seascale but to a group of individuals who were followed up from a time when they attended school in that parish to a fixed time (mid-1986) when some had reached age 35, and long after many of them had moved away from Seascale. No less than 46% of those born outside Seascale who attended the local authority (the main) school had moved again (out of the parish) before reaching the age of 11 years.[3] Inevitably, therefore, an appreciable contribution to the expected values for leukaemia and non-Hodgkin's lymphoma came from periods spent outside Seascale. Furthermore, the expected numbers that were estimated for these malignancies (0·7) referred only to deaths. The only death (in 1956; case No 1 in the Black report) in a child born in 1947 was excluded as the study covered only children born since 1950. There were, however, also two non-fatal cases (case Nos 2 and 16 in the Black report[6]), and a further two cases (case Nos 12 and 14 in Draper et al[4]) have occurred more recently, both in people born outside Seascale.

The large scale of movement out of Seascale is a feature also of the children who were born there, 40% of whom did not stay long enough to attend a local school at the age of 4 or 5—similar to the proportion of parents coming off the electoral register within five years of their child's birth.[7] Almost all the cases of leukaemia and non-Hodgkin's lymphoma among young people born in Seascale have occurred while they were living there. The only two exceptions (both leukaemia) were diagnosed within a few months of the children moving away. (The corresponding expected value cannot be calculated precisely for this period, but it is most unlikely to have been more than 0·05; $p < 0·01$)

The calendar period covered by the present study (1951–91) is wider than that analysed in the recent study by Draper and his colleagues (1963–90 for ages 0–14, 1969–90 for ages 14–24).[1] For the latter periods, the present study found closely similar incidence rates to theirs, in keeping with the similar methods for calculating the populations: for the entire study period, the age standardised annual incidence for leukaemia (all types) and non-Hodgkin's lymphoma was 412·4 per million at ages 0–14 and 218·9 per million at ages 15–24.

Exposures in the high external radiation category occurred only to the fathers of three of the 11 cases in Seascale (or four of 13 if the cases associated with Seascale are included). Even if inspection of the data is allowed to widen the definition of high exposure from 100 mSv to 90 mSv or over, such cases represent only about half the total—namely, six out of 11, or seven out of 13 if the associated cases are included. If the remaining five cases without appreciable paternal preconceptual radiation had been the only cases in Seascale, they would still have represented a significant excess (expected 1·09, $p < 0·01$) and clearly one that cannot be explained on the basis of such radiation. A different explanation must therefore be invoked for these cases. Suggested explanations for the overall excess in Seascale include some unidentified chemical leukaemogen[9] and an (infective) epidemic promoted by the unusual population mixing in an isolated area of high social class,[10] though only for the latter does any independent evidence exist.[10-14] Though it is possible that two separate causes of leukaemia and non-Hodgkin's lymphoma have operated in Seascale, the appeal to scientific parsimony of searching for a single cause cannot lightly be dismissed.

The suggestion that paternal preconceptual radiation could explain the excess of leukaemia and non-Hodgkin's lymphoma in Seascale[2] is not supported by the present study. If there is a single dominant cause for this excess, the association shown by a subgroup with paternal preconceptual radiation, unless partly due to chance, points to an indirect (or conceivably an interactive) relation with the true cause. Some commonality with the excess near Britain's other large remote nuclear site at Dounreay has been strongly suggested,[15] so that the absence of any association there with paternal radiation[14 16] makes an interactive relation[17] most unlikely. If it had been clear from the outset that the association with paternal preconceptual radiation was present only in a subgroup of the excess cases, this association must inevitably have seemed less striking as hypotheses with such a basis are well known often to be unreliable.

I am grateful to Dr A Slovak, chief medical officer, British Nuclear Fuels, and Dr G Green, chief medical officer, Atomic Energy Authority Technology, for details of paternal radiation exposures; Charles Stiller and the Childhood Cancer Research Group for incidence rates at ages 0–14; the Office of Population Censuses and Surveys for cancer incidence rates at ages 15–24 for the period 1962–85; Ms Janette Wallis for clerical help; and Ms Sally Price for secretarial help.

1 Draper GJ, Stiller CA, Cartwright RA, Craft AW, Vincent TJ. Cancer in Cumbria and in the vicinity of the Sellafield nulcear installation, 1963–90. *BMJ* 1993;**306:**89–94.
2 Gardner MJ, Snee MP, Hall AJ, Powell CA, Downes S, Terrell JD. Results of case-control study of leukaemia and lymphoma among young people near Sellafield nuclear plant in west Cumbria. *BMJ* 1990;**300:**423–9.
3 Gardner MJ, Hall AJ, Downes S, Terrell JD. Follow up study of children born elsewhere but attending school in Seascale, west Cumbria (schools cohort). *BMJ* 1987;**295:**819–22.
4 Gardner MJ, Snee MP. Leukaemia and lymphoma among young people near Sellafield. *BMJ* 1990;**300:**678.
5 Kinlen LJ. Leukaemia and lymphoma among young people near Sellafield. *BMJ* 1990;**300:**677.
6 Black D for the Independent Advisory Group. *Investigation of the possible increased incidence of cancer in west Cumbria.* London: HMSO, 1984. (Black report.)
7 Gardner MJ, Hall AJ, Downes S, Terrell JD. Follow up study of children born to mothers resident in Seascale, west Cumbria (birth cohort). *BMJ* 1987;**295:**822–7.
8 Draper GJ, Stiller CA, Cartwright RA, Craft AW, Vincent TJ. Correction: Cancer in Cumbria and in the vicinity of the Sellafield nuclear installation, 1963–90. *BMJ* 1993;**306:**761.
9 Evans HJ. Leukaemia and radiation. *Name* 1990;**345:**16–7.
10 Kinlen L. Evidence for an infective cause of childhood leukaemia: comparison of a Scottish new town with nuclear reprocessing sites in Britain. *Lancet* 1988;**ii:**1323–7.
11 Kinlen LJ. Evidence from population mixing in British new towns 1946–85 of an infective basis for childhood leukaemia. *Lancet* 1990;**336:**577–82.
12 Kinlen LJ, Hudson C, Stiller C. Contacts between adults as evidence for an infective origin of childhood leukaemia: an explanation for the excess near nuclear establishments in west Berkshire? *Br J Cancer* 1991;**64:**549–54.
13 Kinlen LJ, Hudson C. Childhood leukaemia and poliomyelitis in relation to military encampments in England and Wales in the period of national military service 150–63. *BMJ* 1991;**303:**1357–62.
14 Kinlen LJ, O'Brien F, Clark K, Balkwill A, Matthews F. Rural population mixing and childhood leukaemia: effects of the North Sea oil industry in Scotland, including the area near Dounreay nuclear site. *BMJ* 1993;**306:**743–8.
15 Committee on the Medical Aspects of Radiation in the Environment. *Investigation of the possible increased incidence of leukaemia in young people near the Dounreay Nuclear Establishment, Caithness, Scotland.* London: HMSO, 1988 (COMARE, 2nd report.)
16 Urquhart JD, Black RJ, Muirhead MJ, Sharp L, Maxwell M, Eden OB, *et al.* Case-control study of leukaemia and non-Hodgkin's lymphoma in children in Caithness near the Dounreay nuclear installation. *BMJ* 1991;**302:**687–92.
17 Greaves MF. The Sellafield childhood leukaemia cluster: are germline mutations responsible? *Leukaemia* 1990;**4:**391–6.

41: Investigation of the possible increased incidence of cancer in west Cumbria (Black report)

Report of the Independent Advisory Group

Chairman: SIR DOUGLAS BLACK

Chapter 2: Epidemiological evidence and recommendations

BACKGROUND

2.1 Our initial concern was to establish whether or not there was an increased incidence or cluster of cancer, particularly in young people, in the area around Sellafield. The word cluster, which has a technical meaning related to a concentration of cases in space and time, will not be used in this chapter because we are concerned with an extended time period.

2.2 Mr Cutler, the producer of the YTV film, told us that his original intention had been to look at the effects of occupational exposure to radiation in the nuclear power industry, and that initially he had approached BNFL at Sellafield with this in mind. BNFL had already published preliminary epidemiological studies on their workers (Clough 1983) and they agreed to co-operate. However, the attention of the YTV team was drawn to a number of children with leukaemia in Seascale. This led them to change the direction of their investigation, and to concentrate on the general population living near Sellafield.

2.3 The YTV study was carried out in an epidemiologically unconventional manner, cases of childhood cancer being identified by talking to local inhabitants and to the parents of affected children. Local registers were searched for deaths of children and death certificates obtained to establish the cause of death.

2.4 By proceeding in this way the YTV team collected information for the years 1956–83 on seven young people with leukaemia who were under 22 years old at diagnosis, and living in Seascale. Using census data they estimated that there was approximately a 10-fold higher incidence of leukaemia among children under 10 years old in Seascale when compared to the national incidence figures; this statement is based on five cases (Cutler 1983a).

2.5 The YTV team identified 25 young people under 22 years old with cancer in Millom rural district dying or diagnosed between 1954 and 1983, including the seven children with leukaemia in Seascale. These included 6 other young people with leukaemia, 2 children with lymphoma in Seascale, 3 young men with testicular teratoma in Millom town, 3 children with brain tumours (one from Seascale), 3 children with sarcomas (one from Seascale), and 1 child with a kidney tumour (Urquhart 1983).

2.6 The YTV team claimed that the above findings demonstrated "a significant high excess of cancer and particularly leukaemia in children under 18 years old in the five coastal parishes south of Windscale in the last 25 years and, in the absence of any readily apparent cause, the *possibility* of a link with environmental radioactivity from Windscale's discharges must be seriously investigated" (Cutler 1983b).

2.7 In a later television programme in April 1984 the YTV team claimed that there was an excess of cancer deaths among persons aged from 15–24 years in Maryport, a town to the north of Sellafield. They also referred to a further child in Seascale recently diagnosed as having cancer.

2.8 YTV had perforce to use unconventional and unsystematic methods to ascertain their cases. One of our tasks was to check the validity of their results. This included preparing, from official records where possible, a list of young people resident in the area who, since 1950, have died from cancer or have been diagnosed as suffering from cancer.

2.9 An exaggeration of the problem might have arisen in the way that the above data were used because the age group reported was defined by the ages of the discovered cases (paragraph 2.4). This is exemplified also in the statement in paragraph 2.6 with the choice of the age of 18 years as the upper limit. A statistically sounder method is first to define the age range of interest (0–14 years of age is most commonly used for childhood cancer) and then to ascertain the number of cases which fall within this defined range.

2.10 Selection of specific geographical areas for study on the basis of cases of cancer discovered in them may also lead to an artificial result. This can be seen by considering what would happen if there were four cases of leukaemia diagnosed in a particular town. The four (or fewer) streets where the four cases lived would each have a "high" incidence of leukaemia, while all the other streets would have a zero incidence. This result would be a true description of the incidence of leukaemia in the different streets of the town. However it might reflect, not an aetiological influence peculiar to those streets, but merely the fact that four cases of leukaemia cannot occur in more than four streets. Similarly, if parishes are selected for study because cases of cancer are known to have occurred there, it is not surprising if the incidence of cancer in those parishes is found to be unusually high. The same comments apply to similar selection of certain calendar years, disease categories, and age ranges for study.

2.12   Seascale is not a typical west Cumbrian village. We were told that the Ministry of Supply and the United Kingdom Atomic Energy Authority (UKAEA) built much of the accommodation in the village to house its staff before and at the time that the Windscale *piles* were under construction in 1952. We believe that BNFL continues to own a significant proportion of the houses. These are rented mainly to young graduates, who are a mobile population, possibly more likely to be working with radioactive material than the average BNFL employee.

2.13   We were also told that the population of Seascale was more mobile than that of many adjacent villages. This could affect the estimated incidence of cancer in various ways. For instance, the annual size of the population is not known accurately as censuses are only undertaken every 10 years. This results in uncertainty about the numbers to be used in each age group to calculate rates or expected numbers of cases. Also, when considering the effect of a local environmental carcinogen on the incidence of malignant disease in such an area, the latent period between exposure and the development of malignancy can result in under-ascertainment due to emigration of cases. Such population movement is of particular importance when considering the incidence of cancers with long latent intervals between exposure and diagnosis, such as were found for solid tumours in those exposed following the dropping of atom bombs at Hiroshima and Nagasaki.

2.17   All of the fathers of the seven Seascale leukaemia cases, and three of the fathers of the five Seascale cases of other cancers worked at BNFL. These are not unexpected proportions given the predominance of BNFL employees resident in Seascale.

Chapter 6: Conclusions and recommendations

6.1   Our group was set up following a programme produced by YTV, and shown on the national network on Tuesday 1 November 1983. The programme alleged that there had been an excess of young people with leukaemia and other cancers in the neighbourhood of the Windscale plant for reprocessing nuclear fuel situated on BNFL's Sellafield site. The whole programme aroused considerable local and national concern.

6.2   The hypothesis in the television programme that the proximity of Sellafield to the village of Seascale could be a factor in producing cases of childhood leukaemia is not one which can be categorically dismissed, nor on the other hand is it easy to prove.

6.3   In the course of our inquiries we were made aware of what were considered by local doctors and others to be additional unusual concentrations of people with leukaemia, other tumours, and Down's syndrome. The mortality and cancer registry statistics which we examined in chapter 2 included some material concerning older age groups and other cancers and did not support the suggestion that there was any unusual incidence of cancer in people aged over 24 or in other areas of west Cumbria. Down's syndrome falls outside our terms of reference and for this reason we have not examined in detail the evidence relating to the incidence of Down's syndrome in Maryport. We do, however, believe that the matter might be investigated further by detailed studies of maternal age-specific rates of the incidence of congenital disease in the population of the area.

6.4   The number of children who have developed leukaemia in a 30 year period in Seascale was less than 10. This is a relatively small number of cases. Because of uncertainty about the size of the population from which they are drawn the true incidence of leukaemia cannot be determined precisely. The fact that the final estimate of health risk has to be based on data which include those used to raise the hypothesis makes assessment of the significance of the observed incidence of leukaemia difficult. However, taking west Cumbria as a whole, mortality from childhood cancer is near to the national average, particularly for cancers other than leukaemia, but this does not exclude local pockets of high incidence.

6.5   In the northern children's cancer registry region, which contains 765 wards, Seascale had the third highest "lymphoid malignancy" rate during 1968–82 in children under 15 years of age in one study (this excess being entirely due to an increased incidence of leukaemia). Also, Millom rural district (which includes Seascale) had the second highest rate among 152 comparable-sized rural districts in England and Wales, ranked according to mortality from leukaemia among people under the age of 25 during 1968–78. Mortality rates for other diseases in the local population, either of children or adults, are not unusual. In particular the overall mortality rate for young people under 25 in Millom rural district is within normal limits (chapter 2).

6.6   The Sellafield site contains a nuclear operation which is unique in the United Kingdom in terms of scale and complexity. The Windscale plant reprocesses not only the radioactive materials which are generated locally from the Calder Hall power station, but also materials brought from other nuclear power stations in the UK and imported from Italy and Japan (the imported material representing around 10% of the total material handled). The radioactive materials introduced into the plant contain a complex mixture of radioactive and non-radioactive chemicals. In order to reprocess this material and separate out the isotopes of value, large scale physicochemical operations have to be undertaken. The unwanted radioactive materials (gaseous, liquid, and solid) then have to be converted into a form suitable for either safe storage or planned disposal (chapter 3).

6.7   While there is ample evidence of a real and sophisticated concern with the safe operation of the plant, which after all must be a major concern of those who work there, it has to be said that some of the plant was installed many years ago.

6.8   In any complex system there resides the possibility of human error. This was exemplified by the incident in November 1983 shortly after we started our inquiries. Even without such error, the possibility of accident remains, as in the 1957 fire. However, the risks to the public of the Sellafield operation should not be judged against the standard of "total or absolute safety", which is quite unattainable in any human activity. A more realistic standard of comparison would be to the overall risks to the public from public transport or from deriving energy from coal or oil. The fact that no operation can be made absolutely safe does not conflict with the desirability, indeed the necessity, of making it as safe as is practicable.

6.9   Population exposure to radiation is at present inferred from environmental measurements of radionuclides in air, soil, and food. This can only accurately reflect actual exposure if all possible routes from the environment to man are considered and if transfer factors used to calculate doses from environmental levels of radiation are known with certainty (chapter 4).

6.10   It is impossible to establish for certain the situation with regard to environmental levels of radiation around Sellafield 20 or 30 years ago, and we shall never know the actual doses received by those children subsequently contracting leukaemia. In addition one cannot completely exclude the possibility of unplanned discharges which were not detected by the monitoring programmes and yet delivered a significant dose to humans via an unsuspected route.

6.11   Subject to the uncertainties described above, the NRPB provided us with a "best estimate" of the average radiation dose to the red bone marrow received by a model population of the young people in Seascale. We then made a "worst-case" assumption that leukaemia in under 20 year-olds in England and Wales is entirely due to the dose of background radiation received by the red bone marrow, and on this basis we estimated the risk from low dose rate radiation exposure. Using this risk estimate and a simple relationship between dose and effect, we were able to calculate the number of additional deaths from leukaemia in under 20 year-olds in Seascale that might be attributable to the additional dose their red bone marrow received from the discharges from the Sellafield site up to 1980. The number of deaths from leukaemia thus calculated is not sufficient to account for the deaths actually observed in Seascale, being around 20% of the number expected from background radiation (chapter 4, paragraph 4.45).

6.12 These calculations do not support the view that the radiation released from Sellafield was responsible for the observed incidence of leukaemia in Seascale and its neighbourhood. However, it is important to stress the unavoidable uncertainties on dose in this situation, and the model we have used does not exclude other possibilities.

6.13 We have found no evidence of any general risk to health for children or adults living near Sellafield when compared to the rest of Cumbria, and we can give a qualified reassurance to the people who are concerned about a possible health hazard in the neighbourhood of Sellafield. However there are uncertainties concerning the operation of the plant, which were highlighted in the Nuclear Installations Inspectorate report of the November 1983 incident, and also problems attendant on the functioning of a plant, part of which has been long in service. There are further questions concerning the adequacy of the controls over present permitted levels for discharges; the quantitative assesment of apparent excesses of cancer; and possible genetic risks. During our investigations we also found some evidence of lack of co-ordination between the various agencies with an interest in this industry and considering its impact on the health of the community (chapter 4).

Recommendations

6.14 In the interests of enhancing public safety, we believe that these matters should be addressed, and we therefore make the following recommendations. Our terms of reference relate mainly to epidemiological aspects of the problem, but we could not avoid the consideration of other matters during the investigation, in some of which we are unable to claim any special expertise.

I—EPIDEMIOLOGICAL (CHAPTER 2)

Recommendation 1
A study should be carried out on the records of those cases of leukaemia and lymphoma which have been diagnosed among young people up to the age of 25, resident in west Cumbria. These cases should be compared with suitable controls in respect of factors that could be relevant to the development of leukaemia and lymphoma.

Recommendation 2
A study should be carried out of the records on all children born since 1950 to mothers resident in Seascale at the time of birth. Its main purpose would be to examine cancer incidence and mortality among those children, including cases which might have occurred after moving from Seascale.

Recommendation 3
A study should be considered of the records of school children who have attended schools in the area.

Recommendation 4
The northern children's cancer registry should be asked to re-analyse their data using 1961, 1971, and 1981 population census data where appropriate. Also stratification for age at diagnosis, and grouping by electoral ward at birth (as well as at diagnosis), should be undertaken to determine the contribution these factors make to the incidence of leukaemia at Seascale.

Recommendation 5
We were impressed by the amount of data made available to us, and feel that encouragement should be given to an organisation such as OPCS or MRC to co-ordinate centrally the monitoring of small area statistics around major installations producing discharges that might present a carcinogenic or mutagenic hazard to the public. In this way early warning of any untoward health effect could be obtained.

II—HEALTH IMPLICATIONS OF RADIOACTIVE DISCHARGES (CHAPTER 4)

Recommendation 6
More attention should be concentrated on measuring doses of radiation actually received by members of the public in west Cumbria and in other relevant areas (including control areas) using whole body monitors, cyto-genetic techniques, and measurements of urinary and faecal radionuclides as appropriate and feasible. Much of such work is best carried out at a local level, but the ultimate responsibility for seeing that this type of monitoring is carried out should lie with the health departments so that it may be systematically and properly co-ordinated throughout the United Kingdom.

Recommendation 7
More work should be carried out on:
(a) the gut transfer factors at present used, especially for children, with special attention being paid to radionuclides where this factor is believed to be low, and to organic forms of radionuclides;
(b) the metabolic differences between adults and children with a view to improving the models used;
(c) studies on children's habits in relation to the possibility that unknown critical pathways exist which are peculiar to children;
(d) comparisons of the biological effects of low dose rate irradiation from α emitters with the biological effects from β and γ emitters both in vitro and in vivo.

Recommendation 8
Where discharge authorisations are considered, particular attention should be paid to the upper limit placed on discharges over short periods of time, to the removal of solvent from discharges, the adequacy of filter systems to remove particulate material, and to the limits imposed on specific radio-nuclides.

Recommendation 9
There should be a critical review of the necessity for discharges of α as well

as β/γ emitters in discharges from BNFL Sellafield site to be significantly in excess of those from similar plant in other countries.

III REGULATORY MECHANISMS (CHAPTER 4)

Recommendation 10

The controls imposed upon BNFL by government, and the ways in which these are reviewed should be revised so that:

(a) reviews of the authorisations take place more frequently;

(b) greater emphasis is placed on the collection and consideration of relevant epidemiological data and any other human data relevant to the possible health consequences of discharges;

(c) there is formal consultation by the authorising department with health departments and NRPB on the possible health consequences of discharges;

(d) the responsibility for monitoring and for interpretation of the results of monitoring this potentially serious environment pollutant should be more clearly defined by government; these results of monitoring need to be considered in their entirety on a regular basis by a designated body *with significant health representation*, thus enabling decisions on action with regard to the control of permitted discharges to take account of all relevant factors.

42: Committee on Medical Aspects of Radiation in the Environment (COMARE): first report

The implications of the new data on the releases from Sellafield in the 1950s for the conclusions of the *Report on the Investigation of the Possible Increased Incidence of Cancer in West Cumbria* (Black report).

Chairman: M BOBROW

Chapter 5: Conclusions

5.1   The new information from Dr Jakeman and from BNFL shows that there were substantial releases of radioactivity from Sellafield in the early 1950s of which the Black Advisory Group were not aware (III(a) and III(b)). In particular a release of the order of 20 kg of uranium oxide to atmosphere starting in 1954/5.

5.2   The way in which these data came to light is unsatisfactory and undermines our confidence in the adequacy and completeness of the available data. Although we accept that every reasonable effort has been made to ensure completeness of the information now available to us we feel that the monitoring programme and record keeping for the 1950s were such that we cannot be certain that all releases have now been recognised.

5.3   We therefore consider that the level of uncertainty about the information available and about the risk to the population from the Sellafield discharges is now greater than at the time of publication of the Black report.

5.4   We would like to thank Dr Jakeman for this valuable contribution in correcting the available information relating to these early discharges and in bringing this information to our notice.

5.5   We believe that the dose and risk estimates presented by NRPB represent a reasonable picture based on conventional assumptions in the field of radiation protection. However, we have reservations about the conventional framework. A very complex chain of reasoning, involving many uncertainties, is necessary to go from the release data and the sparse environmental monitoring data to a prediction of any possible adverse health effects.

5.6 The multitude and complexity of assumptions needed in order to make the dose and risk assessments are topics to which we wish to return at a later date.

5.7 Notwithstanding the above complexity, we note that the increased doses during the 30 year period between 1950 and 1980 are still well below the doses that are estimated to have been received, during this period, by the population from natural background and from nuclear weapons testing fallout combined.

5.8 The NRPB analysis[18] concludes that 0·1 additional cases of leukaemia would be expected from all sources of radiation in the Seascale study population; Dr Jakeman[13] suggests 0·08 cases in the 200 children born in Seascale during 1950–55; Dr Chamberlain[21] suggests the NRPB calculations tend to overestimate the risk, while calculations using the risk estimates employed in the Black Advisory Group report based on assumptions with regard to the effects of background radiation suggest 0·16 additional cases of leukaemia due to the Sellafield discharges in all those born in Seascale between 1945 and 1980 and resident there until 1980 or their 20th birthday. It should be noted that these calculations of risks do not refer to comparable populations and therefore cannot be directly compared.* However none of them are sufficient alone to explain the observed leukaemia rate in Seascale village.

5.9 The NRPB calculations show that the new data on releases and the change in the gut transfer factor for actinides, increases the dose from the Sellafield discharges to the population in the vicinity of Sellafield from high and low LET radiation by different amounts: up to twofold for low LET radiation and up to four-fold for high LET radiation depending upon the time and duration of residence in Seascale.

5.10 These increased doses are still well below those that would readily explain the observed cases of leukaemia in Seascale using conventional risk estimates. Thus the substance and essential conclusions of the Black Advisory Group report remain unchanged. In order to reach different conclusions it would be necessary to assume either that the calculated doses received or the tissue sensitivity of young persons are at present radically underestimated.

5.11 It is possible that important releases occurred in the past but went unrecorded or undetected by the rudimentary monitoring carried out in the early years. The events since the publication of the Black report increase our concern with this possibility, although it cannot be quantified. This emphasises and underlines our concern regarding the uncertainty with regard to the validity of any conclusions.

5.12 It is possible, within this broad band of uncertainty, to exclude environmental radiation or indeed any other factor as a contributory cause of the cases of leukaemia observed at Seascale, although we stress that there is no firm evidence for the existence of any causal relation between environmental radiation and these leukaemias.

5.13 It is most important to ensure that calculations of dose and risk in relation to future emissions are not hindered by lack of adequate monitoring data or lack of appropriate epidemiological data.

5.14 We are informed that great improvements have been made in monitoring programmes, and that such improved methods have been employed for a long time. We advise Government, however, that they should satisfy themselves as to the adequacy of the current monitoring programme at or near all such installations.

5.15 While we hope that the additional epidemiological data being obtained will clarify the situation further; we must also say that as we shall never know the actual average doses received by the population that the cases are drawn from and, as was pointed out in the Black report (para 6.10), as we shall never know the actual doses received by those children who contracted leukaemia, it is likely that we shall never be able to establish with certainty whether there is any relation between the cases of leukaemia in Seascale and the radioactive discharges from the Sellafield site.

*We understand that more comparable risk estimates for the 1950 cohort will shortly be published by Dr Jakeman[14] and in appendix E of the NRPB addendum to R 171, which we have not seen. For the 1950 cohort the risk of developing radiation-induced leukaemia from the discharges is calculated as 1:33000 by NRPB[18] and 1:14000 by Dr Jakeman[14]. The calculations we have repeated based on the Black report lead to an estimated risk for the same cohort of 1:8000 from the Sellafield discharges plus the Windscale fire.

43: Committee on Medical Aspects of Radiation in the Environment (COMARE): second report

Investigation of the possible increased incidence of leukaemia in young people near the Dounreay Nuclear Establishment, Caithness, Scotland

Chairman: MARTIN BOBROW

Chapter 4

2 ISSUES ADDRESSED

4.10 The issues discussed in the previous chapters raise a number of questions which we need to consider further in reaching our conclusions.

4.11 Does the statistical evidence suggest that the incidences of leukaemia amongst young people living near Dounreay is increased to an extent unlikely to be explained by chance? This question is covered in section 3 which reviews the statistical evidence presented in chapter 2.

4.12 If so, what could be the cause? Could the estimated doses to the local population from the authorised radioactive discharges from the Dounreay site acccount for the leukaemia excess using conventional methods of assessment? In considering this question we review:

  i. The evidence on which dose estimates are based.

  ii. The evidence on which risk assessments are based.

This question is addressed in section 4 which considers the dosimetry evidence presented in chapter 3.

4.13 If the estimated doses from the authorised radioactive discharges, based on conventional assumptions, cannot explain the excess leukaemia incidence, is there any other way in which authorised discharges could be responsible? For instance:

  i. Unrecognised pathways in the environment.

ii. Incorrect assumptions about the risk from high LET radiation.

iii. Incorrect assumptions about target issues for leukaemogenesis.

In section 5 we speculate about these possible mechanisms.

4.14   If it is not the authorised discharges to the environment could it be some aspect of occupational radiation exposure related to site activity? For instance:

i. Preconception effect due to exposure of gonads in workers.

ii. Exposure to families of workers from unrecognised pathways via workers.

These points are discussed in section 6.

4.15   Alternatively could it be something other than losing radiation? For instance:

i. Chemicals used on the site.

ii. A population effect due to workers for the Dounreay site moving into the area.

iii. Non-ionising radiation.

These points are considered in section 7.

4.16   Finally in section 8 we considered whether the leukaemia excess could be due to an infectious agent such as a virus.

4.17   In the rest of this chapter we have addressed the questions outlined above. Having considered these points we shall give a brief overview in section 9 and frame our conclusions and recommendations in subsequent chapters.

6 RADIATION EXPOSURE RELATED TO SITE ACTIVITY

4.58   We are aware of the fact that many of the people who live near Sellafield and Dounreay are workers at the nearby installations. We have limited data on the parental occupation of some of the cases in the Dounreay area (para 2.15), but in the absence of more detailed information on the proportion of children whose parents have at some time worked at Dounreay, we cannot evaluate these data. They do however, raise the possibility that the excess of childhood leukaemia could be partly related to parental occupation at the nuclear installation. There is no direct evidence for this but there are two possible mechanisms by which such an effect could theoretically be mediated.

Preconception effect

4.59   Some data, based on animal experiments,[19] suggest that preconception parental exposure can, in some circumstances, lead to malignancy in offspring by inducing genetic mutation. There is no evidence of this from the limited data available in humans, but the possibility that parents occupationally exposed to radiation may be at above average risk of having children with leukaemia needs to be explored.

Unrecognised pathways via workers

4.60   It is conceivable that minute amounts of radioactive material carried home (eg by dust on clothing) may accumulate and lead to exposure of infants in some unforeseen way.

4.61   Both of these mechanisms by which parental occupational exposure would be implicated are speculative. However, in view of the difficulty in accounting for the observed leukaemia excess by known and accepted mechanisms, the possibilities of either a preconception effect in workers or unrecognised pathways via workers should be investigated.

7 OTHER FACTORS RELATED TO THE SITE

Chemicals

4.62   We are aware of the possibility that there may be an explanation other than radiation. There are other known causes of leukaemia—for example, chemicals such as benzene.[20] UKAEA told us that the use of potentially hazardous chemicals at DNE was on a small scale and subject to normal industrial controls. Nevertheless this possibility needs to be considered.

Population effect

4.63   Another possibility is that the leukaemia incidence may not reflect a local causative agent, but may be related to a specific characteristic of the type of population resident in the area. Both Seascale and Thurso are relatively isolated communities, which have experienced a large influx of scientific, professional, and technical staff and skilled craftsmen to work in the nuclear installations, and their social composition is therefore unusual.

9 OVERVIEW

4.66   In this chapter we conclude that there is evidence of a raised incidence of leukaemia in young people near Dounreay, but that the authorised radioactive discharges from the site are too low to account for this using conventional dose and risk estimates. We have considered a number of possible explanations:

   i. Mechanisms by which the authorised discharges could still be implicated including novel pathways in the environment, incorrect assumptions for high LET radiation, and uncertainty in the choice of target tissue.
   ii. Occupational exposure of workers which could theoretically cause a preconception effect due to parental exposure, or exposure of workers' families by novel pathways via workers.
   iii. Other factors not related to radiation including chemicals, a demographic effect, or viruses.

The possibility that one of these factors or a combination of these factors could be important cannot be ruled out.

Chapter 5: summary and conclusions

1 LEUKAEMIA INCIDENCE

5.1   The incidence of leukaemia among young people age 0–24 living in the vicinity of the Dounreay establishment has been examined in detail, using a number of different areas and time periods for which data are available.

5.2   It must be emphasised that the number of individuals with this disease, in this, as in any comparable area, is small. This causes a degree of uncertainty in any analyses and conclusions. Nevertheless, the best possible efforts must be made to reach firm conclusions.

5.3   Over the complete time-period (1968–1984), and considering the full area within 25 km of Dounreay, six cases of leukaemia were registered among young people aged 0–24 years. This is twice the number expected on the basis of national rates, but the difference does not achieve statistical significance ($p = 0.079$).

5.4   Other comparisons were made varying the geographical area. We regard the results with caution because the boundaries chance to fall close to the homes of the cases. Nevertheless the results showed a statistically significant excess of leukaemia near Dounreay. For example, over the full time period there were excesses greater than threefold both in the area within 12.5 km of Dounreay ($O/E = 3.26$, $p = 0.02$) and in the KW14-7 postcode sector, which contains Dounreay ($O/E = 3.74$, $p = 0.0061$).

5.5   It is notable that all six cases have been registered in the final six year study period (1979–1984). This number of cases would occur by chance only very infrequently ($O/E = 6.50$, $p = 0.00039$). For the same period, in the area within 12.5 km of Dounreay the incidence ratio (O/E) was 10.18 ($p = 0.00016$). Because these results are unexpected and were obtained by inspection of the data they must be regarded with caution. However, we note that these are extreme results and this is a remarkable observation.

5.6   While the geographical areas and time periods chosen for study do affect the observations made, we do not consider that the above estimates of leukaemia incidence in the Dounreay area are artefacts of the selection of geographical or temporal boundaries. No one set of boundaries and time periods is correct and the results must be considered as a whole. In our opinion, the full range of comparisons made by Information and Statistics Division provide clear evidence of a significant excess of leukaemia in young people.

5.7   During the full time period of study (1968–1984) there were two additional cases of leukaemia which had been inappropriately registered as non-Hodgkin's lymphoma (NHL). These two cases could not be included in our analysis of leukaemia incidence because comparable data were not available for the rest of Scotland. However, when leukaemia and NHL incidence were considered together there was a significant excess in the full Dounreay area over the full time period (O/E = 2·07, p = 0·039) in addition to the other boundaries chosen.

5.8   Although chance effects cannot ever be completely ruled out, we are mindful of the fact that a raised incidence of this particular disease at these ages has already been reported near Sellafield, the only other nuclear reprocessing plant in the UK. Notwithstanding the differences between the sites and their surrounding areas and local circumstances, the fact that there is clear evidence of an excess incidence of leukaemia in young people in the areas around both sites makes it less likely that these are chance occurrences.

2 ENVIRONMENTAL RADIATION

5.9   To assess the possible relation between the raised leukaemia incidence and radiation from the Dounreay site we have considered the release of radioactive material from Dounreay. We deal with information on authorised discharges and accidental releases, and information from measurements in the environment.

Authorised discharges

5.10 Authorised discharges of radioactivity from the Dounreay site over the years has been of a relatively low order in comparison with Sellafield. The airborne discharges have been somewhat below those from most nuclear power generating installations and between one and two orders of magnitude below those from the Sellafield reprocessing plant. However, some of the radionuclides discharged to both air and sea are actinides which emit high LET radiation and these are discharged from both Sellafield and Dounreay in a much higher proportion than from nuclear power generating plants.

5.11   Recorded discharges of total radioactivity have been overwhelmingly to the sea, being up to three orders of magnitude greater than those to the air.

5.12   Judging from the details provided to us, the estimates of activity in the discharges used when measurements were not available have been sufficiently cautious to suggest that the totals reported for the authorised discharges are probably an over-estimate.

Accidental releases

5.13   The United Kingdom Atomic Energy Authority presented us with details of accidental releases which contained low levels of radioactivity. A few were reflected in transient slight increases in environmental levels. The total activity from recorded accidental releases appears to have added only minimally to total emissions.

Environmental monitoring

5.14 Marine monitoring, including measurements of radioactivity in seafood, has been carried out by the Ministry of Agriculture, Fisheries and Food (MAFF) on a regular basis since 1958. The levels, in general, were about an order of magnitude below those close to Sellafield, although varying in terms of individual radionuclides. Levels measured have generally, but with a few exceptions, been below those estimated by the NRPB on the basis of recorded discharges, confirming that the cautious assumptions made in the estimation procedure generally tend to overestimate the dose.

5.15 Air monitoring at places remote from the site, using high volume samplers, was introduced as part of a research programme in 1980 at a time when fallout had become relatively low. Analyses have confirmed the reported levels of discharges to air from Dounreay in this recent period. These data have also confirmed the National Radiological Protection Board (NRPB) modelling assumptions. These monitors were not in place for earlier years to confirm discharge levels, and none were placed in the local centre of population, Thurso. However, passive deposition collectors were in place from before 1970. These do not provide quantitative data but would have been sensitive to changes in radioactivity levels in the environment.

5.16 Despite the lack of sufficient land-based environmental monitoring data to confirm in detail the figures for discharges to air throughout the period, there is no real likelihood that discharges to air could be so much higher than those reported as to alter the assessment of the final dose and risk to any significant degree.

Estimates of radiation dose based on known radiation discharges

5.17 Estimates of radiation dose to young people resident in Thurso, have been made by NRPB using conventional dose modelling procedures. Reported discharges for Dounreay contribute only a small proportion of the total estimated dose from all forms of radiation, including natural background, medical radiation, and nuclear weapons test fallout.

5.18 Estimates of dose to specified target tissues in human beings are derived from models based largely on experimental work in animals because it is, in general, difficult to get data from humans. There are therefore major uncertainties concerning both the estimates of dose to specified tissues in the fetus and infant and the choice of tissues relevant to leukaemogenesis early in life.

Estimates of risk to the general population

5.19   Estimates made by NRPB of the risk of leukaemia in Thurso attributable to total radiation dose (from all sources) and employing NRPB's risk coefficients, suggest that the total risk of radiation induced leukaemia in an estimated 4550 young people resident in Thurso between 1950 and 1984 will have been well below 1 case, (0·34) and the risk attributable to discharges very small indeed (0·005).

5.20   There are many uncertainties associated with estimating the risk of radiation induced leukaemia in young people. The human evidence available indicates that exposure *in utero* may be of great importance with regard to the development of leukaemia in children. On present estimates the risk to the fetus and to infants from the discharges from the Dounreay site would not account for the excess of leukaemia observed in the population living in the area surrounding the site. However, the data concerning the risk of leukaemia following low level exposure *in utero* and in infancy are limited. Furthermore, these data are largely confined to exposure to low LET radiation, whereas high LET radiation contributes about 20% of the estimated dose from Dounreay discharges. Although there are differences in the particular radionuclides present, high LET radiation also contributes to the dose from natural background and fallout.

5.21   A comparison of patterns of leukaemia incidence and doses from nuclear weapons test fallout or background radiation, suggests that errors in general risk factors for both low LET and high LET, are most unlikely to be so high that radiation doses from discharges could account for the observed excess incidence of leukaemia. However, there is limited knowledge about the physical and chemical forms of the radionuclides concerned, their distribution in the body, and the relevant target tissues for leukaemogenesis, particularly for children. We therefore cannot exclude the possibility that some features of discharges could generate much higher doses to target organs than the present estimates would suggest.

3   OCCUPATIONAL EXPOSURE

5.22   We were told of some isolated occasions when small amounts of radioactivity attributable to the site were detected off-site. Though we have no expertise in this area, this suggests to us that safeguards against inadvertent transfer off-site have not always been totally effective.

5.23   We have no evidence as to whether, at either Sellafield or Dounreay, the excess of childhood leukaemia is partly related to parental occupation at the nuclear installations but this is a matter which must be investigated at Dounreay as is under way at Sellafield.

4   OTHER FACTORS RELATED TO DOUNREAY

5.24   We have been told that chemicals known to be potentially hazardous

412

are used at the plant on only a small scale under normal industrial controls. We are not aware of any evidence that these could be responsible for cases of childhood leukaemia in the neighbourhood

5.25   As in the area around Sellafield the social class composition of the local population is unusual, consisting of a relatively high population of professional and technical staff and skilled tradesmen, together with their families.

5 CHANCE

5.26   The raised incidence of leukaemia in young people close to Dounreay could be a "chance" occurrence in the sense of the individual cases having no common industrial origin. However, it is less likely to be by chance that such an occurrence would take place around Dounreay and Sellafield, the two installations in the United Kingdom involved in nuclear fuel reprocessing.

6 FINAL CONCLUSION

5.27   There is evidence of a raised incidence of leukaemia among young people living in the vicinity of Dounreay. There are differences between Dounreay and Sellafield, principally a difference of one or more orders of magnitude in discharge levels. However, the evidence of a raised incidence of leukaemia near Dounreay, taken in conjunction with that relating to the area around Sellafield, tends to support the hypothesis that some feature of the nuclear plants that we have examined leads to an increased risk of leukaemia in young people living in the vicinity of those plants. Conventional dose and risk estimates suggest that neither authorised nor accidental discharges could be responsible. There are, however, uncertainties about dose and risk calculations, especially with respect to exposure of the fetus and small child, high LET emissions and prolonged low-level exposure.

5.28   The Committee have considered a number of alternative explanations, including other mechanisms by which the authorised discharges could be implicated; the possibility that parental occupational exposure could be relevant; and the possibility that factors other than radiation could be important. However, in the Committee's view the evidence does not point to any particular explanation, and therefore all possible explanations need to be investigated further. Although chance cannot be entirely dismissed as an explanation of the raised incidence of childhood leukaemia in the vicinity of Dounreay, we consider that it is now less likely than when Sellafield was considered in isolation.

5.29   We are very conscious of the fact that many of our difficulties stem from a general lack of knowledge of the fundamental biological processes involved in leukaemogenesis, and in the behaviour of radionuclides in young people. If these processes were better understood, it is possible that the problems in the locality of Dounreay would be seen in a much clearer perspective. Continuing support and encouragement of basic medical and scientific research is vital. We will therefore make recommendations for further research in these areas. If the leukaemia findings are not a consequence of chance and there is an effect on leukaemia risk related to the Sellafield and Dounreay operations, there must be a mechanism, potentially discoverable and remediable. The findings so far are sufficient to warrant an intensified programme of investigation.

44: Committee on Medical Aspects of Radiation in the Environment (COMARE): third report

Report on the Incidence of Childhood Cancer in the West Berkshire and North Hampshire area, in which are situated the Atomic Weapons Research Establishment, Aldermaston and the Royal Ordnance Factory, Burghfield.

Chairman: M BOBROW

3.47 The nuclear installations operate radiological protection regimes which are specifically designed to limit worker's exposure to radiation to internationally accepted levels. However, there are possible mechanisms by which occupational exposure in adults could theoretically be relevant to the induction of childhood cancer, such as a preconception effect in workers or unrecognised pathways of exposure via workers. Both of these mechanisms, which were discussed in our second report, are highly speculative. However, in view of the difficulty in accounting for the childhood cancer and leukaemia excess, the possibility that parents occupationally exposed to this type of radiation may be at above average risk of having children with leukaemia or cancer, needs to be explored, if only to be excluded.

Chapter 4: Conclusions

CHILDHOOD CANCER INCIDENCE

4.1 There is a small but statistically significant increase in registration rates for childhood leukaemia in the age group 0–14 over the period 1972–1985, in the areas within 10 km of AWRE Aldermaston and ROF Burghfield, compared with both the national rates and the regional rates for Oxford and Wessex.

4.2 In the same areas, there is also a small but statistically significant increase in registration rates for other childhood cancers in the age group 0–14 over the period 1971–1982, compared with national rates.

4.3 These areas lie within the West Berkshire and the Basingstoke and North Hampshire Health Authorities. The registration rates for leukaemia and other cancers in the age group 0–14 in the whole of the West Berkshire and the Basingstoke and North Hampshire Health Authorities also show a statistically significant increase compared with national rates.

4.4 Within the age group 0–14, the elevated registration rates for leukaemia and other cancers, whether considered separately or combined, are confined to the 0–4 year age group. This result applies to the areas within 10 km of the installations and also to areas covered by the whole of these two district health authorities. However, this result needs to be interpreted with caution as the observation was not predicted in advance and only came to light following inspection of these data.

4.5 There is evidence that areas within 10 km of AWRE Aldermaston and ROF Burghfield have had higher registration rates of total childhood cancer in the age group 0–14 than those areas beyond 10 km, but still within the same two district health authorities. However, this is only statistically significant in the age group 0–4 for leukaemia and for total cancers.

4.6 We have considered the possibility that these increased registration rates could be explained by local variation in the completeness of cancer registration; in our judgement this is unlikely to provide the entire explanation.

4.7 We are unable to assess the precise extent to which the increased registration rates for childhood cancer in the area within 10 km of AWRE Aldermaston and ROF Burghfield are unusual, because comparable registration data for childhood cancer in similar small areas in the rest of England and Wales are not yet available.

4.8 In the area within 10 km of AERE Harwell, the available evidence shows no increase in registration rates for childhood leukaemia in the age group 0–14, over the period 1971–1982 compared with national rates. In the same area and for the same time period, there is a statistically significant excess of other cancers in the age group 10–14, compared with national rates, but this result should be treated with caution as it has been obtained by inspection of the data. For the age group 0–14 the registration rates for other cancers in this area are not significantly raised above national rates.

Radiation exposure and dose assessment

4.9 We have considered the estimated radiation doses to the local population from authorised and accidental atmospheric discharges from AWRE Aldermaston, ROF Burghfield, and AERE Harwell. We judge that these atmospheric discharges are much too low to account for the increase in childhood cancer incidence in the area, even allowing for the uncertainties involved in any estimation of radiation dose. The estimated doses from the liquid discharges have, as far as we can ascertain, also been extremely low. We consider it most unlikely that the liquid discharges could cause a sufficient increase in radiation levels to account for the observed increase in childhood cancer incidence in the area.

4.10   We cannot exclude completely the existence of some hitherto unknown and unexpected route by which some individuals could be exposed to increased levels of radiation. Such speculative pathways, including those involving radiation workers, should be explored.

Other factors

4.11   We have also considered factors other than radiation exposure, including chemical carcinogens, demographic phenomena, and viruses. Although we recognise the considerable importance of these factors we are not aware of any specific evidence that these are responsible for the increased incidence of childhood cancer in this area.

MAIN CONCLUSION

4.12   There is a small but stastically significant increase in the incidence of childhood leukaemia and other childhood cancers in the vicinity of AWRE Aldermaston and ROF Burghfield. In our judgement, the authorised and accidental radioactive discharges from AWRE Aldermaston, ROF Burgh-field, and AERE Harwell are far too low to account for the observed increase in childhood cancer incidence in the area. We have considered a number of possible explanations for these findings, including other mechanisms by which radiation may be involved, but we do not have sufficient evidence to point to any one particular explanation and it is possible that a combination of factors may be involved.

4.13   The findings set out in this report, taken with those in previous reports[13] indicate that there is a statistically significant increase in the incidence of childhood leukaemia in the vicinities of Sellafield, Dounreay, and Aldermaston and Burghfield. We cannot exclude completely the possibility that these observations are a consequence of chance or due to the selection of the sites referred to us for our enquiries. However, if there is a link between these installations and childhood leukaemia, it follows that there must be a mechanism for such an association, which should be potentially discoverable and remediable. The findings of this report, together with those of our previous reports, warrant further investigation to clarify the situation.

4.14   We have now completed three reports to Government. Our experi-ence so far leads us to the conclusion that the distribution of cases of childhood leukaemia, or other childhood cancer, around individual nuclear installations cannot be seen in a proper context in the absence of comparable information about the general pattern throughout the rest of the UK. We will therefore make recommendations for further work on the geographical distribution of childhood cancer on a nationwide basis and urge that high priority be given to their implementation.

Chapter 5: Recommendations to government

5.1   We make the following specific recommendations to Government in addition to those already made in our second report.[3]

RECOMMENDATION 1

We have already recommended that case control studies of young people registered as cases of childhood cancer, in the vicinity of those nuclear installations which we have studied, should be undertaken. We have recommended that in these studies particular attention should be paid, where possible, to: the occupations of all members of the relevant households; the history of the exposure of the parents and the children to radiation and potentially carcinogenic chemicals; the children's place of birth; and details of any change of residence.
We now recommend that:
  i. Around Aldermaston and Burghfield, a sample survey of the levels of radionuclides in household dust should be carried out in association with the case control study.
  ii. In association with the case control studies, consideration should be given to the feasibility of monitoring radionuclides in whole body or specific tissues of leukaemic children and appropriate controls. Such studies, where practicable, should be directed towards the determination of the presence or absence of radiologically significant quantities of radionuclides.

RECOMMENDATION 2

We reiterate Recommendation 3 of our second report that epidemiological studies should be set up to consider any possible effects on the health of the offspring of parents occupationally exposed to radiation. We recommend that consideration be given to broadening the scope of such studies to include the health of children of all employees at the nuclear installations we have studied.

RECOMMENDATION 3

The OPCS report on cancer and nuclear installations[7] and our own inquiries, have highlighted a number of problems with the National Cancer Registration Scheme. We recommend that urgent consideration should be given to the validity of cancer registration data, the form and completeness of which is currently variable in quality. In addition, the following specific improvements, which we urged in our second report, should be made:

i. We recommend that high priority be given to the completion of the postcoded childhood cancer registration database for England and Wales, and to ensuring that this database is accurate and complete. As the survival rate for leukaemia and other cancers continues to improve, accurate registration data are becoming an increasingly important part of the information required for the analysis of childhood cancer incidence.

ii. We recommend that high priority be given to the work already under way to enable data on childhood cancer to be analysed by place of birth of the child, as well as by place of residence at time of diagnosis.

RECOMMENDATION 4

We recommend that studies of the geographical distributions of childhood cancer incidence on a nationwide basis be carried out as the data in Recommendation 3 become available. These studies will provide essential information on the distribution of cases of childhood cancer throughout the UK, thus enabling the patterns found around nuclear sites to be seen in the context of patterns in the rest of the UK.

RECOMMENDATION 5

We consider it unlikely that useful information will emerge from further detailed investigations of alleged increased childhood cancer incidence around individual nuclear installations. Such investigations will be difficult to interpret until the results of the studies outlined in Recommendation 4 are available. We recommend that once the results of these national studies are available, this Committee should be asked to participate in a review of the evidence relating to the incidence of childhood cancer around nuclear installations. In the meantime, priority should be given to the recommendations set out in this report, completion of the outstanding recommendations in the Black report[1] and the recommendations in our second report.

45: Leukaemia near nuclear power plant in Massachusetts

Letter to the *Lancet*

RICHARD W CLAPP, SIDNEY COBB, C K CHAN, BAILUS WALKER JUNIOR

Your 17 October issue (*Lancet* 1987; ii:924) carried a note about the latest review of cancer around nuclear installations in Britain. We observed an increased incidence of leukaemia, particularly myelogenous leukaemia, in a five town area in Massachusetts during the years 1982–84. One of those towns (Plymouth) is the site of a commercial nuclear power plant that began operations in late 1972 and from which releases of various isotopes in late 1974 and 1975 have been recorded (figure).

The standard incidence ratios for all haematopoietic and reticuloendothelial system (ICD 169) neoplasms, all types of leukaemia combined, and all types of leukaemia minus chronic lymphocytic leukaemia are presented in table I. The standard rates from which the standard incidence ratios were calculated are the statewide rates for Massachusetts for 1982–84. These are for all ages combined, although it is of interest that the excess was in adults and the elderly, not in those under 25 as noted in British data. The most striking excess was for myelogenous leukaemia in males.

We calculated age-adjusted morbidity odds ratios, comparing the incidence in the five coastal towns with that in the surrounding communities in south eastern Massachusetts. The rationale for this was that there might be a registration effect whereby patients from these towns might be more likely to be diagnosed and reported to the Massachusetts cancer registry than patients in the state as a whole. A further consideration is the fact that about 90% of the patients from the five town area and the rest of south eastern Massachusetts are captured in a regional registry system (Healthstat Inc). It might be argued that the diagnostic and coding conventions used by this regional registration system differed from those used in

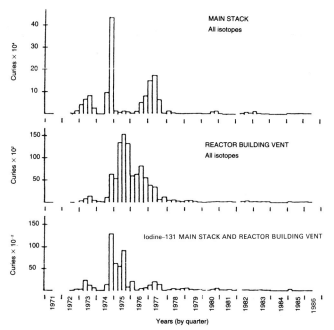

Airborne radioactive effluents from Pilgrim I nuclear reactor in Plymouth, Massachusetts, by quarter, 1972–86. Source: Boston Edison semi-annual effluent reports to USNRC.)

hospitals elsewhere in Massachusetts, although we know of no evidence to support this. The odds ratios comparing the incidence in the five town area and the two comparison areas for the four year period 1982–85 are presented in table II. We conclude that a registration effect is not a plausible explanation for the apparent excess in the five town area for this time period.

As the nuclear power plant is on the coast and as the reported releases of radioactive effluents are too small to produce a doubling of myelogenous

TABLE I—*Incidence of haematological malignancies (ICD 169) in five Massachusetts coastal towns, 1982–84*

Diagnosis	Male	Female	Total
All*	31/18·1 (171)	21/15·2 (138)	52/33·4 (156; 118 to 206)
Leukaemia	22/12·1 (182)	12/9·3 (129)	34/21·4 (159; 113 to 224)
Leukaemia minus chronic lymphocytic leukaemia	19/9·4 (203)	8/7·6 (106)	27/16·9 (160; 108 to 237)
Myelogenous leukaemia	13/5·2 (252)	6/4·8 (126)	19/9·9 (191; 120 to 304)

*All haematopoietic and reticuloendothelial system neoplasms.
Results are shown as observed/expected (and standard incidence ratios, with 95% confidence intervals for totals).

TABLE II—*Adjusted odds ratios and confidence intervals for haematopoietic and reticuloendothelial system neoplasms in five coastal towns compared with south eastern Massachusetts and the state, 1982–85*

	South eastern Massachusetts	Massachusetts
Males	1·52 (35); 1·06 to 2·18	1·56; 1·09 to 2·20
Females	1·19 (28); 0·80 to 1·76	1·35; 0·93 to 1·98
Total	1·38 (63); 1·06 to 1·81	1·49; 1·15 to 1·95

Numbers in parentheses refer to nos of cases

leukaemia in residents of the towns, we must postulate a mechanism by which airborne releases are contained in a coastal pattern. Such a meteorological mechanism is well known to weather observers,[1] and, in this instance, could contain airborne effluents and recycle them over the immediate coastal area. No other series of towns along the Massachusetts coast has had similar increases in leukaemia or in the myelogenous subtype.

Clearly, more detailed modelling of the meteorological conditions in the mid-1970s is needed before dose estimates could be made. Nevertheless, these descriptive data are suggestive and will be followed up by more investigations and more intensive observation of cancer incidence trends around this and other US nuclear power plants.

1 Field F. *Dr Frank Field's weather book.* New York: Putnam, 1901.

46: Childhood leukaemia mortality before 1970 among populations near two United States nuclear installations

Letters to the *Lancet*

JOHN R GOLDSMITH

In light of the findings of Forman *et al* of a possible excess in leukaemia among children living near certain British nuclear installations,[1] I have examined data from the United States for populations living near similar installations. The data are from the "mortality by county by year" file for the period 1950–79, initiated by the National Cancer Institute, and now available from the Environmental Protection Agency, Health Effects Research Laboratory, Research Triangle Park, North Carolina 27711, USA.

Data on mortality attributed to leukaemia by decade was examined for both sexes for the ages 0–9 years for white populations living in two counties adjacent to the Hanford, Washington installation (Benton and Franklin), and two counties adjacent to the Oakridge, Tennessee installations (Anderson and Loudon). The results are shown in the table.

There was significant excess in the four counties in the decade 1950–59, a non-significant excess in 1960–69, and a deficiency in 1970–79. The use of state rates for generating expected values would have made no important difference in the results.

Without further investigation I cannot say if these findings reflect the impact of direct radiation exposure, indirect exposure through parents with occupational exposures, or some other factors. One hypothesis is a deficiency of herd immunity, suggested by Kinlen to explain the excess leukaemia in Seascale, United Kingdom.[2] As these US counties were formerly sparsely populated, the Kinlen hypothesis could be relevant to these data.

Leukaemia mortality at ages 0–9 years in four counties near two major US nuclear facilities by decade

County	1950–59		1960–69		1970–79	
	Observed	Expected*	Observed	Expected*	Observed	Expected*
Washington						
Benton	8	6·65	6	6·24	3	4·17
Franklin	4	2·01	4	2·18	2	1·39
Tennessee						
Anderson	13	6·65	8	5·16	2	2·57
Loudon	3	2·28	3	1·76	1	1·05
Total	28	17·59	21	15·34	8	9·18
Poisson p	0·013		0·098		0·700	

* Expected numbers derived from local populations and US rates.

Before too much reassurance is taken from the deficiency in childhood leukaemia mortality in 1970–79, it should be noted that case-fatality rate for childhood leukaemia fell sharply over the three decades; leukaemia incidence may be a more suitable current indicator of possible effects of radiation exposure.

A systematic study of cancer mortality in the vicinity of US nuclear installations is being undertaken by Dr Seymour Jablon (National Cancer Institute).

This work has been undertaken in response to a request by the European Regional Office of the World Health Organisation and was made possible by a visiting scientist appointment to the Health Effects Research Laboratory, US Environmental Protection Agency.

1 Forman D, Cook-Mozaffari P, Darby S. *et al.* Cancer near nuclear installations. *Nature* 1987;**329**:499–505.
2 Kinlen L. Evidence for an infective cause of childhood leukaemia: comparison of a Scottish new town with nuclear reprocessing sites in Britain. *Lancet* 1988;**ii**:1323—27.

SAMUEL MILHAM JUNIOR

Professor Goldsmith (8 April, p 793) describes increased leukaemia mortality in the years 1950–59 in four United States counties adjacent to two

Births and employment, Benton and Franklin counties, Washington

Year	Births*	Employment (June) at Hanford Project†
1950	1886	14 349
1954	2667	21 563
1959	1948	10 920

*Washington state annual vital statistics summaries.
†Donald M Beck (personal communication).

nuclear facilities. There are a number of other similar United States nuclear facilities. How were these two facilities selected for study? I cannot comment on the Tennessee county data, but I think that, in the two Washington counties, the 0–9 age group was probably underestimated in 1951–59. The US county mortality data cited by Goldsmith used census data (for 1950 and 1960) and linear interpolation to estimate the intercensal populations. There were more births in Benton and Franklin counties and more people employed at the nuclear facility in 1954 than at the beginning or end of the decade (table), suggesting that linear interpolation might underestimate the population at risk and expected leukaemia deaths. In any event, the Benton and Franklin county leukaemia mortality is not significantly raised in the 1950–59 decade (observed 12, expected 8·66; $p > 0·05$).

Goldsmith also cautions that little reassurance should be taken from the deficit of leukaemia cases seen in 1970–79 as leukaemia case-facility rates have fallen sharply over time. Any decrease in the case-fatality rate should be reflected not only in the observed but also in the expected mortality values cited. The leukaemia mortality deficit seen in 1970–79, therefore, requires as much explanation as the purported 1950–59 excess.

JOHN R GOLDSMITH

Counties adjacent to Oakridge, Tennessee, and Hanford, Washington, were selected because these two facilities were the earliest to be activated and thus might closely resemble the British installations near which excess childhood leukaemia has been reported. In the vicinity of Los Alamos, New Mexico, which was another possibility, county boundaries had been changed, but it was less of a production facility anyway.

The birth and employment figures provided by Dr Milham do raise a question of possible underestimation of the population at risk. Incidence data are available on a year to year basis: if birth and population data were available on the same basis this matter could be resolved. Milham is right that 12 observed leukaemia deaths when 8·66 are expected is not significant. I never implied it was.

There are two possible reasons for the preference for incidence data in view of the decline in case-fatality rates. The decline may be attributable to improved treatment, and the quality of diagnosis and treatment could well be better at a given time in communities such as Richland (the community adjacent to the Hanford works) and Oakridge than in communities where the level of education attained by the population has not been as high. Secondly, the numbers of incident cases will tend in recent years to be substantially greater than the number of fatalities, thus giving greater statistical power to morbidity analyses than to mortality analyses. The mortality deficit in 1970–79 is far smaller than the excess in 1950–59, and I do not think it requires explanation. If we assume that recognition and treatment are fairly stable over time, and consistent for the locations generating both observed and expected numbers, of course a drop in case-fatality will lead to a drop in both observed and expected mortality.

The issue of temporal trend gains in importance as British data indicate that, during 1970–79, the incidence of leukaemia at ages 0–9 years remains somewhat high near some nuclear installations.[1] The mortality data for the four United States counties, such as they are, suggest that whatever may have been associated with the mortality excess of 1950–59 is no longer active in 1970–79.

My objective in calling attention to the US data, preliminary as they are, was to indicate that the association observed first in the Sellafield areas and then, to a lesser extent, near other British installations may have had its counterpart in other countries. On the basis of information from a central registry for childhood tumours at the University of Mainz in Germany, Demuth[2] has reported a significant excess incidence of leukaemia at ages 0–15 years during 1980–87 for residents within a 20 km radius of a nuclear installation at Wurgassen.

One must be cautious about attaching importance to excesses over arbitrary periods and distances in view of some uncertainties about distribution aspects of rare diseases. Some examples are presented in the second report of the Committee on Medical Aspects of Radiation in the Environment[3] for childhood leukaemia near the Dounreay nuclear establishment in Scotland.

1 Cook-Mozaffari PJ, Ashwood FL, Vincent T, Forman D, Alderton M. *Cancer incidence and mortality in the vicinity of nuclear installations England and Wales 1959–1980*. London: HMSO, 1987. (Office of Population Censuses and Surveys, studies on medical and population subjects no 51, microfiche table 2.)

2 Demuth M. *Leukamiemorbiditat bei Kindern und Jugendlichen in der Umgebung des Kernkraftwerkes Wurgassen. Die Wirkung niedriger Stahlendosen auf den Menschen.* Symposium, University of Munster, 1988.
3 Committee on Medical Aspects of Radiation in the Environment (chairman M Bobrow). *Investigation of possible increased incidence of leukaemia in young people near the Dounreay Nuclear Establishment, Caithness, Scotland.* London: HMSO, 1988. (COMARE 2nd report.)

47: Cancer near the Three Mile Island nuclear plant: radiation emissions

MAUREEN C HATCH, JAN BEYEA, JERI W NIEVES, MERVYN SUSSER

As a public charge, cancers among the 159 684 residents living within a 16 km (10 mile) radius of the Three Mile Island nuclear plant were studied relative to releases of radiation during the 28 March 1979 accident as well as to routine plant emissions. The principal cancers considered were leukaemia and childhood malignancies. Estimates of the emissions delivered to small geographical study tracts were derived from mathematical dispersion models that accounted for modifying factors such as wind and terrain; the model of accident emissions was validated by readings from off site dosimeters. Incident cancers among area residents for the period 1975–85 (n = 5493) were identified by a review of the records at all local and regional hospitals; trends in cancer rates before and after the accident were examined. For accident emissions, the authors failed to find definite effects of exposure on the cancer types and population subgroups thought to be most susceptible to radiation. No associations were seen for leukaemia in adults or for childhood cancers as a group. For leukaemia in children, the odds ratio was raised, but cases were few (n = 4), and the estimate was highly variable. Moreover, rates of childhood leukaemia in the Three Mile Island area are low compared with national and regional rates. For exposure to routine emissions, the odds ratios were raised for childhood cancers as a whole and for childhood leukaemia, but confidence intervals were wide and included 1·0. For leukaemia in adults there was a negative trend. Trends for two types of cancer ran counter to expectation. Non-Hodgkin's lymphoma showed raised risks relative both to accident and to routine emissions; lung cancer (adjusted only indirectly for smoking) showed raised risks relative to accident emissions, routine emissions, and background γ radiation. Overall, the pattern of results does not provide convincing evidence that radiation releases from the Three Mile Island nuclear facility influenced cancer risk during the limited period of follow up.

48: Background γ radiation and childhood cancers within 10 miles of a United States nuclear plant

MAUREEN HATCH, MERVYN SUSSER

In the light of some recent reports concerning childhood leukaemia near nuclear installations, we examined rates of cancer in children in relation to background γ ray exposure. Data from a national monitoring programme around nuclear facilities were used to map the distribution of background γ radiation for 69 small geographical subunits (average population 2300) within 10 miles of one US nuclear plant. An association was found for incidence of childhood cancers as a whole (odds ratio = 2·4; 95% confidence limits 1·2 to 4·6). For leukaemias specifically, the odds ratio was also high (2·4), but 95% confidence limits were very wide (0·5 to 12·9). Analyses adjusting for sociodemographic characteristics of study tracts (population density and income) gave similar results; data on other risk factors were not available.

Conventional risk models would not predict a detectable increase in childhood cancer from background γ radiation, particularly not an increase of this magnitude. The large effect for solid tumours as well as leukaemias is also somewhat counter to expectation. As a priori the association we observed was unlikely, it is important to know if similar trends in childhood cancer with background radiation are seen in other areas before rejecting chance or bias as an explanation for the result.

49: Childhood leukaemia around the La Hague nuclear waste reprocessing plant

J F VIEL, S T RICHARDSON

The incidence of childhood leukaemia around nuclear facilities has been a topic of much public attention and epidemiological investigation. The Sellafield and Dounreay nuclear waste reprocessing plants have been particularly investigated. A similar reprocessing plant has been operating in La Hague, Normandy, since 1966, several years after Sellafield was commissioned. The amount of radioactive effluent discharged has been much lower than that from Sellafield (the maximum annual discharge in the years to 1980 was 1592 887 GBq in 1975). The main radionuclides released are ruthenium-106, cerium-144 (up to 1980), caesium-137, and antimony-125. Discharges from Sellafield and La Hague differ in their isotope contents: Sellafield releases 10 to 160 times more ^{137}Cs and La Hague four times more ^{125}Sb.

Mortality for the periods 1968–78 and 1979–86 was provided by the Institute National de la Santé et de la Recherche Médicale, which records all the medical causes of deaths in France centrally. Three age groups were examined: 0–4 years, 5–14 years, and 15–24 years. We studied all electoral wards (around 10 000 inhabitants) that had half or more of their area within a specified radius of the nuclear plant. Radiuses of 10 km, 20 km, and 35 km were chosen before the analyses, so 10 wards were included in the study. The expected numbers of

431

Mortality from leukaemia around La Hague nuclear reprocessing plant according to age, period of study, and distance from plant

Period of study and distance from plant	0–4 Years		5–14 Years		15–24 Years	
	Observed deaths	Standardised mortality ratio (%)	Observed deaths	Standardised mortality ratio (%)	Observed deaths	Standardised mortality ratio (%)
1968–78:						
<10 km	0	0	0	0	0	0
10–<20 km	2	109	0	0*	5	250
20–<35 km	0	0	3	111	0	0
1979–86:						
<10 km	0	0	0	0	1	467
10–<20 km	2	203	2	94	1	38
20–<35 km	1	149	2	123	2	115

*p<0·05.

cases of leukaemia (International Classification of Diseases (8th revision) codes 204–207; 9th revision codes 204–208) were estimated by applying the age specific rates for the département de la Manche for 1968–78 and 1979–86 to the 1975 and 1982 census populations of the predefined areas. Results were analysed by two tailed tests based on a Poisson distribution.

Only one death occurred in the area closest to the nuclear installation between 1968 and 1986 (table). Only one standardised mortality ratio was significantly different from one: the ratio for the age group 5–14 living 10–20 km from the plant during 1968–78 showed a decreased risk (observed number of deaths = 0, expected = 3·935). Because of the number of tests carried out (table) one of the tests would be expected to yield a significant result ($p < 0·05$) on the basis of chance.

The standardised mortality ratio for all the age groups, periods, and areas was 89% (observed number of deaths = 21, expected = 23·6) and was not significant (95% confidence interval 0·55 to 1·36). Furthermore, no significant trend between the two periods was found.

50: Cancer around Pilgrim nuclear plant, Massachusetts

SETH SHULMAN

A United States study shows an increase in the incidence of leukaemia among adults who lived and worked close to the Pilgrim nuclear power plant in Massachusetts in 1978–83.* That news is certain to intensify the debate over links between cancer incidence and exposure to a low level of radiation, given that the study follows a United States National Cancer Institute study that found no increased incidence in cancer deaths around nuclear facilities and British data showing a cluster of cases of childhood leukaemia around the Sellafield nuclear plant (see *Nature* 1990; **347**:216 and 343, 679).

The Pilgrim study, carried out by the Massachusetts Department of Public Health, examined the incidence of leukaemia in persons living and working in 22 communities situated near the plant, taking into account how close to the plant they lived and worked and for how long. Although a fourfold incidence in leukamia was found in people who lived within 10 miles of the plant in the period 1979–83, no relation between leukaemia cases and proximity to the plant was found during 1983–86. Leukaemia normally occurs at a rate of 2–3 cases per 100 000 population; the Pilgrim study was triggered by data suggesting that the rate close to the plant was double the Massachusetts average.

Assuming that it takes five years for leukaemia to develop, the 1979–83 increase in leukaemia incidence can be linked to a period of higher than normal emission of airborne radionuclides from the Pilgrim plant during the mid-1970s. Such emissions reduced considerably after 1978.

Three years ago, the Pilgrim plant was described by federal officials as "the worst run" nuclear plant in the United States. But even during the periods of increased air emissions, the levels of radiation to which residents were exposed are believed to have been well within the Nuclear Regulatory Commission's limit of 5 mSv (500 millirem) a year. At least since 1980, exposure levels are believed to have been within the Environmental Protection Agency's more stringent limit of 0·25 mSv (25 millirem) a year.

Officials at Boston Edison, the utility that operates the Pilgrim plant, criticise the timing and methods of the study. But Daniel Hoffman, a researcher at the US Centers for Disease Control who led the committee that reviewed the results, called the study "well designed, impressive, and surprising". Hoffman stressed that the Pilgrim study is one of the first to correct for confounding factors and says that it "suggests strongly that there may be increased risk levels [from radiation] at levels of exposure far lower than we would expect".

Through interviews, the Pilgrim study collected detailed data about the 313 subjects involved and the length of time they had lived and worked near the plant. The researchers tracked all types of adult leukaemia except chronic lymphocytic leukaemia (because it is widely considered to be the only type of leukaemia not associated with radiation). Confounding factors including occupation, age, tobacco consumption, and social status were taken into account, along with such factors as the proximity of toxic waste dumps and the origin of the drinking water. During the 1979–83 period, the researchers could even show that the likelihood of developing leukaemia was linked to where and for how long people lived in the area.

Robert Knorr, one of the study's two principal investigators, stressed the differences between the Pilgrim study and the National Cancer Institute's recent mortality study. The Pilgrim study focused on a much smaller and more specific geographical area than did the National Cancer Institute's study, which drew only on county data that would not detect highly local increases in cancer. The Pilgrim study also looked at the incidence of disease rather than at mortality only.

After the results of the study were released, people living close to the plant flooded a state telephone "hotline" number with calls. Massachusetts' governor, Michael Dukakis, has asked for the state to adopt the strictest radiation emission standard in the country, which would limit exposure of those living near nuclear plants to 0·1 mSv (10 millirem) a year. State researchers have already begun studies on the incidence of childhood leukaemia near the Pilgrim plant and of leukaemia among workers at the plant.

*Southeastern Massachusetts Health Study Final Report: *Investigation of Leukaemia Incidence in 22 Massachusetts Communities 1978–1986.* Massachusetts Department of Public Health, Division of Environmental Health Assessment, October 1990.

51: Overall mortality and cancer mortality around French nuclear sites

CATHERINE HILL, AGNÈS LAPLANCHE

Higher than expected mortality from leukaemia has been observed in the population under the age of 25 living around Sellafield and Dounreay, nuclear reprocessing plants in the United Kingdom. We report the results of a similar study for the population residing around nuclear sites in France. The number of leukaemia deaths was 58, comparable to the 62 in control areas, and slightly less than the 67 expected from national mortality statistics. Twelve deaths due to Hodgkin's disease were observed around nuclear sites; this is about twice the number of Hodgkin's deaths observed in control areas and twice the number expected from national mortality statistics. This observation must, however, be interpreted in the light of the fact that several causes of death were studied, increasing the play of chance.

The two tables show that our results confirm Viel and Richardson's study of leukaemia mortality around La Hague (chapter 48), which used geographical units with populations seven times larger than in our study. The excess leukaemia observed around nuclear sites in the United Kingdom is not observed around French nuclear sites, although the same methodology was used as in chapter 12.

The amount of radioactive effluent discharged might have been higher around Sellafield and Dounreay than around French installations (see chapter 48). The excess leukaemia observed in the United Kingdom could also be attributed to

TABLE I—*Observed and expected number of deaths and standardised mortality ratios (SMRs) by cause, around nuclear sites and in control areas*

Cause of death	Exposed			Control		
	Observed	Expected	SMR (%)*	Observed	Expected	SMR (%)*
All malignancies	166	171·7	97	160	157·2	102
Brain (malignant)	6	14·5	41†	13	13·4	97
Brain (unspecified)	16	14·2	113	15	13·3	113
Lung	2	2·1	94	5	1·9	263
Hodgkin's disease	12	6·1	197†	5	5·6	89
Other lymphomas	16	15·5	103	9	14·2	63
Myelomas	0	0·3	0	0	0·3	0
Leukaemias	58	66·9	87	62	61·2	102
Lymphoid leukaemias	13	19·0	68	14	17·4	80
All causes	3064	3093·7	99	2828	2772·2	102

* Statistical methods: Standardised mortality ratios, in the exposed population were compared to 100 and to SMRs in the exposed population by two tailed tests assuming Poisson distribution.

† $p = 0·02$ (two sided test).

TABLE II—*Number of person years, observed and expected number of leukaemia deaths, and standardised mortality ratios (SMRs) by sex, age, type of installation, and distance from nuclear installations*

Characteristics	Person years in thousands	Observed	Expected	SMR (%)
Sex				
Male	1486	34	39·6	86
Female	1406	24	27·4	88
Age				
0–4	583	13	13·9	93
5–9	588	12	17·5	69
10–14	613	7	13·6	52
15–19	589	16	12·4	129
20–24	519	10	9·6	105
Installation				
Reprocessing	1576	30	36·7	82
Other	1316	28	30·2	93
Distance in km				
<5	260	5	6·1	82
5–9·9	982	21	22·7	93
10–12·9	373	4	8·5	47
13–15·9	748	17	17·3	92
16–21	530	11	12·3	90
Total	2892	58	66·9	87

some characteristic common to Sellafield and Dounreay, but not shared by French installations, for instance a rapid increase of population leading to viral infections (see chapter 13), or some unknown factor shared by existing and potential nuclear sites in the United Kingdom (see chapter 17).

52: Cancer rates after the Three Mile Island nuclear accident and proximity of residence to the plant

MAUREEN C HATCH, SYLVAN WALLENSTEIN,
JAN BEYEA, JERI W NIEVES, MERVYN SUSSER

In the light of a possible link between stress and cancer promotion or progression, and of previously reported distress in residents near the Three Mile Island nuclear power plant, we attempted to evaluate the impact of the March 1979 accident on community cancer rates.

Proximity of residence to the plant, which related to distress in previous studies, was taken as a possible indicator of accident stress; the pattern in cancer rates after the accident was examined in 69 "study tracts" within a 10 mile radius of Three Mile Island, in relation to residential proximity.

A modest association was found between proximity and cancer rates after the accident (odds ratio 1·4; 95% confidence interval 1·3 to 1·6). After adjusting for a gradient in cancer risk prior to the accident, the odds ratio contrasting those closest to the plant with those living farther out was 1·2 (95% confidence interval 1·0 to 1·4). An increase in cancer rates near the Three Mile Island plant after the accident was notable in 1982, persisted for another year, and then declined. Radiation emissions, as modelled mathematically, did not account for the observed increase.

Interpretation in terms of accident stress is limited by the lack of an individual measure of stress and by uncertainty about whether stress has a biological effect on cancer in humans. An alternative mechanism for the cancer increase near the plant is through changes in care seeking and diagnostic practice arising from concern after the accident.

53: Cancer in populations living near nuclear facilities

A survey of mortality nationwide and incidence in two states, USA

SEYMOUR JABLON, ZDENEK HRUBEC,
JOHN D BOICE JUNIOR

Reports from the United Kingdom have described increases in leukaemia and lymphoma among young persons living near certain nuclear installations. Because of concern raised by these reports, a mortality survey was conducted in populations living near nuclear facilities in the United States. All facilities began service before 1982. Over 900 000 cancer deaths occurred 1950–84 in 107 counties with or near nuclear installations. Each study county was matched for comparison to three "control counties" in the same region. There were 1·8 million cancer deaths in the 292 control counties during the 35 years studied. Deaths due to leukaemia or other cancers were not more frequent in the study counties than in the control counties. For childhood leukaemia mortality, the relative risk comparing the study counties with their controls before plant start up was 1·08, whereas after start up it was 1·03. For leukaemia mortality at all ages, the relative risks were 1·02 before start up and 0·98 after. For counties in two states, cancer incidence data were also available. For one facility, the standardised registration ratio for childhood leukaemia was increased significantly after start up. However, the increase also antedated the operation of this facility. The study is limited by the correlational approach and the large size of the geographical areas (counties) used. It does not prove the absence of any effect. If, however, any excess cancer risk was present in the United States counties with nuclear facilities, it was too small to be detected with the methods employed.

54: Incidence of childhood malignancies in the vicinity of West German nuclear power plants

JÖRG MICHAELIS, BIRGIT KELLER,
GÜNTER HAAF, PETER KAATSCH

The incidence of childhood malignancies in 20 areas surrounding major nuclear installations is compared with the incidence in matched control regions. The study is based on the registry of childhood malignancies in the Federal Republic of Germany and includes 1610 cases which were diagnosed before 15 years of age from 1980 to 1990. The relative risk was 0·97 for all malignancies and 1·06 for acute leukaemia in all regions within a 15 km radius of an installation. Increased relative risk for acute leukaemia before 5 years of age and for lymphomas was observed in subgroups, especially in regions close (<5 km) to installations that started operation before 1970. Most of this increase was attributable to an unexpectedly low incidence in the control regions, which could not be explained by analysing possible confounding factors. Using the same control regions, a comparable and even more pronounced increase of relative risks was observed in regions where nuclear power plants have been projected.

55: Paternal radiation exposure and leukaemia in offspring: the Ontario case-control study

JOHN R McLAUGHLIN, WILL D KING,
TERENCE W ANDERSON, E AILEEN CLARKE,
J PATRICK ASHMORE

A study was conducted in regions of Ontario, Canada, that had an operating nuclear facility to test the hypothesis that there is an association between childhood leukaemia and the occupational exposure of fathers to ionising radiation before a child's conception. Cases were children (aged 0–14) who died of leukaemia or were diagnosed as having leukaemia from 1950 to 1988 and were born to mothers residing in the vicinity of an operating nuclear facility. Eight controls per case were identified from birth certificates, matched by date of birth and residence at birth. There were 112 cases and 890 controls. Paternal radiation exposure was determined by a record linkage to the Canadian National Dose Registry. The analyses showed that six fathers of cases and 53 fathers of controls had had a total whole body dose greater than 0.0 mSv before the child's conception, resulting in an odds ratio of 0.87 (95% confidence interval 0.32 to 2.34). There was no evidence of an increased risk of leukaemia in relation to any exposure period (lifetime, six months, or three months before conception) or exposure type (total whole body dose, external whole body dose, or tritium dose), except for radon exposure in uranium miners, which had a large odds ratio that was not significantly different from the null value. The findings of this study do not support the hypothesis that childhood leukaemia is associated with the occupational exposure of fathers to ionising radiation before conception.

Index